Watch surgical videos from *Endothelial Keratoplasty* online at MediaCenter.thieme.com!

Simply visit MediaCenter.thieme.com and, when prompted during the registration process, enter the code below to get started today.

5D47-95XQ-8K96-B225

	WINDOWS	MAC	TABLET
Recommended Browser(s)**	Recent browser versions on all major platforms and any mobile operating system that supports HTML5 video playback ** *all browsers should have JavaScript enabled*		
Flash Player Plug-in	Flash Player 9 or Higher* * *Mac users: ATI Rage 128 GPU does not support full-screen mode with hardware scaling*		Tablet PCs with Android OS support Flash 10.1
Recommended for optimal usage experience	Monitor resolutions: • Normal (4:3) 1024×768 or Higher • Widescreen (16:9) 1280×720 or Higher • Widescreen (16:10) 1440×900 or Higher DSL/Cable internet connection at a minimum speed of 384.0 Kbps or faster WiFi 802.11 b/g preferred.		7-inch and 10-inch tablets on maximum resolution. WiFi connection is required.

f Find us on **Facebook**   *Connect with us on Facebook® for exclusive offers.*

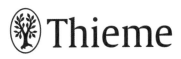

Endothelial Keratoplasty

Mastering DSEK, DMEK, and PDEK

Amar Agarwal, MS, FRCS, FRCOphth
Professor of Ophthalmology
Ramachandra Medical College
Chairman and Managing Director
Dr. Agarwal's Eye Hospital & Eye Research Centre
Chennai, India

Terry Kim, MD
Professor of Ophthalmology
Duke University School of Medicine
Chief, Cornea and External Disease Division
Director, Refractive Surgery Service
Duke University Eye Center
Durham, North Carolina, USA

592 illustrations

Thieme
New York • Stuttgart • Delhi • Rio de Janeiro

Executive Editor: William Lamsback
Managing Editor: Elizabeth Palumbo
Director, Editorial Services: Mary Jo Casey
Production Editor: Torsten Scheihagen
International Production Director: Andreas Schabert
International Marketing Director: Fiona Henderson
International Sales Director: Louisa Turrell
Director of Sales, North America: Mike Roseman
Senior Vice President and Chief Operating Officer: Sarah Vanderbilt
President: Brian D. Scanlan
Printer: Everbest Printing Co.

Library of Congress Cataloging-in-Publication Data

Names: Agarwal, Amar. | Kim, Terry.
Title: Endothelial keratoplasty : mastering DSEK, DMEK, and PDEK /
[edited by] Amar Agarwal, MS, FRCS, FRCOphth, professor of
ophthalmology, Ramachandra Medical College, chairman and
managing director, Dr. Agarwal's Eye Hospital, Chennai, India, Terry
Kim, MD, professor of ophthalmology, chief, Cornea and External
Disease Service, director, Refractive Surgery Service, Duke
University Medical Center, Durham, NC.
Description: New York : Thieme, [2017] | Includes bibliographical
references. Identifiers: LCCN 2016057980 (print) | LCCN
2016059316 (ebook) | ISBN 9781626234512 (print) | ISBN
9781626234529 (e-book) | ISBN 9781626234529 (e book)
Subjects: LCSH: Cornea–Surgery. | Cornea–Transplantation. |
  Eye–Surgery.
Classification: LCC QM511 .E63 2017 (print) | LCC QM511 (ebook) |
DDC
                    617.7/19059–dc23
LC record available at https://lccn.loc.gov/2016057980

Copyright © 2017 by Thieme Medical Publishers, Inc.

Thieme Publishers New York
333 Seventh Avenue, New York, NY 10001 USA
+1 800 782 3488, customerservice@thieme.com

Thieme Publishers Stuttgart
Rüdigerstrasse 14, 70469 Stuttgart, Germany
+49 [0]711 8931 421, customerservice@thieme.de

Thieme Publishers Delhi
A-12, Second Floor, Sector-2, Noida-201301
Uttar Pradesh, India
+91 120 45 566 00, customerservice@thieme.in

Thieme Publishers Rio de Janeiro, Thieme Publicações Ltda.
Edifício Rodolpho de Paoli, 25º andar
Av. Nilo Peçanha, 50 – Sala 2508
Rio de Janeiro 20020-906 Brasil
+55 21 3172-2297 / +55 21 3172-1896

Cover design: Thieme Publishing Group
Typesetting by DiTech Process Solutions

Printed in China by Everbest Printing Co.   5 4 3 2 1

ISBN 978-1-62623-451-2

Also available as an e-book:
eISBN 978-1-62623-452-9

Important note: Medicine is an ever-changing science undergoing continual development. Research and clinical experience are continually expanding our knowledge, in particular our knowledge of proper treatment and drug therapy. Insofar as this book mentions any dosage or application, readers may rest assured that the authors, editors, and publishers have made every effort to ensure that such references are in accordance with **the state of knowledge at the time of production of the book.**

Nevertheless, this does not involve, imply, or express any guarantee or responsibility on the part of the publishers in respect to any dosage instructions and forms of applications stated in the book. **Every user is requested to examine carefully** the manufacturers' leaflets accompanying each drug and to check, if necessary in consultation with a physician or specialist, whether the dosage schedules mentioned therein or the contraindications stated by the manufacturers differ from the statements made in the present book. Such examination is particularly important with drugs that are either rarely used or have been newly released on the market. Every dosage schedule or every form of application used is entirely at the user's own risk and responsibility. The authors and publishers request every user to report to the publishers any discrepancies or inaccuracies noticed. If errors in this work are found after publication, errata will be posted at www.thieme.com on the product description page.

Some of the product names, patents, and registered designs referred to in this book are in fact registered trademarks or proprietary names even though specific reference to this fact is not always made in the text. Therefore, the appearance of a name without designation as proprietary is not to be construed as a representation by the publisher that it is in the public domain.

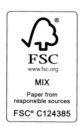

To a great friend and surgeon, William Trattler

Contents

Video Contents

Foreword

It is a great pleasure, a privilege, and also an honor to write the foreword for the groundbreaking book *Endothelial Keratoplasty: Mastering DSEK, DMEK, and PDEK*, edited by Amar Agarwal and Terry Kim.

The scientific and educational quality of the book is ensured by the prolific and inexhaustible publications from both editors in the fields of cornea, cataract, refractive surgery, and anterior segment of the eye. Dr. Amar Agarwal has edited over 70 books in ophthalmology since 1998, with many original contributions, such as pre-Descemet endothelial keratoplasty (PDEK), which is covered in the book. In addition, Dr. Terry Kim's academic accomplishments include, along with over 200 journal articles in the peer-reviewed literature, being the editor and author of some of the most important textbooks on corneal diseases and cataract surgery.

Endothelial keratoplasty (EK) represents a very hot topic as a new and rapidly evolving field for corneal surgeons. This is a fascinating area with different surgical procedures that have revolutionized corneal transplantation because they provide important benefits for patient care. In this book, Drs. Agarwal and Kim have gathered the most distinguished leaders from around the world who have themselves provided the most important contributions to the emerging field of EK.

The book includes 23 chapters, which are didactically divided. The first part of the book covers the basics and includes the surgical anatomy chapter from Dr. Harminder Dua, who had described the novel corneal layer that is especially relevant for these procedures. Dr. Gerrit Melles, who is acknowledged as "the Father of modern EK,"

provides, with his great team of collaborators, the history of EK and insights for the future with the nonkeratoplasty concepts of hemi-Descemet membrane EK and Descemet membrane endothelial transfer.

The book is intended for corneal surgeons, designed to provide the reader with the essentials for starting and mastering EK. The section on surgical techniques presents the descriptions for all EK procedures along with a surgical DVD. The section on EK in special situations includes, among other very challenging situations, a chapter on glaucoma by Dr. Francis Price, one of the world's foremost experts on EK. The book's final section reviews optical coherence tomography as a diagnostic technology for EK as well as complications that arise in Descemet stripping automated EK and pre-Descemet EK. The last chapter provides a thorough discussion of the contributions of eye banks in obtaining and preparing grafts for corneal surgeons.

In summary, Dr. Agarwal and Dr. Kim are to be commended for their work in editing this book, which is anticipated as a "must read" for any practicing corneal surgeon.

Renato Ambrósio, Jr., MD, PhD
Founder and Scientific Coordinator
Rio de Janeiro Corneal Tomography and
Biomechanics Study Group
Associate Professor of Ophthalmology
Federal University of São Paulo and
Pontific Catholic University
Rio de Janeiro, Brazil

Preface

As endothelial keratoplasty has revolutionized the surgical management of disorders related to the corneal endothelium, this book has been written to provide ophthalmologists and corneal surgeons with a comprehensive tool both for reading and for teaching. We believe that the information presented here is essential to successful learning.

The aim of the endothelial keratoplasty procedure is to maintain and enhance the cornea's most remarkable property—the transmission of light in the visible part of the spectrum—and this book is a step toward achieving this goal for our patients. The step-by-step chapters clarify the concepts and are organized and presented in four sections: Basics; Surgical Techniques; Endothelial Keratoplasty in Special Situations; and Surgical Outcomes, Complications, and Future Trends.

This book provides the necessary instructional information on Descemet stripping endothelial keratoplasty (DSEK), which has been practiced widely, and also Descemet membrane endothelial keratoplasty (DMEK), which is an evolving technique. The book also presents pre-Descemet endothelial keratoplasty (PDEK), which has itself evolved as a lexicon of various endothelial keratoplasty subtypes. The videos accompanying the book give viewers a better understanding of the surgical techniques described.

Although it was our idea to write a book on endothelial keratoplasty, it would have remained only a dream without our contributors. We are deeply grateful for their excellent contributions; the debt we owe them is beyond measure.

Amar Agarwal, MS, FRCS, FRCOphth
Terry Kim, MD

About the Editors

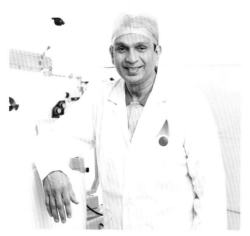

Amar Agarwal, MS, FRCS, FRCOphth
Chairman and Managing Director
Dr. Agarwal's group of eye hospitals and Eye Research
    Center
Chennai, India
Past President—International Society of Refractive Surgery
    (ISRS)
Secretary General—Indian Intraocular Implant and
    Refractive Society (IIRSI)

Amar Agarwal is the pioneer of phakonit—phako with a needle incision technology. This technique became popularized as bimanual phaco, microincision cataract surgery (MICS), or microphaco. He is the first to remove cataracts through a 0.7 mm tip with the technique called microphakonit. He has also developed no-anesthesia cataract surgery and FAVIT, a new technique to remove dropped nuclei. The air pump, which was a simple idea of using an aquarium pump to increase the fluid into the eye in bimanual phaco and coaxial phaco, has helped prevent surge. This provided the basis for various techniques of forced infusion for small-incision cataract surgery. Dr. Agarwal has also discovered a new refractive error, called aberropia. He has been the first to perform a combined surgery of microphakonit (700 μm cataract surgery) with a 25-gauge vitrectomy in the same patient, thus using the smallest incisions possible for cataract and vitrectomy. He is also the first surgeon to implant a new mirror telescopic intraocular lens (IOL) (LMI) for patients with age-related macular degeneration. He has been the first in the world to implant a glued IOL. In this procedure, a posterior chamber (PC) IOL is fixed in an eye without any capsules by using fibrin glue. The Malyugin Ring (MicroSurgical Technologies) for small-pupil cataract surgery was also modified by him, as the Agarwal modification of the Malyugin Ring for miotic pupil cataract surgeries with posterior capsular defects. Dr. Agarwal's eye hospital has performed for the first time an anterior segment transplantation in a 4-month-old child with anterior staphyloma. He has also developed the technique of IOL scaffold, in which a three-piece IOL is injected into an eye between the iris and the nucleus to prevent the nucleus from falling down in PC ruptures. He has combined glued IOL and IOL scaffold in cases of PC rupture where there is no iris or capsular support and termed the technique the glued IOL scaffold. Dr. Agarwal's eye hospital has also performed for the first time a glued endocapsular ring in cases of subluxated cataract.

Pre-Descemet endothelial keratoplasty, or PDEK, was developed by Dr. Agarwal. In this procedure the pre-Descemet layer and the Descemet membrane with endothelium are transplanted en bloc in patients with diseased endothelium. Dr. Agarwal's eye hospital has performed for the first time contact lens–assisted collagen cross linking (CACXL), a new technique for cross linking thin corneas. The hospital has also worked on developing endoilluminator-assisted Descemet membrane endothelial keratoplasty (E-DMEK). Dr. Agarwal has designed the new instrument called the trocar anterior chamber maintainer, which is now used in complicated cases to help with infusion through the anterior chamber and works like a trocar cannula.

Dr. Agarwal has performed more than 150 live surgeries at various conferences. His videos have won many awards at the film festivals of the American Society of Cataract and Refractive Surgery, the American Academy of Ophthalmology, and the European Society of Cataract and Refractive Surgeons. He has written more than 70 books, which have been published in various languages, including English, Spanish, and Polish. At his center, he trains doctors from around the world in various procedures, including phaco, bimanual phaco, LASIK, and retinal surgery.

Dr. Agarwal is the chairman and managing director of Dr. Agarwal's group of eye hospitals, which has 70 eye hospitals around the world. He can be contacted at dragarwal@vsnl.com. The hospital website is http://www.dragarwal.com.

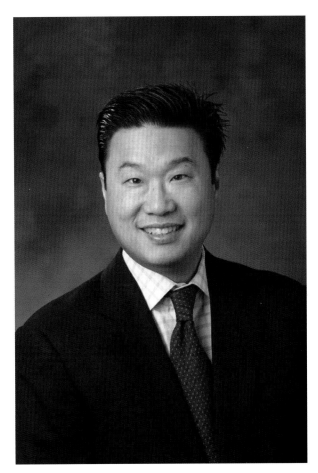

Terry Kim, MD
Professor of Ophthalmology
Duke University School of Medicine
Chief, Cornea and External Disease Division
Director, Refractive Surgery Service
Duke University Eye Center

Dr. Terry Kim, Professor of Ophthalmology at Duke University Eye Center, received his medical degree from Duke University School of Medicine and completed his residency and chief residency in ophthalmology at Emory Eye Center. He continued with his fellowship training in cornea, external disease, and refractive surgery at Wills Eye Hospital. He was then recruited to Duke University Eye Center, where he serves as principal and coinvestigator on a number of clinical trials and research grants from the National Institutes of Health and other institutions. Dr. Kim was formerly the director of the Residency Program and Ophthalmology Fellowship Program and currently serves as chief of the Cornea and External Disease Division and director of the Refractive Surgery Service.

Dr. Kim's academic accomplishments include his extensive publications in the peer-reviewed literature, which include over 200 journal articles, textbook chapters, and scientific abstracts. He is also editor and author of three well-respected textbooks on corneal diseases and cataract surgery. Dr. Kim has delivered over 200 invited lectures, both nationally and internationally. He has been the recipient of the Achievement Award and the Senior Achievement Award from the American Academy of Ophthalmology (AAO). His clinical and research work has earned him honors and grants from the National Institutes of Health, Fight for Sight/Research to Prevent Blindness, Heed Ophthalmic Foundation, Alcon Laboratories, and Allergan. Dr. Kim is also continually listed in *Best Doctors in America, Best Doctors in North Carolina*, and *America's Top Ophthalmologists*. He has been voted by his peers as one of the 250 most prominent cataract and intraocular lens surgeons in the country by *Premier Surgeon*, as one of the "135 Leading Ophthalmologists in America" by *Becker's ASC Review*, and as one of the "Top 50 Opinion Leaders" by *Cataract and Refractive Surgery Today*.

Dr. Kim serves on the governing board for the American Society of Cataract and Refractive Surgery (ASCRS) as chair of the Cornea Clinical Committee, on the Annual Program Committee for the AAO, and on the executive committee and board of directors for the Cornea Society. He was recently inducted into the International Intra-Ocular Implant Club and is consultant to the Ophthalmic Devices Panel of the Food and Drug Administration. Dr. Kim also sits on the editorial board for several peer-reviewed journals and trade publications, including *Cornea, Journal of Cataract and Refractive Surgery, Ocular Surgery News, Eyeworld, Cataract & Refractive Surgery Today, Premier Surgeon, Review of Ophthalmology, Advanced Ocular Care*, and *Topics in Ocular Antiinfectives*. As Consultant Ophthalmologist for the Duke men's basketball team, Dr. Kim provides medical and surgical care for the players, coaches, and staff, which has been featured on the *Discovery Channel* and in *The Wall Street Journal*.

Contributors

Amar Agarwal, MS, FRCS, FRCOphth
Professor of Ophthalmology
Ramachandra Medical College
Chairman and Managing Director
Dr. Agarwal's Eye Hospital
Chennai, India

Ashvin Agarwal, MS
Director
Dr. Agarwal's Eye Hospital
Chennai, India

Athiya Agarwal, MD, DO
Director
Dr. Agarwal's Eye Hospital
Chennai, India

Brandon Daniel Ayres, MD
Co-Director for Cornea Fellowship
Wills Eye Hospital
Bala Cynwyd, Pennsylvania, USA

Dimitri T. Azar, MD, MBA
Dean
College of Medicine
Distinguished University Professor and BA Field Chair of
  Ophthalmologic Research
Professor of Ophthalmology, Pharmacology and
  Bioengineering
University of Illinois at Chicago
Chicago, Illinois, USA

Brandon James Baartman, MD
Resident Opthalmologist
Cleveland Clinic Cole Eye Institute
Cleveland, Ohio, USA

Lamis Baydoun, MD, FEBO
Head of NIIOS Academy
Corneal Surgeon
Netherlands Institute for Innovative Ocular Surgery (NIIOS)
Melles Cornea Clinic
Rotterdam, The Netherlands

Isabel Dapena, MD, PhD
Head of Medical Department
Corneal Surgeon
Netherlands Institute for Innovative Ocular Surgery (NIIOS)
Melles Cornea Clinic
Rotterdam, The Netherlands

William J. Dupps, Jr., MD, PhD
Staff
Ophthalmology, Biomedical Engineering and Transplant
Cole Eye Institute and Lerner Research Institute, Cleveland
  Clinic
Cleveland, Ohio, USA

Rachel L.R. Gomes, MD
Ophthalmologist
Federal University of Sao Paulo (UNIFESP)
Sao Paulo, Brazil
New England Eye Center
Boston, Massachusetts, USA
Hospital de Olhos Paulista
Sao Paulo, Brazil

Joelle A. Hallak, PhD
Assistant Professor
Executive Director
Ophthalmic Clinical Trials and Translational Center
Department of Ophthalmology
University of Illinois at Chicago
Chicago, Illinois, USA

Soosan Jacob, MS, FRCS, DNB
Director and Chief
Dr. Agarwal's Refractive and Cornea Foundation
Dr. Agarwal's Eye Hospital
Chennai, India

Bennie H. Jeng, MD
Professor and Chair
University of Maryland School of Medicine
Department of Ophthalmology and Visual Sciences
Baltimore, Maryland, USA

Thomas John, MD
Clinical Associate Professor
Loyola University at Chicago
Chicago, Illinois, USA

Kenneth R. Kenyon, MD
Clinical Professor
Tufts/New England Eye Center
Harvard Medical School
Shepens Eye Research Institute
Cornea Consultants International
Marion, Massachusetts, USA

Michelle J. Kim, MD
Resident
Duke University Eye Center
Durham, North Carolina, USA

Terry Kim, MD
Professor of Ophthalmology
Chief, Cornea and External Disease Service
Director, Refractive Surgery Service
Duke University Medical Center
Durham, North Carolina, USA

Dhivya Ashok Kumar, MD, FICO
Senior Consultant
Dr. Agarwal's Eye Hospital
Chennai, India

W. Barry Lee, MD
Partner
Eye Consultants of Atlanta
Medical Director
Georgia Eye Bank
Atlanta, Georgia, USA

Salvatore Luceri, MD, FEBO
Cornea Fellow
Netherlands Institute for Innovative Ocular Surgery (NIIOS)
Rotterdam, The Netherlands

Gerrit R.J. Melles, MD, PhD
Director
Netherlands Institute for Innovative Ocular Surgery (NIIOS)
Melles Cornea Clinic
Rotterdam, The Netherlands

Yuri McKee, MD
Corneal and Refractive Surgeon
Swagel Wootton Hiatt Eye Center
Mesa, Arizona, USA

Priya Narang, MS
Director
Narang Eye Care and Laser Centre, Ahmedabad
Navrangpura
Ahmedabad, Gujarat, India

Ashiyana Nariani, MD, MPH
Clinical Associate
Duke University Eye Center
Durham, North Carolina, USA

Claudia E. Perez-Straziota, MD
Private Practice
Atlanta, Georgia, USA

Francis W. Price, Jr., MD
Founder and President
Price Vision Group
Indianapolis, Indiana, USA

Marianne O. Price, PhD
Executive Director
Cornea Research Foundation of America
Indianapolis, Indiana, USA

Christopher S. Sáles, MD, MPH
Assistant Professor of Ophthalmology
Weill Cornell Medical College
New York, New York, USA
Associate Medical Director
Lions VisionGift
Portland, Oregon, USA

Evan D. Schoenberg, MD
Cornea, Cataract, and Refractive Surgeon
Georgia Eye Partners
Atlanta, Georgia, USA

Matthew Shulman, MD
PGY3 Resident
Department of Ophthalmology and Visual Sciences
University of Maryland School of Medicine
Baltimore, Maryland, USA

Mark A. Terry, MD
Director
Corneal Services, Devers Eye Insitute
Scientific Director
Lions VisionGift
Professor of Clinical Ophthalmology
Oregon Health Sciences University
Portland, Oregon, USA

Peter Wu, MD
Cornea Clinical Fellow
Department of Ophthalmology
University of Illinois at Chicago
Chicago, Illinois, USA

Part I

Basics

1 Anatomy of the Cornea and Pre-Descemet Layer

Dhivya Ashok Kumar and Amar Agarwal

1.1 Introduction

Cornea, the anteriormost refractive surface is the major refractive component of the eye. The normal vertical and horizontal diameter is about 11.5 mm and 12 mm, respectively. The radius of curvature is 7.8 mm anteriorly and 6.5 mm posteriorly. It measures about 0.52 to 0.54 mm thick in the center. Human corneal ultrastructure can be divided into five different layers, namely the epithelium, the Bowman layer, the stroma, the Descemet membrane layer, and the endothelium (▸ Fig. 1.1).[1,2] Recently a new layer has been noted that varies from normal stroma by a few histological characteristics, and it has been popularly termed as pre-Descemet layer (PDL) or Dua layer.[3]

1.2 Corneal Ultrastructure

1.2.1 Epithelium

The most superficial layer, present in contact with the tear film layer is made up of stratified squamous nonkeratinized cells. There are five to six layers and three types. The lowermost cells are columnar basal cells that are attached to the underlying basement membrane with hemidesmosomes. The wing cells occupy the layer above the basal cells and are usually two to three layers thick. The outermost layer consists of squamous cells that possess microvilli or plicae for adhesion with the overlying tear film.

1.2.2 Bowman Layer

Bowman layer is an acellular, basement membrane layer, formed by randomly arranged collagen fibrils. Constituents of this layer are believed to be synthesized and secreted by both epithelial cells and stromal keratocytes. Collagen fibrils in this layer are smaller than those of the stroma. Collagen types I, V,

and VII are some of the types of collagen present in this layer, along with proteoglycans.

1.2.3 Stroma

The stroma forms the major portion of the cornea. It is made up of regularly arranged collagen fibrils spaced by proteoglycans, namely dermatan sulphate and keratin sulphate. It also contains the modified fibroblasts named keratocytes. Lumican and keratan are the core proteins of keratan sulfate proteoglycan. Collagen types I, V, VI, and XII are distributed widely in the lamellae.

1.2.4 Pre-Descemet Layer, or Dua Layer

This layer has been recently identified by Dua et al as it showed few differences from normal corneal stroma.[3] It measured about $10.15 \pm 3.6 \, \mu m$ (▸ Fig. 1.2) thick (range 6.3–15.83 μm) in Dua et al's study.[3] It was observed to consist of five to eight thin lamellae of tightly packed collagen bundles that were oriented in longitudinal, transverse, and oblique directions. In immunohistochemistry staining, CD34 was negative in the PDL, which showed the lack of keratocytes in this layer, unlike in the stroma. Collagen types IV and VI seemed to be more positive for PDL compared with the corneal stroma. Another report shows the separation of PDL to be randomly arranged cleavages in collagen layers measuring 4.5 to 27.5 μm with a variable presence of keratocytes.[4]

Descemet Membrane

This is a defined sheet of collagen (▸ Fig. 1.3) with an anterior banded and a posterior nonbanded zone. This is a specialized basement membrane of the endothelium that lies in front of the endothelial cells. It is approximately $10 \pm 2 \, \mu m$ thick.

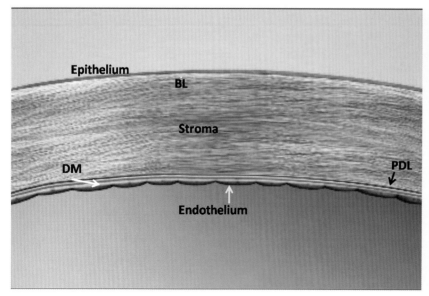

Fig. 1.1 Anatomical layers of the cornea. BL, Bowman layer; DM, Descemet membrane; PDL, pre-Descemet layer.

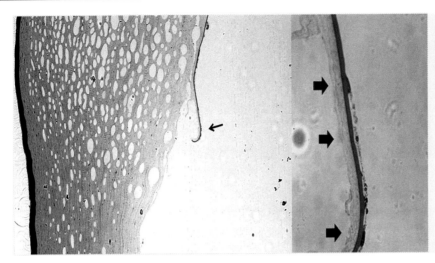

Fig. 1.2 Pre-Descemet layer (PDL) seen in histo-pathological section. Arrows demonstrate the PDL layer with the Descemet layer and the endothelial complex.

Endothelium

The endothelium is a monolayer of hexagonal cells arranged in a mosaic pattern (▶ Fig. 1.4). The average density of corneal endothelial cells at birth is approximately 4000 cells/mm^2. There are active pumps present in the endothelial cells that function continuously for nurturing the corneal layers and maintaining transparency.

1.3 Isolation of Pre-Descemet Layer

The PDL layer can be harvested by pneumatic dissection, which involves injecting air from the limbus into the midperipheral stroma of the donor cornea with a 30-gauge needle. The type 1 large bubble, which starts from the center and is well circumscribed and thicker, is the complex containing endothelium, Descemet membrane, and PDL (▶ Fig. 1.5). The bubble with PDL extends to the periphery approximately 7 to 8.5 mm and does not usually go beyond 9 mm. The overlying Descemet membrane layer can be peeled, and the bubble of PDL stays intact due to its fibrous nature. The type 1 bubble was known to withstand pressure up to 1.4 bars as compared to an isolated Descemet membrane bubble, which popped at 0.6 bars (▶ Fig. 1.6). The bubble can also be separated using viscoelastic or storage medium. The findings from an additional study that evaluated the cleavage plane of Descemet membrane after dissection provided the evidence for the existence of a physiological cleavage plane between the interfacial matrix, the anteriormost adhesive zone of the Descemet membrane, and the corneal stroma, suggesting a relatively weak attachment that can be disconnected by mechanical forces.[5]

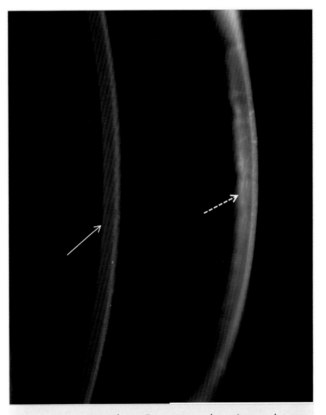

Fig. 1.3 Descemet membrane. Descemet membrane in normal cornea (solid arrow). Abnormal thickened Descemet membrane and associated folds with posterior stromal edema (dotted arrow).

1.4 Applied Anatomy of Corneal Layers

1.4.1 Epithelium

The epithelium's unique functions include light refraction, protection, transmittance, and survival over an avascular bed. The function of light refraction is obtained by its smooth, wet apical surface and its extraordinarily regular thickness. The layer traverses the high sensory nerve supplies that terminate in the suprabasal and squamous cells. The epithelium has a high regenerative or proliferative property and grows centripetally from the existing limbal stem cells. The layer protects the cornea from external injury, pathogens, and fluid loss. The mitogenic activity takes place in the basal cells and moves apically. The apical surface has microplicae and a glycocalyx that help in tear film adhesion for forming the smooth ocular surface (▶ Fig. 1.7). Persistent

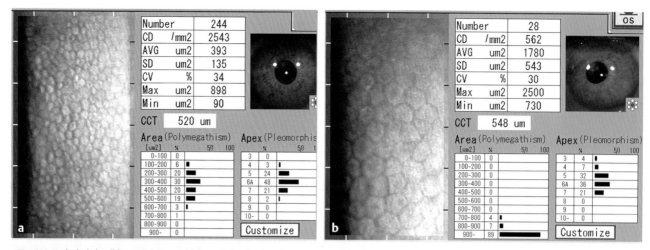

Fig. 1.4 Endothelial cell layer. **(a)** Normal hexagonal cells. **(b)** Endothelial cells showing polymegathism (enlarged cell area).

Table (a):

Number		244
CD	/mm2	2543
AVG	um2	393
SD	um2	135
CV	%	34
Max	um2	898
Min	um2	90
CCT	520 um	

Area (Polymegathism) [um2]	%		Apex (Pleomorphism)	%
0-100	0		3	0
100-200	6		4	3
200-300	20		5	24
300-400	30		6A	48
400-500	20		7	21
500-600	19		8	2
600-700	3		9	0
700-800	1		10-	0
800-900	0			
900-	0		Customize	

Table (b):

Number		28
CD	/mm2	562
AVG	um2	1780
SD	um2	543
CV	%	30
Max	um2	2500
Min	um2	730
CCT	548 um	

Area (Polymegathism) [um2]	%		Apex (Pleomorphism)	%
0-100	0		3	4
100-200	0		4	7
200-300	0		5	32
300-400	0		6A	36
400-500	0		7	21
500-600	0		8	0
600-700	0		9	0
700-800	4		10-	0
800-900	7			
900-	89		Customize	

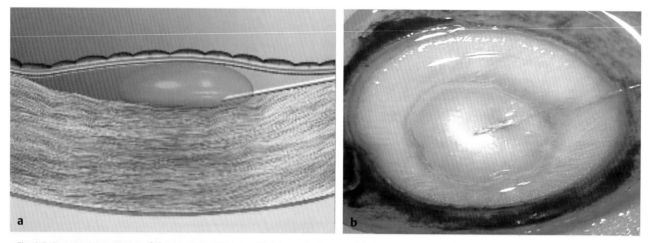

Fig. 1.5 Pneumatic separation of the pre-Descemet layer. **(a)** Schematic diagram. **(b)** Ex vivo pneumatic dissection performed in a donor cornea with air in the 30-gauge needle. Note the type 1 central big bubble being formed.

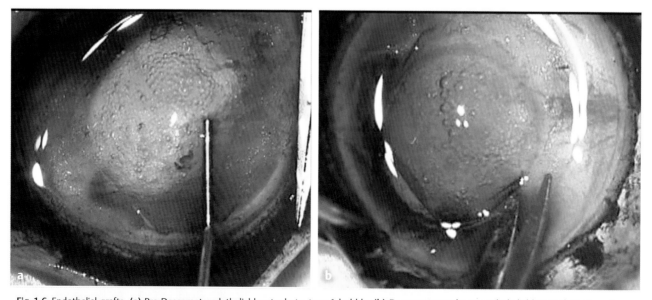

Fig. 1.6 Endothelial grafts. **(a)** Pre-Descemet endothelial keratoplasty, type 1 bubble. **(b)** Descemet membrane endothelial keratoplasty, type 2 bubble.

epithelial defect can happen in chronic ocular surface problems or upper eyelid or tear film abnormalities.

1.4.2 Bowman Layer

This layer has a protective function between the epithelium and stroma (▶ Fig. 1.7).

1.4.3 Stroma

The stroma of the human eye contains 200 to 250 lamellae. Lamellae in the middle and posterior regions of the stroma are arranged at approximate right angles, whereas those in the anterior stroma are arranged at less than right angles. The small diameter of the collagen fibrils and their close, regular packing creates a lattice or three-dimensional diffraction grating.[6] The

lattice theory of Maurice suggests the ability of the cornea to scatter 98% of the falling light with equal spacing of collagen fibrils.[7] The whole of the corneal stroma or partial lamellar stroma can be damaged due to corneal trauma, inflammation, infection, or surgery, leading to corneal opacity.

Keratoplasty techniques (▶ Fig. 1.8) have evolved over the time period from full thickness to individual layer transplantation. Penetrating keratoplasty includes the transplantation of all the layers of stroma along with the endothelium.[8] Lamellar keratoplasties involve customized corneal layers being transplanted.[9,10,11] Deep anterior lamellar keratoplasty, posterior lamellar keratoplasty, anterior lamellar keratoplasty, and Descemet stripping endothelial keratoplasty are some of the prevalent procedures. Because the stroma is highly antigenic, the risk of rejection has been known to occur more often in penetrating rather than lamellar keratoplasties.[12]

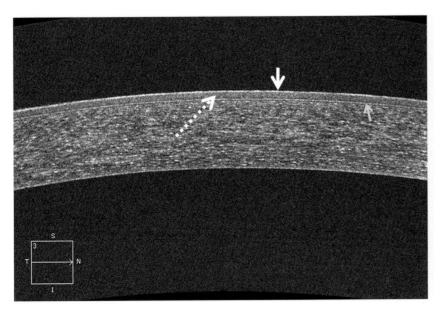

Fig. 1.7 Optical coherence tomography showing the tear film–epithelial interface (solid arrow), normal epithelium (dotted arrow), and Bowman layer (yellow arrow).

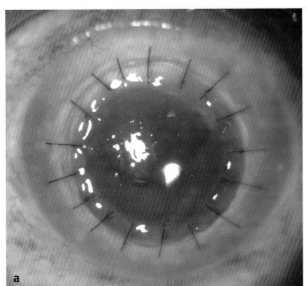
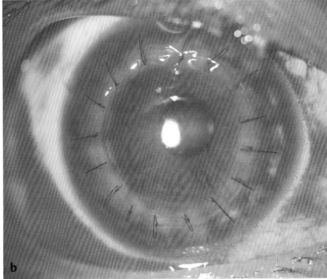

Fig. 1.8 Keratoplasties procedure. **(a)** Penetrating. **(b)** Deep anterior lamellar.

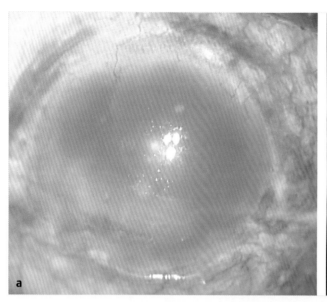
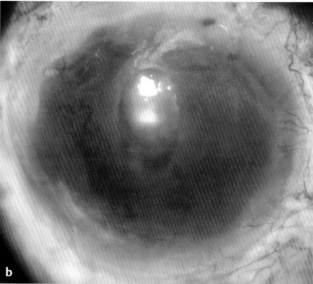

Fig. 1.9 Pre-Descemet endothelial keratoplasty. (a) Preoperative decompensated cornea. (b) Postoperative.

1.4.4 Pre-Descemet Layer

The discovery of this layer has given rise to a new technique using this layer in corneal endothelial disease. The plane between the PDL and stroma has been exploited in generating the pre-Descemet endothelial keratoplasty (PDEK) surgery (► Fig. 1.9).[13] The additional PDL along with Descemet membrane will provide strength for the graft handling during surgery. Posterior stromal pathologies, such as acute hydrops in keratoconus or descemetocele after chronic infection, may also seem to be related to the changes in PDL as a part of the original pathologies in progressive disease. The PDL and Descemet membrane layer complex can be obtained from any age group, unlike the isolated Descemet layer that is often retrieved from elderly corneas.[14]

1.4.5 Descemet Layer

Descemet membrane can be torn during cataract surgery (► Fig. 1.10) and can remain detached, which can lead to corneal edema in chronic cases. Descemet membrane along with an endothelial monolayer can be transplanted in eyes with decompensated cornea.[15] This thin layer prevents complications of interface problems associated with thicker grafts. Descemet membrane endothelial keratoplasty (DMEK) is a technique of replacing recipient diseased endothelium with a new, healthy donor Descemet endothelium layer. The Descemet membrane layer is expected to have loose adhesion with the posterior stroma in the aged population, which helps in the easy retrieval of DMEK grafts in elderly patients.

1.4.6 Endothelial Layer

The endothelium is responsible for maintaining the relatively low level of stromal hydration required for corneal transparency. The endothelium has ionic pumps that draw water from the stroma, thus maintaining the highly organized collagen lamellar structure. The pump-leak hypothesis

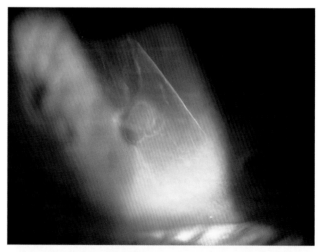

Fig. 1.10 Descemet detachment in a patient after cataract surgery.

states that the rate of fluid leakage into the stroma is balanced by the rate of fluid pumped out of the stroma. The endothelium also secretes components for Descemet membrane.[16] As such, the glucose, amino acids, vitamins, and other elements needed by the epithelial cells and stromal keratocytes must traverse the corneal endothelial monolayer. Loss of endothelial cells (by trauma or dystrophy) or damage to the endothelium (► Fig. 1.11) due to surgery can lead to bullous keratopathy or corneal decompensation. Though endothelial cells have previously been known to be nonproliferative, recent investigations have shown that they possess the property of slow regeneration, and their ability to grow human corneal endothelial cells in tissue culture indicates that these cells retain proliferative capacity that can be harnessed under appropriate conditions.[17,18,19] Hence corneal pathologies involving dysfunction of the endothelium are currently treated by endothelial replacement via a donor cornea.[20,21] Cultured human corneal endothelial cells have

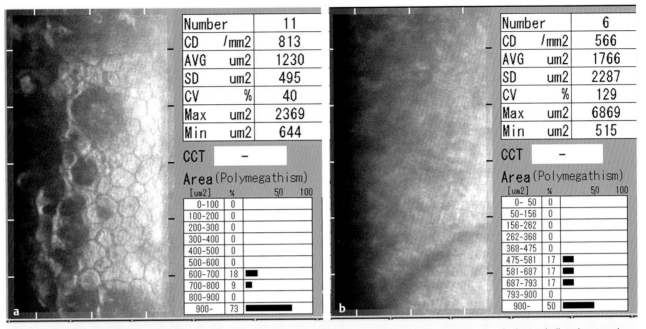

Fig. 1.11 Abnormal endothelial cells. **(a)** Endothelium showing guttate changes. **(b)** Endothelium seen in patient with chronic bullous keratopathy.

been tried for treating corneal decompensation due to endothelial dysfunction.[22] Recently ex vivo studies have shown that corneal endothelial precursors may be an effective strategy for corneal endothelial regeneration.[23]

1.5 Conclusion

Corneal microanatomy has been physiologically fashioned for its functional capability. All individual layers separately and together provide the optical transparency required for its very nature. Disease or disorder in the ultrastructure of any of its component is known to affect its competence. Understanding the intricate details of the fundamental corneal microstructure is indispensable to facing the upcoming newer diseases or refractory chronic disorders. Though the discussion of the entire physiology and applied anatomy of the cornea is beyond the scope of this book, related structural differences have been detailed here. Combined with the thorough knowledge of basic anatomy and biomechanics and aided by recent technological advancements ophthalmologists will surely gain the advantage of diagnosing and managing the corneal diseases at the preliminary stage.

References

[1] Gipson IK. Anatomy of the conjunctiva, cornea, and limbus. In: Smolin G, Thoft RA, eds. The Cornea. Boston, MA: Little, Brown and Company; 1994

[2] Warwick R. Eugene Wolff's Anatomy of the Eye and Orbit. 7th ed. London: Chapman & Hall Medical; 1997

[3] Dua HS, Faraj LA, Said DG, Gray T, Lowe J. Human corneal anatomy redefined: a novel pre-Descemet's layer (Dua's layer). Ophthalmology. 2013; 120 (9):1778–1785

[4] Schlötzer-Schrehardt U, Bachmann BO, Tourtas T, et al. Ultrastructure of the posterior corneal stroma. Ophthalmology. 2015; 122(4):693–699

[5] Schlötzer-Schrehardt U, Bachmann BO, Laaser K, Cursiefen C, Kruse FE. Characterization of the cleavage plane in DESCemet's membrane endothelial keratoplasty. Ophthalmology. 2011; 118(10):1950–1957

[6] Berman E. Cornea. In: Berman E, ed. Biochemistry of the Eye. New York: Plenum; 1991

[7] Maurice DM. The structure and transparency of the cornea. J Physiol. 1957; 136(2):263–286

[8] Nanavaty MA, Wang X, Shortt AJ. Endothelial keratoplasty versus penetrating keratoplasty for Fuchs endothelial dystrophy. Cochrane Database Syst Rev. 2014; 2:CD008420

[9] Cursiefen C, Schaub F, Bachmann B. Update: Deep anterior lamellar keratoplasty (DALK) for keratoconus : When, how and why [in German]. Ophthalmologe. 2016; 113(3):204–212

[10] Chen G, Tzekov R, Li W, Jiang F, Mao S, Tong Y. Deep Anterior Lamellar Keratoplasty Versus Penetrating Keratoplasty: A Meta-Analysis of Randomized Controlled Trials. Cornea. 2016; 35(2):169–174

[11] Acar BT, Akdemir MO, Acar S. Visual acuity and endothelial cell density with respect to the graft thickness in Descemet's stripping automated endothelial keratoplasty: one year results. Int J Ophthalmol. 2014; 7(6):974–979

[12] Abudou M, Wu T, Evans JR, Chen X. Immunosuppressants for the prophylaxis of corneal graft rejection after penetrating keratoplasty. Cochrane Database Syst Rev. 2015; 8:CD007603

[13] Agarwal A, Dua HS, Narang P, et al. Pre-Descemet's endothelial keratoplasty (PDEK). Br J Ophthalmol. 2014; 98(9):1181–1185

[14] Agarwal A, Agarwal A, Narang P, Kumar DA, Jacob S. Pre-Descemet Endothelial Keratoplasty With Infant Donor Corneas: A Prospective Analysis. Cornea. 2015; 34(8):859–865

[15] Ham L, Balachandran C, Verschoor CA, van der Wees J, Melles GR. Visual rehabilitation rate after isolated descemet membrane transplantation: descemet membrane endothelial keratoplasty. Arch Ophthalmol. 2009; 127(3):252–255

[16] Gipson IK, Joyce N. Anatomy and cell biology of the cornea, superficial limbus, and conjunctiva. In Albert and Jakobiec's Principles and Practice of Ophthalmology. 3rd ed. Philadelphia, PA: WB Saunders; 2008:423–29

[17] Joyce NC. Proliferative capacity of the corneal endothelium. Prog Retin Eye Res. 2003; 22(3):359–389

[18] Joyce NC, Zhu CC. Human corneal endothelial cell proliferation: potential for use in regenerative medicine. Cornea. 2004; 23(8) Suppl:S8–S19

[19] Engelmann K, Böhnke M, Friedl P. Isolation and long-term cultivation of human corneal endothelial cells. Invest Ophthalmol Vis Sci. 1988; 29 (11):1656–1662

[20] Boynton GE, Woodward MA. Evolving Techniques in Corneal Transplantation. Curr Surg Rep. 2015; 3(2)

[21] Ple-Plakon PA, Shtein RM. Trends in corneal transplantation: indications and techniques. Curr Opin Ophthalmol. 2014; 25(4):300–305

[22] Mimura T, Yamagami S, Yokoo S, et al. Cultured human corneal endothelial cell transplantation with a collagen sheet in a rabbit model. Invest Ophthalmol Vis Sci. 2004; 45(9):2992–2997

[23] Mimura T, Yamagami S, Amano S. Corneal endothelial regeneration and tissue engineering. Prog Retin Eye Res. 2013; 35:1–17

2 History of Endothelial Keratoplasty

Salvatore Luceri, Lamis Baydoun, Isabel Dapena, and Gerrit R.J. Melles

Although the idea of lamellar keratoplasty was introduced 200 years ago, for a long time these techniques were perceived as too complicated to be adopted by contemporary surgeons. After Dr. Eduard Zirm performed the first successful penetrating keratoplasty (PK) in 1905,[1] the full-thickness technique remained the only available treatment for corneal disorders for almost a century. Thus, in eyes with corneal endothelial disease, not only the diseased cell layer but also healthy layers of the cornea were replaced by a full-thickness penetrating transplant.

2.1 Early Work

This also remained the status quo after another attempt was made in the 1950s by Dr. José Barraquer and Dr. Charles Tillett, who introduced the concept of lamellar keratoplasty into clinical practice. They performed the first posterior lamellar endothelial transplant underneath a manually dissected stromal flap that was secured by sutures.[2,3,4] However, the lack of adequate instruments to create thin corneal layers and limited knowledge of endothelial cell physiology resulted in early complications and insufficient functional results[5] that brought further developments of these techniques to a halt. Although in the early 1990s various scientists continued to evaluate the replacement of posterior corneal tissue underneath a sutured stromal flap in experimental animal models,[6] describing a sclerocorneal approach,[7] or trying to standardize flap preparation by using a microkeratome,[8] it was only in 1998 that the first clinically successful case of endothelial keratoplasty (EK) was presented. At that time, PK was still considered the standard of care for unselective treatment of all diseased corneal layers. However, well-known and profound intra- and postoperative complications of this technique could not be sufficiently solved in the past 100 years and still 30 to 50% of indications for PK affected solely the corneal endothelium,[9] resulting in the unnecessary replacement of healthy anterior corneal tissue in treating corneal endothelial disorders. These facts were probably the reason for the following rapid advances and the breakthrough of EK in the following years.

2.2 Endothelial Keratoplasty

The first encouraging successful steps in EK led to refinements that transformed the technique into a less invasive procedure, with thinner transplants, while extinguishing many complications associated with PK and obtaining unexpected and unprecedented clinical outcomes (▶ Fig. 2.1).[10]

In 1998, Melles and colleagues introduced the first successful approach for posterior lamellar keratoplasty (PLK) in humans, in which an *unsutured* donor posterior corneal disc, consisting of posterior stroma, Descemet membrane, and endothelium, was transplanted into the anterior chamber through a limbal incision.[11,12] In 2001, this technique was popularized as deep lamellar endothelial keratoplasty (DLEK) in the United States by Terry and Ousley.[13] This PLK/DLEK technique consisted of a posterior lamellar disc dissected from the recipient cornea through a 9 mm sclerocorneal incision and replaced by an equally sized donor disc. The latter was introduced into the recipient anterior chamber and placed against the recipient posterior cornea secured only by an air bubble, while the patient had to remain in a supine position.[14] In 2000, Melles et al improved the technique by creating a smaller, self-sealing, 5 mm tunnel incision through which the **taco-folded** donor (endothelium, Descemet membrane, and a layer of stroma) was inserted, and then unfolded inside the recipient anterior chamber.[15] This less invasive technique, popularized as **small incision** DLEK, soon proved to provide clinical outcomes surpassing PK while diminishing many PK-associated complications,[16,17,18] but it was still challenging regarding donor and host tissue manual dissection. In 2002, Melles et al further simplified the concept of EK by introducing a technique that facilitated selective removal (**stripping**) of the host diseased corneal Descemet membrane and its endothelium using a reversed Sinskey hook. This step, known as descemetorhexis, was then followed by the insertion of a taco-folded posterior lamellar disc, similar to the one used in PLK/DLEK, which was then positioned onto the denuded host posterior stroma.[19] Price and colleagues later popularized this technique as Descemet stripping endothelial keratoplasty (DSEK).[20,21] At the same time Gorovoy and colleagues facilitated donor preparation by means of an automated microkeratome that enabled standardized dissection of the donor posterior lamella from a corneoscleral button while mounted on an artificial anterior chamber; to differentiate this technique from manually dissected tissue, this procedure was termed Descemet stripping *automated* endothelial keratoplasty (DSAEK).[22]

Facilitating donor tissue preparation by using a microkeratome enabled eye banks to provide precut donor tissue, making DSAEK rapidly accessible to corneal surgeons worldwide.

2.3 Advantages

Advantages of EK over PK included (1) better functional outcomes with faster visual recovery, (2) reduced risk of intraoperative bleeding or infections due to the surgery on a **closed globe** compared to the **open globe surgery** in PK, (3) elimination of suture-related complications with a preserved anterior corneal surface avoiding unpredictable postoperative refractive errors, (4) the lack of a large penetrating wound providing a tectonically stronger globe with reduced risk of traumatic wound dehiscence, and (5) reduced risk of allograft rejection.[23,24] These advantages, together with the techniques' high accessibility, played a key role in the remarkable increase of DSEK/DSAEK procedures over the following years and their implementation as the new gold standard for the treatment of endothelial pathologies.

2.4 Drawbacks

However, the DSEK/DSAEK techniques also had drawbacks, such as expensive donor tissue preparation and varying (suboptimal)

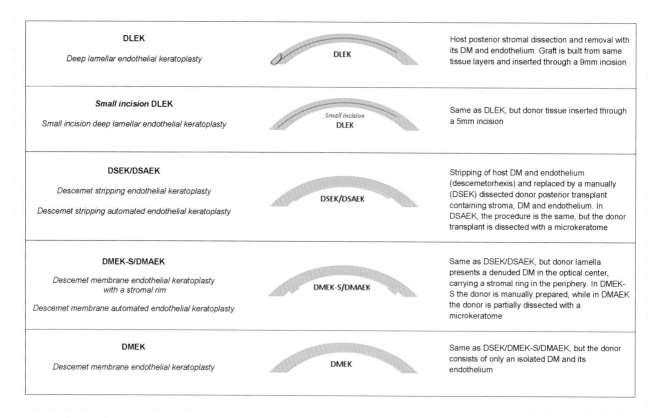

DLEK *Deep lamellar endothelial keratoplasty*	DLEK	Host posterior stromal dissection and removal with its DM and endothelium. Graft is built from same tissue layers and inserted through a 9mm incision
***Small incision* DLEK** *Small incision deep lamellar endothelial keratoplasty*	Small incision DLEK	Same as DLEK, but donor tissue inserted through a 5mm incision
DSEK/DSAEK *Descemet stripping endothelial keratoplasty* *Descemet stripping automated endothelial keratoplasty*	DSEK/DSAEK	Stripping of host DM and endothelium (descemetorhexis) and replaced by a manually (DSEK) dissected donor posterior transplant containing stroma, DM and endothelium. In DSAEK, the procedure is the same, but the donor transplant is dissected with a microkeratome
DMEK-S/DMAEK *Descemet membrane endothelial keratoplasty with a stromal rim* *Descemet membrane automated endothelial keratoplasty*	DMEK-S/DMAEK	Same as DSEK/DSAEK, but donor lamella presents a denuded DM in the optical center, carrying a stromal ring in the periphery. In DMEK-S the donor is manually prepared, while in DMAEK the donor is partially dissected with a microkeratome
DMEK *Descemet membrane endothelial keratoplasty*	DMEK	Same as DSEK/DMEK-S/DMAEK, but the donor consists of only an isolated DM and its endothelium

Fig. 2.1 Schematic diagram of penetrating keratoplasty and the current endothelial keratoplasty techniques. (Reprinted from Melles GRJ, Dapena I. How to Get Started with Standardized 'No-Touch' Descemet Membrane Endothelial Keratoplasty (DMEK). Rotterdam, The Netherlands: Netherlands Institute for Innovative Ocular Surgery; 2014, with permission.)

visual acuity outcomes despite a technically successful surgery owing to thickness irregularities of the donor posterior stroma or stromal interface haze causing optical aberrations (► Fig. 2.2).[25] Visual limitations owing to graft thickness irregularities were addressed by Busin et al when they introduced so-called ultrathin DSAEK grafts, which provided better clinical results than standard DSAEK but still required a costly microkeratome for graft preparation.[26]

2.5 Descemet Membrane Endothelial Keratoplasty

In 1998, Melles and colleagues had already presented the next refinement of EK. With this technique, called Descemet membrane endothelial keratoplasty (DMEK), a selective replacement of a Descemet membrane and its endothelium was achieved (► Fig. 2.2c).[27] After the first DMEK surgeries, performed in 2006, it soon became evident that the near complete restoration of the corneal anatomy provided unprecedented visual outcomes[10,28,29,30] and an even lower risk of allograft rejection.[31,32] Furthermore, with DMEK, the anterior corneal lamella could still be used for deep anterior lamellar keratoplasty, also known as split cornea transplantation, permitting a more efficient use of donor tissue.[33,34,35] Despite these advances, difficulties in tissue preparation, intracameral graft

unfolding, and a relatively high incidence of postoperative graft detachments were perceived as the main obstacles for a widespread application of DMEK.[36]

Studeny et al attempted to facilitate intraoperative handling of the thin DMEK transplant by introducing DMEK-S, in which a graft consisting of only Descemet membrane and endothelium in the central optical portion, supported by a peripheral stromal rim, was manually dissected improving the graft's stability inside the host anterior chamber.[37] Later, Pereira et al and McCauley et al modified the concept of this technique by using a microkeratome for donor graft dissection, a technique popularized as Descemet membrane *automated* endothelial keratoplasty (DMAEK). In fact, DMEK-S/DMAEK provided better visual outcomes when compared with DSEK/DSAEK and were considered as technically less challenging than DMEK. However, a relatively high incidence of graft detachments often required a repeat air injection (rebubbling) to achieve graft adherence.[38,39,40]

In particular technique standardization and reproducibility of DMEK tissue preparation, provision of precut tissue, and standardization of intracameral DMEK graft unfolding solved many difficulties and helped corneal surgeons to take the first steps in DMEK or make the switch from DSEK/DSAEK to DMEK.[41,42,43,44,45]

With increasing experience also graft detachment rates could be reduced significantly as reported by different groups worldwide.[46,47,48]

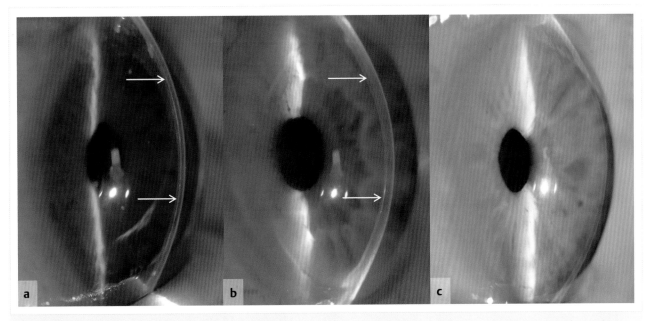

Fig. 2.2 Slit-lamp pictures showing eyes after **(a)** deep lamellar endothelial keratoplasty (DLEK), **(b)** Descemet stripping endothelial keratoplasty (DSEK), and **(c)** Descemet membrane endothelial keratoplasty (DMEK). Note the intrastromal interface (white arrows) clearly seen between the posterior stroma and the thicker DLEK graft and the thinner DSEK graft **(a, b)**, whereas after DMEK **(c)** there is no interface visible, resulting in an almost complete corneal anatomical restoration.

2.6 Conclusion

Nowadays, after a decisive phase of endothelial keratoplasty innovations, posterior lamellar techniques seem to have become the gold-standard for the treatment of corneal endothelial disease, such as Fuchs endothelial corneal dystrophy or aphakic/pseudophakic bullous keratopathy, while PK is reserved for diseases and corneal alterations that affect most of the corneal layers.

In addition, the growing experience with DMEK provided a better understanding of endothelial cell biology and physiology, as well as endothelial cell migration. For example, corneal clearance with good clinical outcomes has been observed in denuded stromal areas that were not covered by Descemet membrane and endothelium.[49,50] Thus the recent evolution in EK may not only simplify existing surgical techniques, allowing for a more efficient use of donor tissue, but may also provide a better understanding of the behavior of the endothelium in corneal endothelial diseases that may lead to alternative future treatment options.

References

[1] Zirm E. Eine Erfolgreiche totale Keratoplastik. Albrecht Von Graefes Arch Ophthalmol. 1906; 54:580–593

[2] Barraquer JI. Queratoplastia: Problemas que plantea la fijacion del injerto. In: 16th Concilium Ophthalologicum Acta. London: British Medical Association; 1951:999–1004.

[3] Barraquer JI. Lamellar keratoplasty. (Special techniques). Ann Ophthalmol. 1972; 4(6):437–469

[4] Tillett CW. Posterior lamellar keratoplasty. Am J Ophthalmol. 1956; 41 (3):530–533

[5] Culbertson WW. Endothelial replacement: flap approach. Ophthalmol Clin North Am. 2003; 16(1):113–118, vii

[6] Busin M, Monks T, Arffa RC. Endokeratoplasty in the rabbit model: A new surgical technique for endothelial transplantation. Ophthalmology. 1996; 103:167

[7] Ko WW, Frueh BE, Shields CK, Costello ML, Feldman ST. Experimental posterior lamellar transplantation of the rabbit cornea. (ARVO abstract). Invest Ophthalmol Vis Sci. 1993; 34:1102

[8] Jones DT, Culbertson WW. Endothelial lamellar keratoplasty (ELK). (ARVO abstract). Invest Ophthalmol Vis Sci. 1998; 39:876

[9] Cursiefen C, Küchle M, Naumann GO. Changing indications for penetrating keratoplasty: histopathology of 1,250 corneal buttons. Cornea. 1998; 17 (5):468–470

[10] Melles GR. Posterior lamellar keratoplasty: DLEK to DSEK to DMEK. Cornea. 2006; 25(8):879–881

[11] Melles GRJ, Eggink FAGJ, Lander F, et al. A surgical technique for posterior lamellar keratoplasty. Cornea. 1998; 17(6):618–626

[12] Melles GRJ, Lander F, Beekhuis WH, Remeijer L, Binder PS. Posterior lamellar keratoplasty for a case of pseudophakic bullous keratopathy. Am J Ophthalmol. 1999; 127(3):340–341

[13] Terry MA, Ousley PJ. Deep lamellar endothelial keratoplasty in the first United States patients: early clinical results. Cornea. 2001; 20(3):239–243

[14] Melles GRJ, Lander F, van Dooren BTH, Pels E, Beekhuis WH. Preliminary clinical results of posterior lamellar keratoplasty through a sclerocorneal pocket incision. Ophthalmology. 2000; 107(10):1850–1856, discussion 1857

[15] Melles GR, Lander F, Nieuwendaal C. Sutureless, posterior lamellar keratoplasty: a case report of a modified technique. Cornea. 2002; 21(3):325–327

[16] Terry MA, Ousley PJ. Small-incision deep lamellar endothelial keratoplasty (DLEK): six-month results in the first prospective clinical study. Cornea. 2005; 24(1):59–65

[17] Terry MA, Ousley PJ. Deep lamellar endothelial keratoplasty visual acuity, astigmatism, and endothelial survival in a large prospective series. Ophthalmology. 2005; 112(9):1541–1548

[18] Ousley PJ, Terry MA. Stability of vision, topography, and endothelial cell density from 1 year to 2 years after deep lamellar endothelial keratoplasty surgery. Ophthalmology. 2005; 112(1):50–57

[19] Melles GR, Wijdh RH, Nieuwendaal CP. A technique to excise the descemet membrane from a recipient cornea (descemetorhexis). Cornea. 2004; 23 (3):286–288

[20] Gorovoy M, Price FW. New technique transforms corneal transplantation. Cataract Refract Surg Today. 2005; 11:55–58

[21] Price FW, Jr, Price MO. Descemet's stripping with endothelial keratoplasty in 50 eyes: a refractive neutral corneal transplant. J Refract Surg. 2005; 21 (4):339–345

[22] Gorovoy MS. Descemet-stripping automated endothelial keratoplasty. Cornea. 2006; 25(8):886–889

[23] Chen ES, Terry MA, Shamie N, Hoar KL, Friend DJ. Precut tissue in Descemet's stripping automated endothelial keratoplasty donor characteristics and early postoperative complications. Ophthalmology. 2008; 115(3):497–502

[24] Price MO, Gorovoy M, Benetz BA, et al. Descemet's stripping automated endothelial keratoplasty outcomes compared with penetrating keratoplasty from the Cornea Donor Study. Ophthalmology. 2010; 117(3):438–444

[25] Tourtas T, Laaser K, Bachmann BO, Cursiefen C, Kruse FE. Descemet membrane endothelial keratoplasty versus descemet stripping automated endothelial keratoplasty. Am J Ophthalmol. 2012; 153(6):1082–90.e2

[26] Busin M, Madi S, Santorum P, Scorcia V, Beltz J. Ultrathin Descemet's stripping automated endothelial keratoplasty with the microkeratome double-pass technique: two-year outcomes. Ophthalmology. 2013; 120(6):1186–1194

[27] Melles GRJ, Rietveld FJR, Pels E, Beekhuis WH, Binder PS. Transplantation of Descemet's membrane carrying viable endothelium through a small scleral incision. ARVO Abstract. Fort Lauderdale, FL:, May 1998

[28] Melles GR, Lander F, Rietveld FJ. Transplantation of Descemet's membrane carrying viable endothelium through a small scleral incision. Cornea. 2002; 21(4):415–418

[29] Melles GR, Ong TS, Ververs B, van der Wees J. Descemet membrane endothelial keratoplasty (DMEK). Cornea. 2006; 25(8):987–990

[30] Melles GR, Ong TS, Ververs B, van der Wees J. Preliminary clinical results of Descemet membrane endothelial keratoplasty. Am J Ophthalmol. 2008; 145 (2):222–227

[31] Dapena I, Ham L, Netuková M, van der Wees J, Melles GR. Incidence of early allograft rejection after Descemet membrane endothelial keratoplasty. Cornea. 2011; 30(12):1341–1345

[32] Anshu A, Price MO, Price FW, Jr. Risk of corneal transplant rejection significantly reduced with Descemet's membrane endothelial keratoplasty. Ophthalmology. 2012; 119(3):536–540

[33] Lie JT, Groeneveld-van Beek EA, Ham L, van der Wees J, Melles GR. More efficient use of donor corneal tissue with Descemet membrane endothelial keratoplasty (DMEK): two lamellar keratoplasty procedures with one donor cornea. Br J Ophthalmol. 2010; 94(9):1265–1266

[34] Heindl LM, Riss S, Laaser K, Bachmann BO, Kruse FE, Cursiefen C. Split cornea transplantation for 2 recipients - review of the first 100 consecutive patients. Am J Ophthalmol. 2011; 152(4):523–532.e2

[35] Heindl LM, Riss S, Bachmann BO, Laaser K, Kruse FE, Cursiefen C. Split cornea transplantation for 2 recipients: a new strategy to reduce corneal tissue cost and shortage. Ophthalmology. 2011; 118(2):294–301

[36] Cursiefen C. Descemet membrane endothelial keratoplasty: the taming of the shrew. JAMA Ophthalmol. 2013; 131(1):88–89

[37] Studeny P, Farkas A, Vokrojova M, Liskova P, Jirsova K. Descemet membrane endothelial keratoplasty with a stromal rim (DMEK-S). Br J Ophthalmol. 2010; 94(7):909–914

[38] Pereira CdaR, Guerra FP, Price FW, Jr, Price MO. Descemet's membrane automated endothelial keratoplasty (DMAEK): visual outcomes and visual quality. Br J Ophthalmol. 2011; 95(7):951–954

[39] McCauley MB, Price MO, Fairchild KM, Price DA, Price FW, Jr. Prospective study of visual outcomes and endothelial survival with Descemet membrane automated endothelial keratoplasty. Cornea. 2011; 30(3):315–319

[40] Kymionis GD, Yoo SH, Diakonis VF, Grentzelos MA, Naoumidi I, Pallikaris IG. Automated donor tissue preparation for Descemet membrane automated endothelial keratoplasty (DMAEK): an experimental study. Ophthalmic Surg Lasers Imaging. 2011; 42(2):158–161

[41] Groeneveld EA, Lie JT, van der Wees J, Bruinsma M, Melles GR. Standardized 'no-touch' donor tissue preparation for DALK and DMEK: harvesting undamaged anterior and posterior transplants from the same donor cornea. Acta Ophthalmol (Copenh). 2013; 91:145–150

[42] Dapena I, Moutsouris K, Droutsas K, Ham L, van Dijk K, Melles GR. Standardized "no-touch" technique for Descemet membrane endothelial keratoplasty. Arch Ophthalmol. 2011; 129(1):88–94

[43] Kruse FE, Laaser K, Cursiefen C, et al. A stepwise approach to donor preparation and insertion increases safety and outcome of Descemet membrane endothelial keratoplasty. Cornea. 2011; 30(5):580–587

[44] Liarakos VS, Dapena I, Ham L, van Dijk K, Melles GR. Intraocular graft unfolding techniques in Descemet membrane endothelial keratoplasty. JAMA Ophthalmol. 2013; 131(1):29–35

[45] Melles GRJ, Dapena I. How to Get Started with Standardized 'No-Touch' Descemet Membrane Endothelial Keratoplasty (DMEK). Rotterdam, Netherlands: Institute for Innovative Ocular Surgery; 2014

[46] Rodríguez-Calvo-de-Mora M, Quilendrino R, Ham L, et al. Clinical outcome of 500 consecutive cases undergoing Descemet's membrane endothelial keratoplasty. Ophthalmology. 2015; 122(3):464–470

[47] Tourtas T, Schlomberg J, Wessel JM, Bachmann BO, Schlötzer-Schrehardt U, Kruse FE. Graft adhesion in Descemet membrane endothelial keratoplasty dependent on size of removal of host's Descemet membrane. JAMA Ophthalmol. 2014; 132(2):155–161

[48] Price MO, Price FW, Jr. Descemet's membrane endothelial keratoplasty surgery: update on the evidence and hurdles to acceptance. Curr Opin Ophthalmol. 2013; 24(4):329–335

[49] Balachandran C, Ham L, Verschoor CA, Ong TS, van der Wees J, Melles GR. Spontaneous corneal clearance despite graft detachment in Descemet membrane endothelial keratoplasty. Am J Ophthalmol. 2009; 148(2):227–234.e1

[50] Dirisamer M, Dapena I, Ham L, et al. Patterns of corneal endothelialization and corneal clearance after Descemet membrane endothelial keratoplasty for fuchs endothelial dystrophy. Am J Ophthalmol. 2011; 152(4):543–555.e1

3 Clinical Investigations and Diagnosis of Endothelial Cell Dysfunction

Joelle A. Hallak, Peter Wu, and Dimitri T. Azar

3.1 Introduction

The corneal endothelium is a transparent single cell layer lining the posterior cornea. It plays an essential role in maintaining stromal fluid balance and transparency. A minimum number of endothelial cells is required to provide adequate endothelial function; endothelial cell density decreases from approximately 3000 to 4000 cells/mm^2 at birth to 2500 cells/mm^2 in late adulthood.[1] Tight junctions among endothelial cells and pump function association with Na+/K+-ATPase and bicarbonate-dependent Mg2+-ATPase are necessary for endothelial functioning.[1]

The currently accepted paradigm is that corneal endothelial cells have limited proliferative potential. Various pathological conditions can lead to damage of the endothelial cells. Neighboring residual cells migrate and spread over the area of endothelial cell injury; they compensate for the endothelial cell loss and maintain corneal deturgescence and corneal transparency. However further endothelial loss will ultimately lead to decompensation of the corneal endothelium, associated with progressive visual impairment.[2]

3.2 Endothelial Cell Dysfunction

It has been shown that the density of the corneal endothelial cells is strongly heritable, with an 82% heredity contribution compared to 18% unique environmental contribution.[3] These genetic and environmental factors may trigger endothelial dysfunction and dystrophies. This chapter reviews the clinical findings and investigations needed for various conditions leading to endothelial cell dysfunction, including Fuchs dystrophy, and posterior polymorphous corneal dystrophy and pseudophakic bullous keratopathy (PBK).

3.2.1 Endothelial Dystrophies

Corneal dystrophies are noninflammatory corneal diseases that affect the cornea, leading to progressive loss of transparency. They have long been clinically classified into three groups: superficial corneal dystrophy, stromal corneal dystrophy, and posterior corneal dystrophy.[4] In 2008, an International Committee for Classification of Corneal Dystrophies classified dystrophies into four groups based on clinical features, pathological exams, and genetic data[5]: (1) epithelial and subepithelial dystrophies, (2) epithelial–stromal transforming growth factor beta induced (TGFBI) dystrophies, (3) stromal dystrophies, and (4) endothelial dystrophies.[4] Fuchs endothelial corneal dystrophy (FECD), posterior polymorphous corneal dystrophy, congenital hereditary endothelial dystrophy, and X-linked endothelial corneal dystrophy are characterized as endothelial dystrophies.

Fuchs Endothelial Corneal Dystrophy

FECD is a slowly noninflammatory progressive disease characterized by loss of endothelial cells that results in edema and loss of vision. Its key features include the presence of central guttae, folds in Descemet's membrane, stromal edema, and microcystic epithelial edema[6] (► Fig. 3.1). Fuchs endothelial dystrophy is the most common endothelial dystrophy, with a prevalence ranging between 4 and 9% in various populations.[7,8,9] A 10-year review from 2005 to 2014 showed that FECD accounted for 22% of corneal transplantations in the United States.[10] It is also more prevalent in females than in males, where females are predisposed to Fuchs dystrophy and develop corneal guttae 2.5 times more frequently than males, progressing to corneal edema 5.7 times more often than males.[11] All layers of the cornea may be affected by FECD. It is characterized by loss of endothelial cells, with thickening and excrescences of the Descemet membrane (guttae) in the central cornea.[4] Development of guttae and the onset of symptoms are more common in the fifth through seventh decades in life. Studies have demonstrated that Fuchs corneas exhibit a 45 to 59% reduction in endothelial cell density compared to healthy corneas.[12,13]

Most of the corneal dystrophies are inherited with an autosomal dominant pattern. Posterior polymorphous dystrophy has been associated with mutations in VSX1, COL8A2, and ZEB1 genes.[4] There is some genetic basis for Fuchs dystrophy. Coding mutations in four genes have been identified to be causal for the FECD phenotype: TCF8, SLC4A11, LOXHD1, and AGBL1.[1] Mutations in two transcription factors (TCF4/E2–2 and TCF8/ZEB-1), one collagen subunit (COL8A2), and two membrane proteins (LOXHD1 and SLC4A11/NaBC1) have been found in Fuchs dystrophy.[9] Except LOXHD1, these mutations appear to converge on the collagen secretion and water pump functions of corneal endothelium.

L450W[14] and Q455K[15] in the COL8A2 are two autosomal dominant mutations reported in early-onset Fuchs dystrophy. COL8A2 is the gene encoding the α2 chain of type VIII collagen. Missense mutations attributing to loss of function in TCF8, a gene encoding the ZEB1 protein, are sufficient to cause late-onset of Fuchs.[16] Additionally single-nucleotide polymorphisms in the TCF4 gene, encoding the E2–2 protein, are thought to result in decreased expression of the protein.[17] E2–2 is a transcription factor known to upregulate TCF8,[18] suggesting that both TCF4 and TCF8 are involved in the same pathway in Fuchs dystrophy development. Additional mutations in SLC4A11 were also identified.

Posterior Polymorphous Corneal Dystrophy

Posterior polymorphous corneal dystrophy (PPCD) encompasses a broad spectrum of corneal and anterior segment

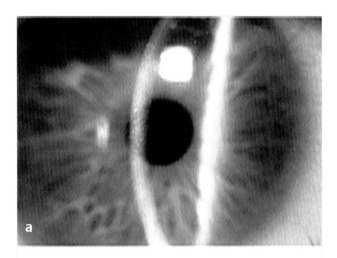

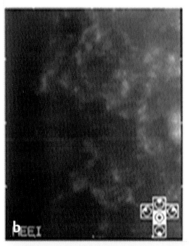

Fig. 3.1 (a) Slit lamp photography showed corneal guttae (OD). Specular microscopy was unable to provide an image of the eye due to corneal edema. (b) Specular microscopy of the left eye (OS) captured multiple guttae, with inability to perform cell counts. (Adapted from Jurkunas U, Azar DT. Potential complications of ocular surgery in patients with coexistent keratoconus and Fuchs' endothelial dystrophy. Ophthalmology 2006;113(12):2187–97.)

abnormalities.[19] This rare dystrophy has a clinical spectrum that ranges from congenital corneal edema to late-onset corneal edema in middle age. PPCD is a bilateral autosomal dominant disease. It has been linked to three chromosomal loci: PPCD1 on chromosome 20p11.2-q11.2, PPCD2 on 1p34.3-p32.3, and PCD3 on 10p11.2. The gene for PPCD1 is unknown, the gene for PPCD2 is collagen type VIII alpha 2 (COL8A2), and the gene for PPCD3 is zinc finger E-box binding homeobox 1 (ZEB1).[19,20,21,22]

The hallmark of PPCD is a vesicular lesion. Examination of the posterior corneal surface will show any or all of isolated grouped vesicles; geographic-shaped, discrete, gray lesions; and broad bands with scalloped edges. On slit lamp examination the vesicular lesions appear as transparent cysts surrounded by a gray halo at the level of the Descemet membrane. By specular microscopy, the vesicular lesions range in diameter from 0.10 to 1.00 mm.[20,21] The endothelial cells between the involved areas may have three appearances: normal-sized cells with a typical mosaic pattern, cells smaller than normal and crowded together, or enlarged pleomorphic cells.[20,21] Diffuse

opacities are also observed, and they may be either small, macular, gray-white lesions or larger sinous lesions at the level of the Descemet membrane.[19] Various degrees of stomal edema, corectopia, and broad iridocorneal adhesions may also be seen.[22]

3.2.2 Pseudophakic and Aphakic Bullous Keratopathy

PBK and aphakic bullous keratopathy (ABK) are corneal diseases caused by endothelial decompensation following cataract surgery in the presence (PBK) or absence (ABK) of intraocular lenses (IOLs). The endothelial density is reduced and a compromised endothelial cell pump leads to overhydration of the cornea.[23] PBK is more likely to occur after anterior chamber IOLs than after posterior chamber IOLs. The incidence of bullous keratopathy induced by anterior chamber IOLs may be up to 10%.[23,24] Other than Fuchs dystrophy, failed corneal grafts, penetrating or blunt trauma, and refractory glaucoma are listed as secondary causes.[23] Visual acuity is reduced in almost all cases. This is due to increased corneal thickness and Descemet membrane folds. Patients may experience discomfort and severe pain following the formation, and rupturing, of epithelial layer bullae. PBK and ABK also predispose to corneal infection and scarring.

Modern techniques of posterior keratoplasty have supplanted corneal transplantation as the gold standard treatment for patients with PBK. Other (historical) alternatives that are rarely used today include anterior stromal puncture, phototherapeutic keratectomy, amniotic membrane transplantation, conjunctival flap, bandage contact lens, and collagen cross-linking.

3.3 Clinical Examination

Corneal guttae are the first sign of Fuchs dystrophy and develop centrally and spread toward the periphery.[22] The guttae initially appear as scattered, discrete, isolated structures, smaller than an individual endothelial cell. Patients at this early stage are not symptomatic. Over time the guttae spread peripherally, the Descemet membrane becomes thickened and irregular, and folds develop secondary to stromal edema. Additional to swelling, blurred vision, foreign body sensation, photophobia, and halo perception may develop. A more advanced FECD may have "buried guttae" centrally.[25]

The epithelium is generally intact in early stages of classic Fuchs dystrophy; however, in severe FECD loss of pump function in the edematous cornea results in anterior migration of fluid through the corneal stroma and the formation of painful epithelial bullae.[1] Microcystic epithelial edema may follow, characterized as a stippled pattern that stands out in sclerotic scatter.[19] An abnormal Bowman layer with diffuse bright reflection and a paucity or absence of nerves are revealed in approximately half of the patients with FECD.[1] An increased center-to-peripheral thickness ratio in the stroma of FECD-affected corneas has been observed versus that in controls.[26] The Descemet membrane in FECD is marked by the presence of a thick posterior banded layer, a posteriormost layer in which collagen fibrils approximately 10 to 20 μm in diameter with 110 μm banding are deposited by the endothelium.[1] This posterior banded layer is approximately 16 μm thick and correlates

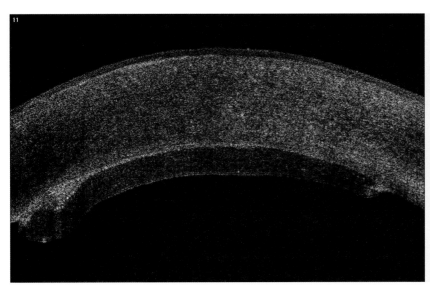

Fig. 3.2 Anterior segment optical coherence tomographic scan of a patient with posterior polymorphous corneal dystrophy (PPMD) who had undergone Descemet stripping automated endothelial keratoplasty. Image reveals recurrence of PPMD at the graft–host interface (white density).

directly with the clinical severity of FECD.[27] Additionally, a fibrillary layer may be present in corneas with severe edemas, described as a posterior collagenous layer.[28,29] Transmission electron microscopy of FCD corneas demonstrates some endothelial cells with cytoplasmic filaments, increased rough endoplasmic reticulum, and cytoplasmic processes, bearing similarity to fibroblasts; intercellular vacuoles remain in areas associated with loss of cells.[29] In end-stage disease, avascular subepithelial fibrous scarring occurs between the epithelium and the Bowman membrane. Peripheral superficial corneal neovascularization can also occur. Irregularity of the surface and loss of transparency further decrease vision.[19]

Patients with PPCD are mainly diagnosed through slit lamp by observing vesicular, band-like, or placoid areas on the posterior corneal surface. In patients with unknown corneal edema, diagnosis is based on light and electron microscopy of the excised buttons obtained during keratoplasty.[6] Specular microscopy may be helpful in differential diagnosis. The involved cells in iridocorneal endothelial syndrome appear as dark areas with a central highlight and light peripheral borders. ▶ Fig. 3.2 shows an anterior segment optical coherence tomographic (AS-OCT) scan of a patient with PPCD who had undergone Descemet stripping automated endothelial keratoplasty. ▶ Fig. 3.2 reveals recurrence of PPCD at the graft–host interface (white density).

3.4 Diagnosis and Testing

Slit lamp examination is an important diagnostic tool in the early stages of endothelial dysfunction. However, the diagnosis and clinical decision prior to surgery are enhanced by resorting to additional tools, including specular microscopy, pachymetry, and optical coherence tomography (OCT). It has become standard practice to use imaging techniques to determine anterior and posterior corneal structure and the cellular abnormalities, which begin early in endothelial dystrophies and before the onset of edema. These characteristics can also help predict outcomes of endothelial keratoplasty and determine the optimal time for intervention.

3.4.1 Specular Microscopy

The first sign of Fuchs dystrophy is observed through slit lamp examination with the presence of guttae. Specular microscopy is helpful in confirming the morphological changes in Fuchs dystrophy and other endothelial dystrophies. Additionally, specular microscopy provides endothelial cell counts, as well as a photographic record. Subtle stromal edema can be observed using sclerotic scatter techniques. ▶ Fig. 3.3 shows the difference in specular microscopy results of a normal patient versus patients with FECD. (▶ Fig. 3.4 and ▶ Fig. 3.5) also show images from the specular microscopy for a patient with iridocorneal endothelial syndrome (▶ Fig. 3.4), and a patient with PBK (▶ Fig. 3.5).

Corneal pachymetry and mapping are used to measure corneal thickness and densitometry, which allows the evaluation of the optical quality of the cornea in different corneal layers and annuli, and corneal irregularities. Anterior Segment Ocular Coherence Tomography (AS-OCT) has been used for guttae analysis and for determining the predictive value of grafts after Descemet membrane endothelial keratoplasty[30] and other methods of corneal transplants.

3.4.2 Ultrasonic and Optical Pachymetry

Ultrasound and optical devices, such as the Scheimpflug Pentacam (Oculus) and Orbscans have been used to study the corneal thickness and irregularities in patients with FECD. In a recent study Alnawaiseh et al quantified Scheimpflug corneal densitometry in patients with FECD. Patients were examined using the Scheimpflug-based Oculus Pentacam. Central corneal thickness, ring-averaged noncentral corneal thickness, and densitometry data in different corneal layers and annuli were extracted and analyzed.[31] This study showed that the total corneal light backscatter at total corneal thickness and at total diameter was significantly higher in the FECD than in controls (FECD group: 28.8 ± 6.7; control group: 24.3 ± 4.1; $P < 0.001$).

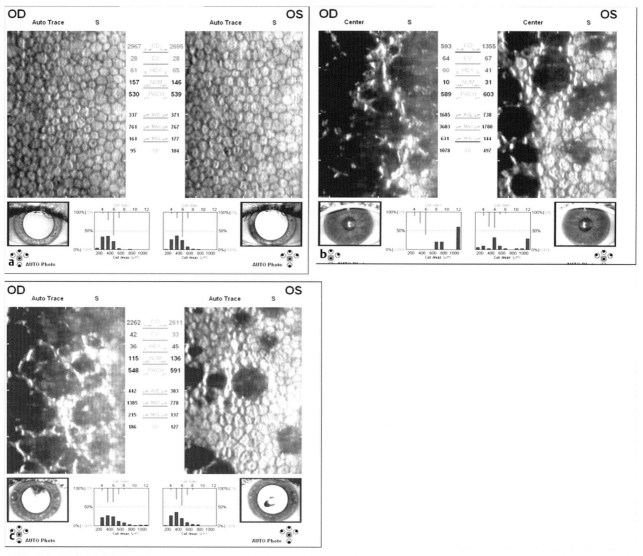

Fig. 3.3 Specular microscopy of **(a)** a patient with normal endothelial cell count and appearance and of **(b, c)** patients with Fuchs endothelial corneal dystrophy in both eyes.

When the corneal surface was divided into concentric annular zones at total corneal thickness, the differences were significant only in the two central annuli ($P < 0.001$). The total corneal light backscatter at total corneal thickness in the central 0 to 2 mm annulus correlated moderately with the central corneal thickness (Pearson's correlation = 0.55, $P < 0.001$).[31]

Brunette et al characterized the three-dimensional corneal shape deformation incurred by FECD and PBK using integrated Orbscan topographic maps. They showed that there is little anterior deformation, whereas the posterior surface presented a significant central bulging toward the anterior chamber. The thinnest point was toward the superior nasal midperiphery. The corneal periphery remained unaffected, except in the final stages.[32]

Wacker K et al determined anterior and posterior corneal higher-order aberrations and backscatter over a range of severity of FECD using Scheimpflug images.[33] FECDs were characterized as mild, moderate, or advanced according to the area and confluence of guttae and the presence of clinically visible

edema. Wavefront errors were derived from Scheimpflug images and expressed as Zernike polynomials through the sixth order over a 6 mm diameter optical zone. Backscatter from the anterior and posterior of the cornea was also measured and standardized to a fixed scatter source. They showed that anterior and posterior corneal higher-order aberrations and backscatter are higher than normal, even in early stages of FECD. The early onset of higher-order aberrations might contribute to the persistence of aberrations and incomplete visual recovery after endothelial keratoplasty.[33]

Amin et al determined the anterior corneal structure and cellular abnormalities that have been associated with visual deficits before and after endothelial keratoplasty in FECD.[34] Slit lamp biomicroscopy, ultrasonic pachymtery, and confocal microscopy were used to assess the presence of guttae and clinically evident edema and measure the corneal backscatter. Stromal cell density and number and presence of abnormal subepithelial cells were determined from confocal images.[34] Similar to the study by Wacker et al,[33] they showed that

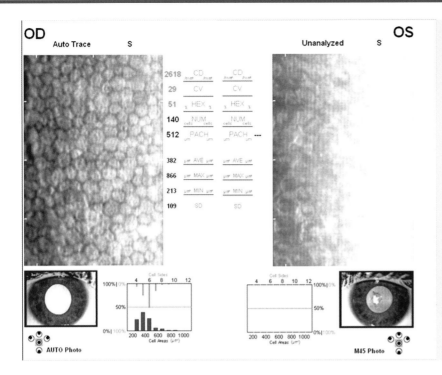

Fig. 3.4 Specular microscopy of a patient with iridocorneal endothelial syndrome of the left eye. This demonstrates the characteristic **dark-light reversal** where the endothelial cells are dark centrally and light in the periphery.

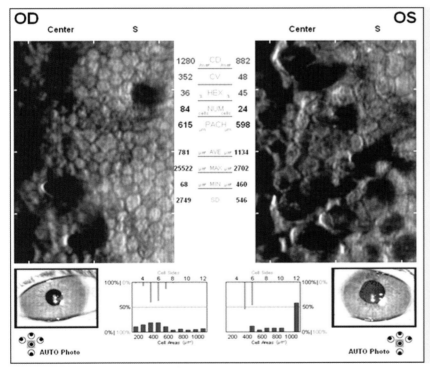

Fig. 3.5 Specular microscopy of a patient with pseudophakic bullous keratopathy of the left eye.

anterior corneal cellular and structural abnormalities begin early in the course of Fuchs dystrophy, where the trends were similar in eyes with, mild, moderate, and advanced Fuchs dystrophy when compared to normal. Regardless of disease severity, stromal cell density and the absolute number of cells in the anterior 10% of the stroma were approximately 29 and 27% lower in patients with FECD when compared to normal patients.[34]

3.4.3 Anterior Segment Ocular Coherence Tomography

AS-OCT is a noncontact imaging device that provides the detailed structure of the anterior eye part of the eyes. ▶ Fig. 3.6 shows the layers of the cornea as displayed by the AS-OCT. ▶ Fig. 3.7 shows an AS-OCT image of postoperative Descemet

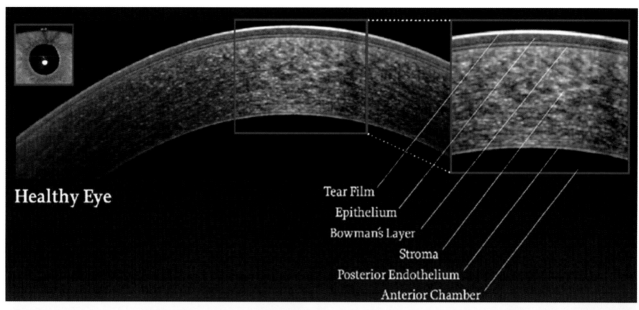

Fig. 3.6 Layers of the cornea as displayed on anterior segment optical coherence tomographic scan.

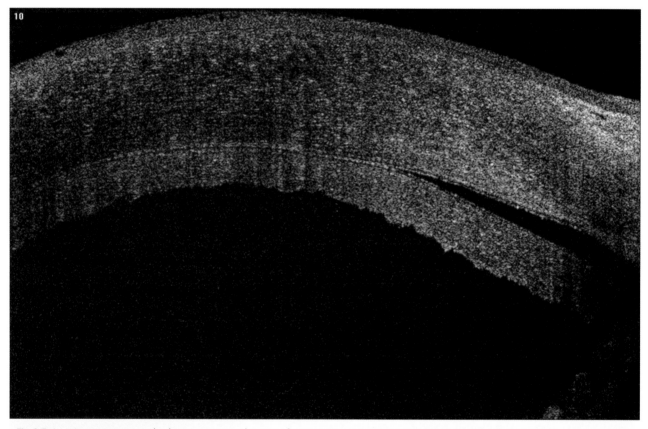

Fig. 3.7 Anterior segment optical coherence tomographic scan of postoperative Descemet stripping automated endothelial keratoplasty reveals inversion of the endothelial graft.

stripping automated endothelial keratoplasty revealing inversion of the endothelial graft. ▶ Fig. 3.8 reveals the correct orientation of the Descemet stripping automated endothelial keratoplasty graft after surgical replacement with a new graft.

▶ Fig. 3.9 shows the AS-OCT of a patient with Fuchs corneal dystrophy, revealing guttae on the endothelial surface. ▶ Fig. 3.10 displays the pachymetry function showing increased corneal thickness in a patient with Fuchs endothelial dystrophy.

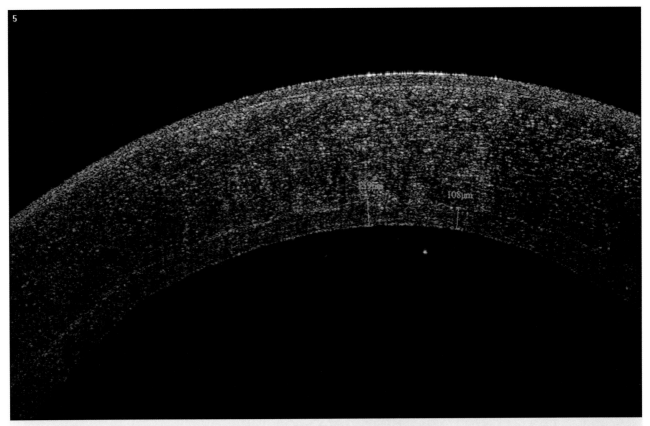

Fig. 3.8 Anterior segment optical coherence tomographic scan of the same eye as the previous photo reveals correct orientation of the Descemet stripping automated endothelial keratoplasty graft after surgical replacement with a new graft.

Yeh et al evaluated the predictive value of early AS-OCT on graft adherence or detachment after Descemet membrane endothelial keratoplasty.[30] Indication for surgery was Fuchs endothelial dystrophy and bullous keratopathy. AS-OCT was performed within the first hour after Descemet membrane endothelial keratoplasty and at 1 week, 1 month, 3 months, and 6 months. Detachments were classified as **none,** ≤⅓ detachment, >⅓ detachment of the total graft surface area, or **complete** detachment. The 1-hour AS-OCT scans showed the best predictive value on 6-month graft adherence status. Graft detachments of >⅓ at 1 hour showed reattachment at 6 months in 25% of the cases, whereas 67.5% of the cases showed a persistent detachment of >⅓ at 6 months, and 12.5% showed a complete detachment.[30]

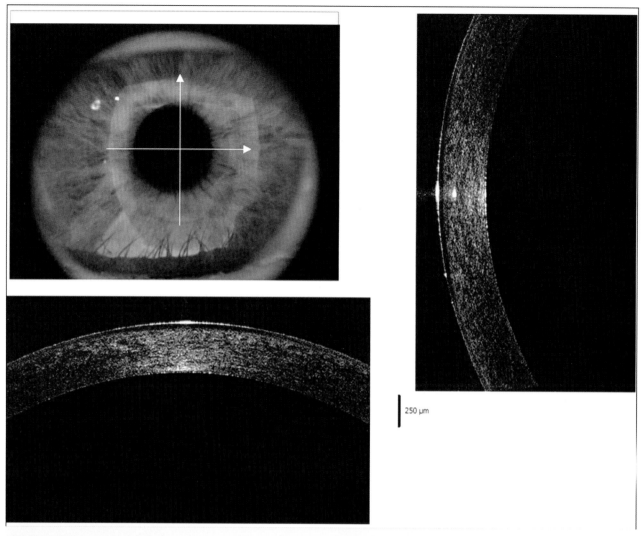

Fig. 3.9 Anterior segment optical coherence tomographic scan of a patient with Fuchs corneal dystrophy, revealing guttae on the endothelial surface.

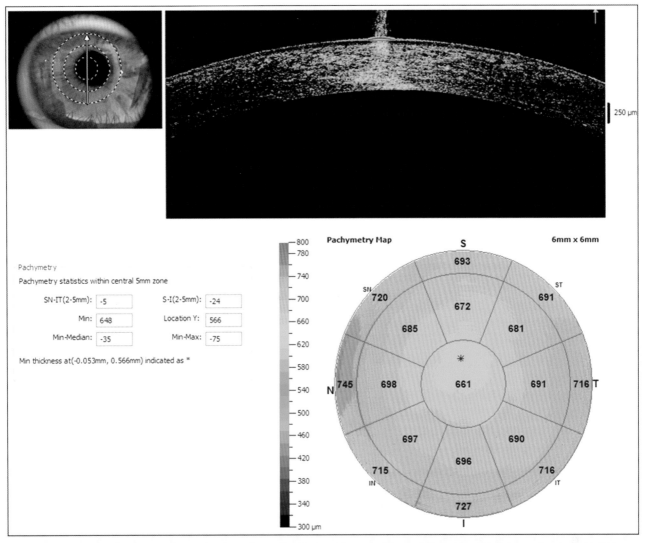

Fig. 3.10 Anterior segment optical coherence tomographic scan pachymetry function showing thickened corneal thickness of patient with Fuchs corneal dystrophy.

References

[1] Eghrari AO, Riazuddin SA, Gottsch JD. Overview of the Cornea: Structure, Function, and Development. Prog Mol Biol Transl Sci. 2015; 134:7–23

[2] Okumura N, Kinoshita S, Koizumi N. Cell-based approach for treatment of corneal endothelial dysfunction. Cornea. 2014; 33(33) Suppl 11:S37–S41

[3] Racz A, Toth GZ, Tarnoki AD, et al. The inheritance of corneal endothelial cell density. Ophthalmic Genet. 2016:1–4

[4] Sacchetti M, Macchi I, Tiezzi A, La Cava M, Massaro-Giordano G, Lambiase A. Pathophysiology of Corneal Dystrophies: From Cellular Genetic Alteration to Clinical Findings. J Cell Physiol. 2016; 231(2):261–269

[5] Weiss JS, Møller HU, Lisch W, et al. The IC3D classification of the corneal dystrophies. Cornea. 2008; 27(27) Suppl 2:S1–S83

[6] Rosado-Adames N, Afshari NA. Corneal endothelium. In: Yanoff M, Duker J, eds. Ophthalmology. 4th ed. Philadelphia, PA: Elsevier, Saunders; 2013: ch. 4.2

[7] Zoega GM, Fujisawa A, Sasaki H, et al. Prevalence and risk factors for cornea guttata in the Reykjavik Eye Study. Ophthalmology. 2006; 113(4):565–569

[8] Kitagawa K, Kojima M, Sasaki H, et al. Prevalence of primary cornea guttata and morphology of corneal endothelium in aging Japanese and Singaporean subjects. Ophthalmic Res. 2002; 34(3):135–138

[9] Zhang J, Patel DV. The pathophysiology of Fuchs' endothelial dystrophy—a review of molecular and cellular insights. Exp Eye Res. 2015; 130:97–105

[10] Park CY, Lee JK, Gore PK, Lim CY, Chuck RS. Keratoplasty in the United States: A 10-Year Review from 2005 through 2014. Ophthalmology. 2015; 122 (12):2432–2442

[11] Krachmer JH, Purcell JJ, Jr, Young CW, Bucher KD. Corneal endothelial dystrophy. A study of 64 families. Arch Ophthalmol. 1978; 96(11):2036–2039

[12] Mustonen RK, McDonald MB, Srivannaboon S, Tan AL, Doubrava MW, Kim CK. In vivo confocal microscopy of Fuchs' endothelial dystrophy. Cornea. 1998; 17(5):493–503

[13] Schrems-Hoesl LM, Schrems WA, Cruzat A, et al. Cellular and subbasal nerve alterations in early stage Fuchs' endothelial corneal dystrophy: an in vivo confocal microscopy study. Eye (Lond). 2013; 27(1):42–49

[14] Gottsch JD, Zhang C, Sundin OH, Bell WR, Stark WJ, Green WR. Fuchs corneal dystrophy: aberrant collagen distribution in an L450W mutant of the COL8A2 gene. Invest Ophthalmol Vis Sci. 2005; 46(12):4504–4511

[15] Biswas S, Munier FL, Yardley J, et al. Missense mutations in COL8A2, the gene encoding the alpha2 chain of type VIII collagen, cause two forms of corneal endothelial dystrophy. Hum Mol Genet. 2001; 10(21):2415–2423

[16] Riazuddin SA, Vithana EN, Seet LF, et al. Missense mutations in the sodium borate cotransporter SLC4A11 cause late-onset Fuchs corneal dystrophy. Hum Mutat. 2010; 31(11):1261–1268

[17] Baratz KH, Tosakulwong N, Ryu E, et al. E2-2 protein and Fuchs's corneal dystrophy. N Engl J Med. 2010; 363(11):1016–1024

[18] Sobrado VR, Moreno-Bueno G, Cubillo E, et al. The class I bHLH factors E2-2A and E2-2B regulate EMT. J Cell Sci. 2009; 122(Pt 7):1014–1024

[19] Weisenthal RW, Streeten BW. Descemet's membrane and endothelial dystrophies. In: Krachmer JH, Mannis MJ, Holland EJ, eds. Cornea. 3rd ed. St. Louis, MO: Mosby/Elsevier; 2011:845–64

[20] Laganowski HC, Sherrard ES, Muir MG. The posterior corneal surface in posterior polymorphous dystrophy: a specular microscopical study. Cornea. 1991; 10(3):224–232

[21] Laganowski HC, Sherrard ES, Muir MG, Buckley RJ. Distinguishing features of the iridocorneal endothelial syndrome and posterior polymorphous dystrophy: value of endothelial specular microscopy. Br J Ophthalmol. 1991; 75 (4):212–216

[22] American Academy of Ophthalmology. Corneal dystrophies and ectasia. In: External Disease and Cornea: Section 8. Basic and Clinical Science Course. San Francisco, CA: Author; 2014–2015:253–87

[23] Siu GD, Young AL, Jhanji V. Alternatives to corneal transplantation for the management of bullous keratopathy. Curr Opin Ophthalmol. 2014; 25(4):347–352

[24] Taylor DM, Atlas BF, Romanchuk KG, Stern AL. Pseudophakic bullous keratopathy. Ophthalmology. 1983; 90(1):19–24

[25] Adamis AP, Filatov V, Tripathi BJ, Tripathi RC. Fuchs' endothelial dystrophy of the cornea. Surv Ophthalmol. 1993; 38(2):149–168

[26] Repp DJ, Hodge DO, Baratz KH, McLaren JW, Patel SV. Fuchs' endothelial corneal dystrophy: subjective grading versus objective grading based on the central-to-peripheral thickness ratio. Ophthalmology. 2013; 120(4):687–694

[27] Bourne WM, Johnson DH, Campbell RJ. The ultrastructure of Descemet's membrane. III. Fuchs' dystrophy. Arch Ophthalmol. 1982; 100(12):1952–1955

[28] Waring GO, III, Rodrigues MM, Laibson PR. Corneal dystrophies. II. Endothelial dystrophies. Surv Ophthalmol. 1978; 23(3):147–168

[29] Iwamoto T, DeVoe AG. Electron microscopic studies on Fuchs' combined dystrophy. II. Anterior portion of the cornea. Invest Ophthalmol. 1971; 10(1):29–40

[30] Yeh RY, Quilendrino R, Musa FU, Liarakos VS, Dapena I, Melles GR. Predictive value of optical coherence tomography in graft attachment after Descemet's membrane endothelial keratoplasty. Ophthalmology. 2013; 120(2):240–245

[31] Alnawaiseh M, Zumhagen L, Wirths G, Eveslage M, Eter N, Rosentreter A. Corneal Densitometry, Central Corneal Thickness, and Corneal Central-to-Peripheral Thickness Ratio in Patients With Fuchs Endothelial Dystrophy. Cornea. 2016; 35(3):358–362

[32] Brunette I, Sherknies D, Terry MA, Chagnon M, Bourges JL, Meunier J. 3-D characterization of the corneal shape in Fuchs dystrophy and pseudophakic keratopathy. Invest Ophthalmol Vis Sci. 2011; 52(1):206–214

[33] Wacker K, Baratz KH, Maguire LJ, McLaren JW, Patel SV. Descemet Stripping Endothelial Keratoplasty for Fuchs' Endothelial Corneal Dystrophy: Five-Year Results of a Prospective Study. Ophthalmology. 2016; 123(1):154–160

[34] Amin SR, Baratz KH, McLaren JW, Patel SV. Corneal abnormalities early in the course of Fuchs' endothelial dystrophy. Ophthalmology. 2014; 121(12):2325–2333

4 Clinicopathology of Corneal Endothelial Diseases

Rachel L.R. Gomes, Thomas John, and Kenneth R. Kenyon

4.1 Introduction

Endothelial keratoplasty has been specifically devised solely to replace a defective corneal endothelial cell population in the concomitant presence of sufficient stromal optical clarity and topographic plus tectonic stability, to thereby support visual recovery. As such, the most appropriate cases for endothelial keratoplasty comprise those several intrinsic or acquired endothelial disorders that do not adversely affect stromal clarity or ocular surface integrity. Here we survey the clinical and pathological features of such primary and secondary corneal endothelial disorders, arranged in accordance with their primary or secondary endothelial dysfunctions as follows:

1. Primary/intrinsic endothelial disorders
   a) Fuchs endothelial dystrophy (FED)
   b) Posterior polymorphous corneal dystrophy (PPCD)
   c) Congenital hereditary endothelial dystrophy (CHED)
   d) X-linked endothelial corneal dystrophy
   e) Iridocorneal endothelial (ICE) syndrome
2. Secondary/acquired endothelial disorders
   a) Postsurgical
      1. Cataract: aphakic and pseudophakic corneal edema, toxic anterior segment syndrome (TASS)
      2. Keratoplasty: immunologic rejection and endothelial attrition/decompensation
      3. Glaucoma: postfiltration surgery (tube shunt), chronic topical medication toxicity
   b) Trauma
      1. Congenital glaucoma
      2. Birth forceps injury
      3. Blunt injury
   c) Postinflammatory and postinfectious: uveitis, keratitis, endotheliitis (herpes zoster ophthalmicus [HZO], herpes simplex virus [HSV], cytomegalovirus [CMV])

4.1.1 Primary/Intrinsic Endothelial Disorders

According to the recent report of the International Committee for the Classification of the Corneal Dystrophies (IC3D),[1] the endothelial dystrophies comprise Fuchs endothelial dystrophy (FED), posterior polymorphous corneal dystrophy (PPCD), congenital hereditary endothelial corneal dystrophy (CHED), and X-linked endothelial corneal dystrophy (XECD). Primary and often inherited abnormalities of the corneal endothelium and Descemet membrane are the common characteristic of this group.

Fuchs Endothelial Dystrophy

Etiology

The most prevalent corneal dystrophy in the United States, FED affects approximately 4% of the population over the age of 40 years[2] and is more frequent and severe in women (3:1). Also common in European populations, it is rare among Asians. Exhibiting a strong inherited predisposition with more than one genetic cause, it is reported that two alleles present in the transcription factor 4 (*TCF4*) gene encoding the E2-2 protein increase the FED risk in homozygotes by up to 30 times.[2] In particular, the TGC trinucleotide repeat expansion in *TCF4* is strongly associated with FED, and a repeat length > 50 is highly specific and predictive for the disease and a predictor of disease risk.[3,4] There is also evidence of significant allelic heterogeneity, with two mutations described in the collagen, type VIII, alpha 2 gene (*COL8A2*). Hence abnormality of solute carrier family 4, sodium borate transporter, member 11 (*SLC4A11*)—a sodium-coupled borate transporter of the human plasma membrane that is also linked with congenital hereditary endothelial dystrophy type 2—is implicated.[5]

Clinical Features

FED is a bilateral but unpredictably progressive corneal disorder, usually appearing by the fifth or sixth decade of life but sometimes earlier. The hallmark clinical findings are minute focal excrescences (guttae) on a thickened Descemet membrane, progressing to generalized stromal and eventually epithelial edema with concomitant decreased visual acuity. With slit lamp biomicroscopy, guttata appear as a glittering golden brown excrescence of the Descemet membrane, and by retroillumination, as minute dewdrops. Because the advent of guttata precedes the development of visual symptoms by many years, serial examination by endothelial specular microscopy and corneal pachymetry is an important means to monitor disease progression.

The dystrophy is classified into four stages: (1) cornea guttata initially central and subsequently diffusely; (2) endothelial decompensation and progressive stromal edema; (3) stromal edema progressing to cause intraepithelial and interepithelial edema, manifest as microcytic and/or bullous keratopathy; and (4) subepithelial fibrosis, scarring, and peripheral superficial vascularization consequent to long-standing chronic edema. Such surface and stromal alterations render stage 4 cases potentially inappropriate for endothelial keratoplasty. ▶ Fig. 4.1, ▶ Fig. 4.2, ▶ Fig. 4.3, ▶ Fig. 4.4, and ▶ Fig. 4.5 show the clinical aspects of different stages of Fuchs dystrophy.

Imaging and Pathology

Confocal microscopy as well as specular microscopy provides relevant information at different FED stages. There is reduction of anterior and eventually stromal cell density.[6] Most critically, endothelial cell population density and uniformity are diminished and guttata increase in frequency depending on disease severity and area of analysis. Corneal innervation can also be altered as total nerve length, total nerve number, and number of main nerve trunks and branches decrease with disease progression.[7]

Both light and electron microscopy disclose dramatic diffuse Descemet membrane thickening with superimposed focal guttate excrescences plus the progressive distortion and attrition of the endothelial cells. ▶ Fig. 4.5 and ▶ Fig. 4.6 show the pathological aspects of the disease.

Posterior Polymorphous Corneal Dystrophy

Etiology

Much less common than FED, PPCD is an autosomal dominant disorder. The genetic locus is heterogenic as the pericentromeric region of chromosome 20 (PPCD1 locus), associated with mutations in *COL8A2* on chromosome 1 (PPCM2 locus) and related to nonsense mutations in the zinc finger E-box binding homeobox 1 gene (*ZEB1* or *TCF8*) on chromosome 10 have been identified.[8,9]

Clinical Features

Small aggregates of vesicles bordered by a gray haze, and gray geographic areas arise at the level of the Descemet membrane and contain round or elliptical vesicular zones, creating a pattern resembling Swiss cheese. Adhesions fusing the iris with the posterior surface of the peripheral cornea can progress to secondary glaucoma.

PPCD is bilateral but extremely asymmetrical such that only one cornea appears clinically affected.[1,10] Most patients remain asymptomatic, and corneal edema is usually absent

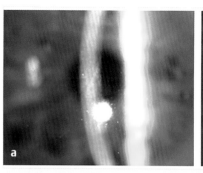
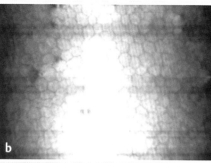
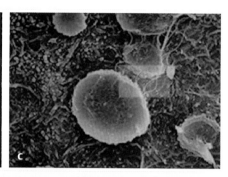

Fig. 4.1 Fuchs endothelial dystrophy. (a) Slit lamp biomicroscopy discloses stromal edema involving the visual axis. (b) In early-stage dystrophy, endothelial specular microscopy clearly resolves relatively normal endothelial cell mosaic of polygonal cells with sporadic guttae evident as focal dark opacities. (c) In an advanced case requiring keratoplasty, scanning electron microscopy of the keratoplasty disc shows multiple guttae as mushroom-like excrescences projecting posteriorly from the exposed surface of the Descemet membrane, which itself has become increasingly fibrotic. No intact endothelial cells are apparent. (× 1000)

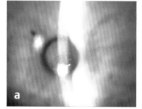
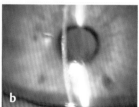
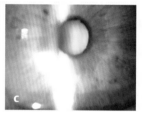

Fig. 4.2 Fuchs endothelial dystrophy. (a–c) Slit lamp biomicroscopy displays various stages of corneal edema as well as cataract. (d) High magnification retroillumination biomicroscopy highlights guttae as glittering golden-brown excrescences of the Descemet membrane having a beaten metal appearance.

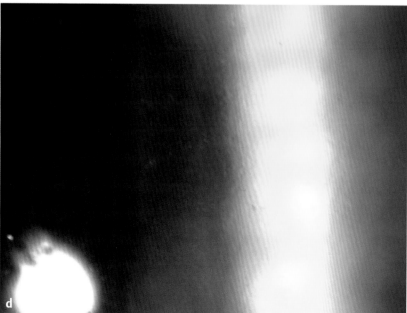

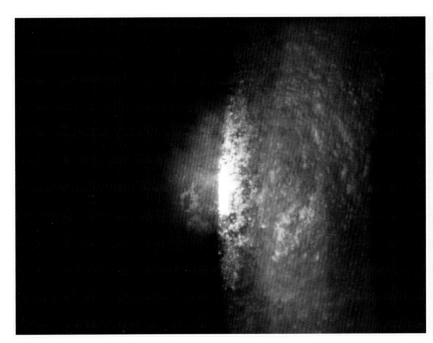

Fig. 4.3 Fuchs endothelial dystrophy. Slit lamp biomicroscopy with high magnification and ret-roillumination highlights guttae as a glittering golden-brown excrescence of the Descemet membrane. (Courtesy of Gustavo A. Novais, MD, PhD.)

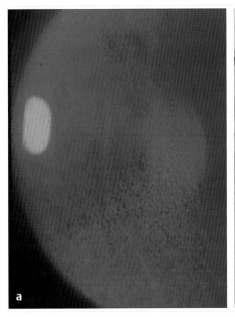
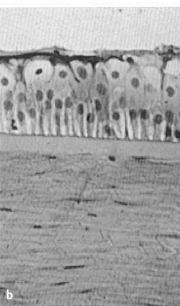

Fig. 4.4 Fuchs endothelial dystrophy. **(a)** Biomicroscopy with fluorescein staining of tear film reveals fine microcytic epithelial edema. **(b)** Light microscopy of anterior cornea exhibits intra- and interepithelial edema, although the Bowman layer and stroma remain intact. (Hematoxylin-eosin, × 400)

or clinically insignificant because the corneal endothelium remains functionally adequate. In cases where endothelial dysfunction is progressive, stromal edema and calcific band keratopathy can develop and are indications for surgical intervention. ▶ Fig. 4.7 and ▶ Fig. 4.8 represent some clinical aspects of PPCD.

Imaging and Pathology

Cornea endothelial vesicular lesions are characterized by rounded dark areas (doughnut-like) with cellular detail centrally. Vesicles may also coalesce and form well-demarcated curvilinear bands appearing to protrude into the anterior chamber, some with central posterior concavity. Endothelial

pleomorphism and polymegathism can also be notable, and, in particular, focal epithelioid mosaicism is evident.[11,12] ▶ Fig. 4.9, ▶ Fig. 4.10, and ▶ Fig. 4.11 show some of the pathological characteristics of PPCD.

Congenital Hereditary Endothelial Dystrophy

Etiology

Although long thought to have both dominant and recessive forms, congenital hereditary endothelial dystrophy (CHED) is now considered solely as a congenital autosomal recessive disorder[1] with mutation of the gene *SLC4A11* in the *20p13* locus.[13]

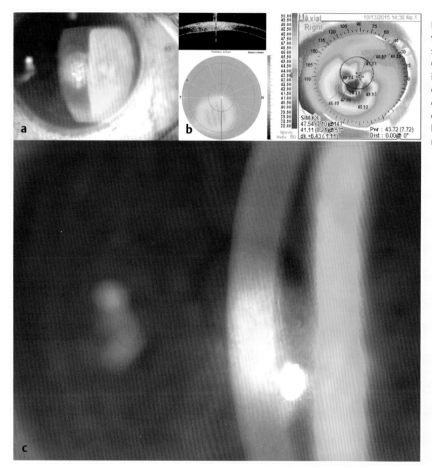

Fig. 4.5 Fuchs endothelial dystrophy. **(a)** Slit lamp view of advanced case with marked epithelial and stromal edema involving the visual axis. **(b)** Optical coherence tomography and topographic imaging highlight corneal thickening and steepening consequent to profound localized stromal edema. **(c)** Biomicroscopy of advanced case with epithelial plus stromal edema, Descemet membrane folds, and, in retroilluminated area (right), numerous focal gutta.

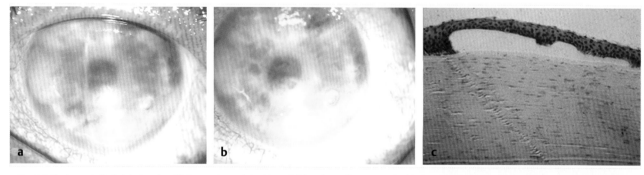

Fig. 4.6 Fuchs endothelial dystrophy. Slit lamp photos **(a)** with and **(b)** without fluorescein highlight epithelial macrobullous edema as well as diffuse stromal swelling and haze plus superficial neovascularization. **(c)** Light microscopy of keratoplasty specimen displays microbullous separation of epithelium from Bowman layer and stroma, consequent to profound epithelial and stromal edema (Hematoxylin-eosin, x300).

Clinical Features

Corneal abnormalities are bilateral but often asymmetric, as profound stromal edema (two to three times normal thickness) varies from diffuse haze to complete opacity with occasional gray spots. The endothelial cell population density is extremely low. Importantly, intraocular pressure (IOP) is not elevated. ▶ Fig. 4.12 shows the clinical and pathological characteristics of CHED.

Imaging and Pathology

Descemet membrane is often diffusely thickened in the posterior nonbanded zone, and focal guttae are never evident. The endothelium is extremely attenuated or altogether absent.

X-Linked Endothelial Corneal Dystrophy

Etiology

This rare X-chromosomal dominant dystrophy is consequent to mutation at locus at *Xq25*.

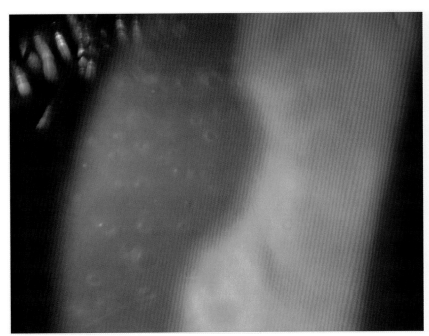

Fig. 4.7 Posterior polymorphous dystrophy. Slit lamp biomicroscopy at high magnification resolves multiple minute, round vesicles at the level of the endothelium. (Courtesy of Gustavo A. Novais, MD, PhD.)

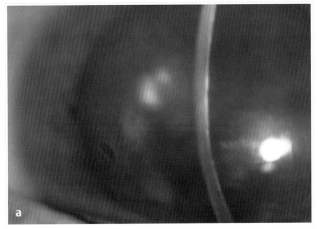

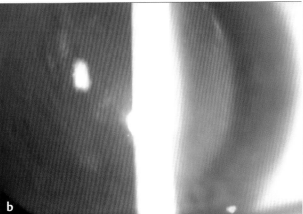

Fig. 4.8 Posterior polymorphous dystrophy. (a) Thin slit beam resolves Descemet membrane thickening. (b) By retroillumination, multiple focal vesicular alterations of the Descemet membrane become apparent.

Clinical Features

Due to the mode of inheritance, males are more severely affected. Females are asymptomatic but evidence endothelial changes reminiscent of moon craters. In males, the abnormalities are similar to those evident in CHED. Advanced cases can also develop band keratopathy.

Iridocorneal Endothelial (ICE) Syndrome: Chandler, Essential Iris Atrophy, Cogan–Reese

Etiology

The ICE syndrome comprises a group of related disorders, all characterized by an abnormal corneal endothelium. It almost always appears unilateral (although with minimal fellow-eye abnormality), manifests in young adulthood, and is more prevalent in women.

The etiology remains unknown, although some studies have related the endothelial cell metaplasia to viral infections (herpes simplex and Epstein–Barr viruses).[14],[15] Additional clarification remains required.[16]

Mechanistically, the abnormal metaplastic endothelial cell layer grows across the anterior chamber angle, and the contraction of this tissue results in angle closure as well as full-thickness iris tissue distortions and defects. In the early stages of the disease, the affected individuals are usually asymptomatic, but with progression, blurred vision, elevated IOP, and/or iris changes become evident. Depending on the relative contributions of corneal, angle, and iris changes, three syndromes are commonly recognized:

1. **Essential iris atrophy**: significant iris traction, thinning, and holes with irregular displaced pupil (▶ Fig. 4.13)
2. **Chandler syndrome**: corneal edema with relatively mild iris changes
3. **Cogan–Reese iris nevus syndrome**: pigmented iris surface nodules, iris atrophy

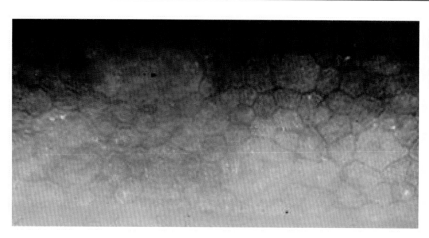

Fig. 4.9 Posterior polymorphous dystrophy. Specular microscopy discloses mosaicism of endothelial cell population as focal clusters of epithelial-appearing cells are interspersed among typical endothelial cells.

Imaging and Pathology

Specular microscopy reveals a population of abnormal endothelial cells, so-called ICE-cells,[17] which are uniquely enlarged, pleomorphic, and epithelial-like and show a light–dark reversal with light cell borders, dark cell interiors, and hyperreflective nuclei.[18] They appear progressively irregular and seemingly relate to the disease stage.[19,20] Abnormally grouped keratocytic clusters may appear in the posterior stroma.[20] Scanning microscopy of a keratoplasty specimen with ICE syndrome is shown in ▸ Fig. 4.14.

4.1.2 Secondary/Acquired Endothelial Disorders

Postsurgical

Cataract: Aphakic and Pseudophakic Corneal Edema

Irreversible corneal endothelial dysfunction resulting in clinically significant bullous keratopathy may occur in approximately 1 to 2% of patients undergoing cataract surgery, thereby representing annually about 2 to 4 million cases worldwide.[21]

The primary cause is the loss of endothelial cells secondary to surgical trauma, in most situations involving older patients with more densely mature cataracts and/or with preexisting corneal endothelial compromise, such as Fuchs endothelial dystrophy. ▸ Fig. 4.15 shows the clinical characteristics of a patient with endothelial dysfunction after cataract surgery. Corneal edema also occurs after multiple surgeries for glaucoma, particularly those involving tube shunts, and intraocular lens (IOL) secondary placement or exchange by either anterior chamber or scleral-fixated posterior chamber IOL. Following intraocular surgery, reduction in the population of Na +, K + adenosine triphosphatase (-ATPase) pumps, predominantly in the corneal endothelium but also in the epithelium, contribute to the development of bullous keratopathy.[21] ▸ Fig. 4.16, ▸ Fig. 4.17, and ▸ Fig. 4.18 describe the pathological aspects of the disease.

Toxic Anterior Segment Syndrome

The toxic anterior segment syndrome (TASS) is an acute and intense sterile inflammation of the anterior segment of the eye following cataract and other anterior segment surgical procedures.[22] Typically developing within 24 hours after surgery, TASS is characterized by corneal edema and anterior chamber hypopyon (▸ Fig. 4.19). Often occurring as a cluster of cases, TASS is distinguished from infectious endophthalmitis by its immediate postoperative onset. A recent study reported an incidence of 0.22%.[23] Several causes of TASS have been proposed, including intraocular solutions with inappropriate chemical composition, concentration, pH, or osmolality; preservatives; denatured ophthalmic viscosurgical devices; enzymatic detergents; bacterial endotoxin; oxidized metal deposits and residues; and factors related to IOLs, such as residues from polishing or sterilizing compounds.[22] Problems with the instrument-cleaning process, especially inadequate flushing of ophthalmic instruments and handpieces, enzymatic detergents, and ultrasound baths, remain the most common associations.[24]

Patients experience often extremely reduced vision, but pain is relatively infrequent. Pancorneal edema and marked anterior segment inflammatory response, frequently with hypopyon and fibrin reaction, are common. Other findings include iris damage with a dilated, irregular, and tonic pupil as well as trabecular meshwork involvement with possible secondary glaucoma.

Following resolution of the acute inflammatory reaction, specular microscopy discloses a major reduction in the endothelial cell population with pleomorphism.[25] If collateral anterior segment damage is otherwise modest, such eyes are appropriate for endothelial keratoplasty, often in conjunction with iridoplasty.

Keratoplasty: Immunologic Rejection and Endothelial Attrition/Decompensation

Following penetrating or endothelial keratoplasty, the long-term loss of corneal clarity due to endothelial cell attrition and subsequent endothelial dysfunction, is an important cause of non-rejection-associated graft failure. Endothelial failure accounts for 15% of all causes of graft failure, against 5 to 18% due to rejection. For favorable prognostic indications, survival of first-time penetrating keratoplasty (PK) is 90% at 5 years and 82% at 10 years.

Etiology

A combination of factors can lead to postkeratoplasty endothelial failure. Donor factors, tissue storage, and preparation

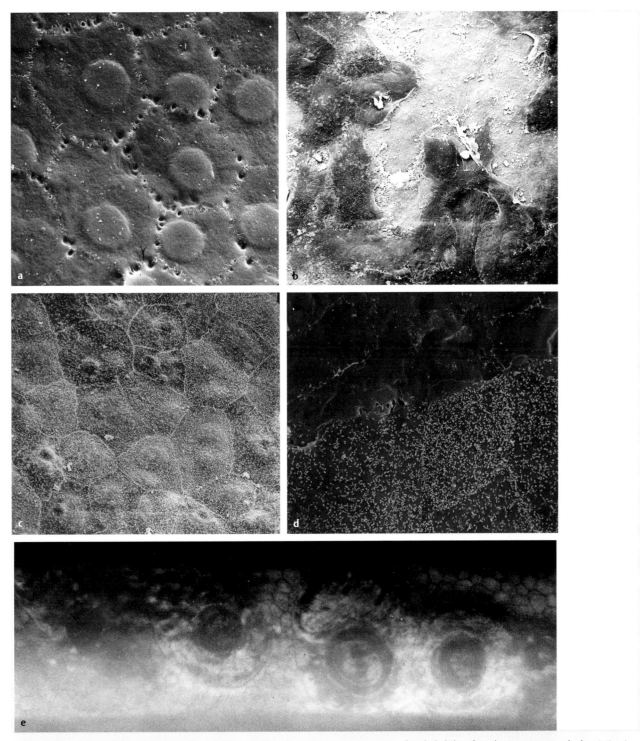

Fig. 4.10 Posterior polymorphous dystrophy. **(a)** Scanning electron microscopy appearance of endothelial surface demonstrates marked variation in cell size (×2000). **(b)** Geographic area of endothelial cell degeneration exposes fibrillar posterior collagen layer. Remaining cells are configured bizarrely, with extended cytoplasmic processes (×540). **(c)** Foci of epithelial-like endothelial cells display distinct surface membrane pattern (×1000). **(d)** At higher magnification, typical polygonal endothelial cells (above) contrast with adjacent epithelial-like cells (below) displaying numerous microvilli (×3000). **(e)** Specular microscopy resolves grouped vesicle-like Descemet membrane thickenings with associated focal abnormalities of underlying endothelial cells as surrounding endothelium retains normal configuration.

techniques, as well as surgical and postoperative host factors, collectively contribute to endothelial cell damage and attrition. In the extremes, primary donor failure comprises immediate postoperative irreversible edema of the graft, whereas chronic endothelial failure progressively occurs several years after keratoplasty. A recent large study detected a significant effect of donor age, and preoperative donor endothelial cell population density (ECD) (favorable if > 2200 cells/mm^2), on endothelial

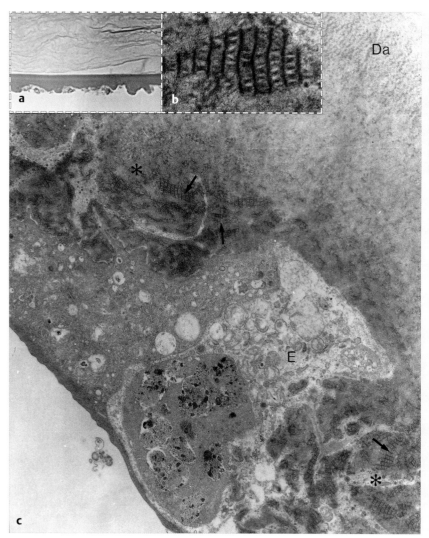

Fig. 4.11 Posterior polymorphous dystrophy. **(a)** Phase contrast photomicrograph of guttate changes in Descemet membrane with many irregularly shaped excrescences and deteriorating endothelial cells (×400). **(b)** Higher magnification transmission electron micrograph of areas indicated by arrows in **(c)** discloses fusiform configuration of long-spacing collagen. **(c)** Ultrastructural details of the lesions as remnants of a degenerating endothelial cell (E) seen between two Descemet membrane excrescences (*).

failure at 5 years following PK.[26] However, other long-term studies have failed to demonstrate an adverse effect of donor age on PK survival.[27]

The term *graft rejection* refers to a specific immunologic response of the host to the donor corneal tissue, as distinct from non-immune-mediated graft failures. Occurring at least weeks to months following technically uncomplicated surgery, the incidence of rejection is greatest in the initial 1 to 2 years following transplant but also sustains a lifetime risk. Acute corneal endothelial rejection involves destruction of grafted endothelial cells by T-lymphocytes, and its clinical outcomes are determined by the success of aggressive steroid treatment in rescuing and preserving a functionally adequate endothelial cell population.

Clinical Features

The clinical signs of graft rejection are either localized or diffuse corneal edema with keratic precipitates confined to the transplanted donor cornea. In some instances, epithelial rejection lines, subepithelial infiltrates, and stromal neovascularization develop. The pathognomonic sign of endothelial rejection is the Khodadoust line, demarcating immunologically damaged endothelium from unaffected endothelium, because in the affected area, endothelial decompensation results in stromal and epithelial edema.[28] ▶ Fig. 4.20, ▶ Fig. 4.21, and ▶ Fig. 4.22 show the clinical aspects of graft rejection and failure.

Imaging and Pathology

In patients with graft rejection the in vivo confocal microscopy shows an increase in activated keratocytes (AKs). Because this finding can predict graft rejection 2 months before the development of clinically evident rejection, it constitutes the first sign of subclinical rejection.[29] The presence of lymphocytes adherent to the graft endothelium is especially dramatic when viewed by confocal or scanning electron microscopy.

The suitability of irreversibly rejected penetrating or endothelial keratoplasty to undergo subsequent endothelial keratoplasty is determined by whether secondary stromal changes (deep neovascularization, scarring, or other opacity involving the visual axis) have developed. Corneas with only stromal edema remain favorable, whereas those with more chronic alterations may require PK.

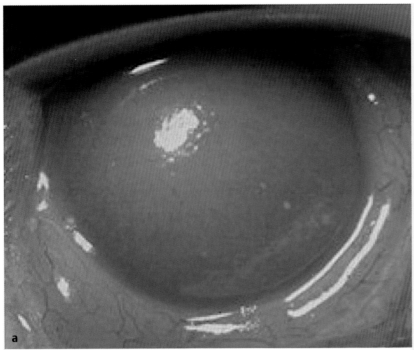

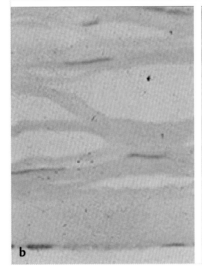

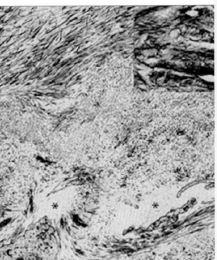

Fig. 4.12 Congenital hereditary endothelial dystrophy. (a) Dense corneal opacity is consequent to profound stromal edema. (b) Light photomicrograph of posterior cornea depicts diffuse uniform thickening of Descemet membrane as a homogeneous acellular layer with marked attenuation of endothelial cell layer evident at extreme lower margin (Hematoxylin-eosin, × 500). (c) By light microscopy (inset, upper right) and transmission electron microscopy (main figure), edematous disruptions (*) of collagen lamellae are resolved (× 400, × 19,000).

Glaucoma: Postfiltration Surgery (Tube Shunt), Chronic Topical Medication Toxicity

Postoperative endothelial cell loss can occur after trabeculectomy and deep sclerectomy (alone and combined with cataract extraction) and is progressive from 3 to 12 months following glaucoma surgery.[30] Protracted IOP may also have adverse effects on the corneal endothelium. Endothelial cell loss is higher after penetrating glaucoma surgery than after nonpenetrating surgery and is especially prevalent following tube shunt placement in the anterior chamber.[31,32]

As such eyes often undergo multiple anterior segment surgical procedures over a prolonged course, the collective results of corneal endothelial attrition not infrequently precipitate irreversible corneal edema. Such corneas are appropriate for endothelial keratoplasty, recognizing the surgical challenges presented, especially in the presence of anteriorly located shunt tubes.

Acetazolamide, a systemic carbonic anhydrase inhibitor, has long been used to reduce IOP. Dorzolamide, the first approved topical carbonic anhydrase inhibitor, accumulates within the cornea, allowing a sustained delivery to the anterior uvea, mainly through scleral and conjunctival routes. However, increased tissue concentrations of carbonic anhydrase inhibitors near corneal endothelium potentially inhibit its HCO_3^--dependent fluid transport and thereby cause corneal edema. The clinically relevant effect of dorzolamide on corneal function remains unclear. Corneal decompensation has been reported in dorzolamide-using patients[33]; however, these eyes had also undergone multiple anterior surgical procedures plus other topical medications. The specific causality of dorzolamide in the etiology of corneal edema therefore remains uncertain.[34] Finally, depending on the study, endothelial cell density of dorzolamide-treated patients either did not change or decreased after treatment.

Traumatic Endothelial Failure

Congenital Glaucoma

Although technically not traumatic, the acute and chronically elevated IOP of congenital glaucoma not only causes corneal edema (potentially reversible when IOP is normalized) but the mechanical deformation of the still elastic neonatal cornea results in overall corneal and globe enlargement (buphthalmos) with potential linear ruptures of the Descemet membrane. As with the acute hydrops phenomenon of keratoconus, the ruptured Descemet edges tend to curl over time and develop a thickened appearance evident on optical coherence tomography (OCT).[35] With IOP control and time, the Descemet membrane ruptures heal and appear as typical horizontal parallel linear tracks (Haab striae). The consequence of the resultant endothelial cell attrition may only later become evident as progressive corneal edema. Such corneas remain favorable for endothelial keratoplasty, presuming IOP control is stable.

Imaging and Pathology

There is a mild reduction of keratocyte density in the mid- and posterior stroma, a particular abnormal "claw-shaped" mor-

phology of stromal nerves, and the presence of discontinuous hyperreflective structures overhanging the endothelial layer at the level of the Descemet membrane. The endothelium

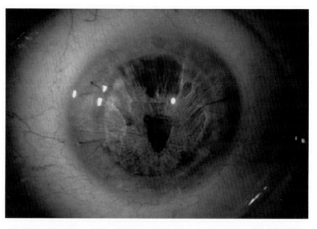

Fig. 4.13 Iridocorneal endothelial syndrome. Essential iris atrophy variant. Following successful keratoplasty for corneal edema, pupillary distortion is consequent to extensive atrophy of superior iris with full-thickness holes.

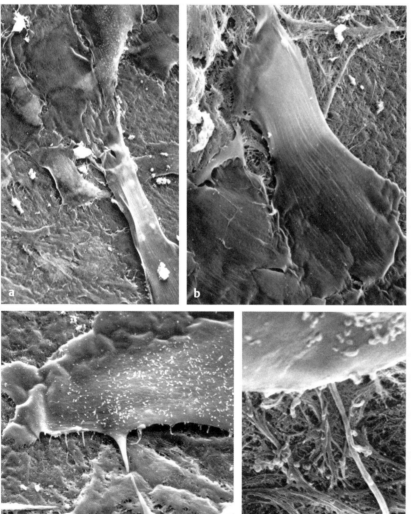

Fig. 4.14 Iridocorneal endothelial syndrome. Scanning microscopy of keratoplasty specimen shows **(a)** extremely attenuated and pleomorphic endothelial cells overlying irregular surface of posterior collagen layer (×550). **(b)** A single endothelial cell has enormously elongated and enlarged its surface area (×1200). **(c)** Another attenuated endothelial cell has extended numerous cytoplasmic processes (×2000). **(d)** At higher magnification, the endothelial cell (above) is observed to rest upon a layer of randomly oriented filaments and fibrils (below) (×15,000).

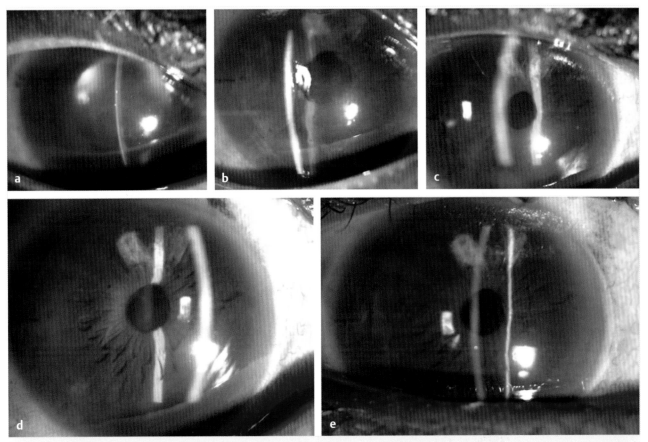

Fig. 4.15 Pseudophakic corneal edema. (a) Slit lamp photograph displays diffuse corneal stromal edema secondary to pseudophakic bullous keratopathy. (b) Five days following Descemet membrane endothelial keratoplasty (DMEK), there is partial corneal clearing, central pupil and inferior peripheral iridectomy. (c) At 3 weeks following DMEK, corneal clearing continues. (d,e) At postoperative months 2 and 11 months, the cornea has retained and maintained crystal clarity.

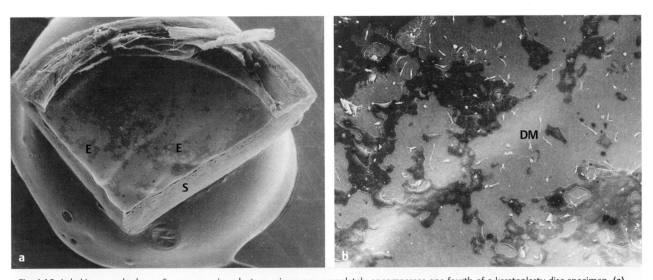

Fig. 4.16 Aphakic corneal edema. Survey scanning electron microscopy completely encompasses one-fourth of a keratoplasty disc specimen. (a) Diffuse reduction of endothelial cell population across entire posterior Descemet surface with only scattered remnants of endothelial cells (E). S, stroma (× 20). (b) Higher magnification of central (a) confirms extensive areas of Descemet membrane (DM) exposed between noncontiguous endothelial cell clusters (× 100).

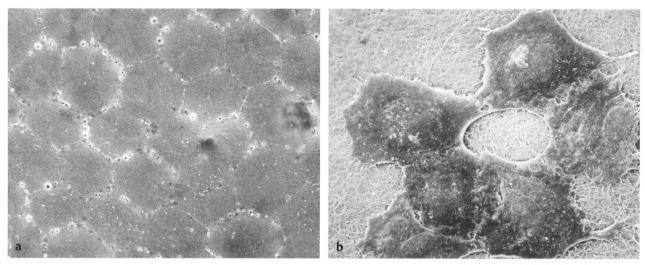

Fig. 4.17 Aphakic corneal edema. **(a)** Normal adult human corneal endothelium demonstrates uniformly hexagonal cells arranged in a continuous monolayer (× 1000). **(b)** Aphakic corneal edema at same magnification features remaining endothelial cells as extremely flattened and attenuated. The exposed surface of the posterior collagenous layer appears as a fibrous feltwork (× 1000).

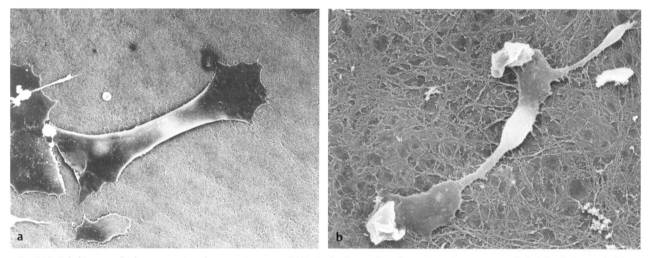

Fig. 4.18 Aphakic corneal edema, scanning electron microscopy. **(a)** Typically distorted configurations of remaining endothelial cells (× 1000). **(b)** Degenerating endothelial cell and randomly interwoven pattern of posterior collagenous layer (× 2000).

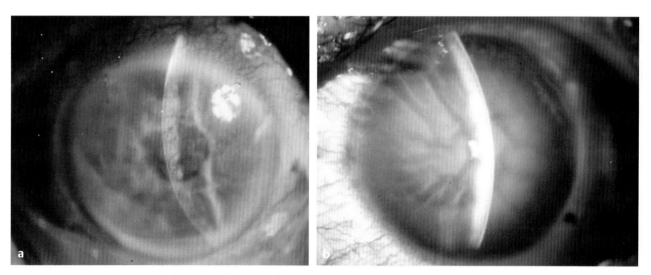

Fig. 4.19 Toxic anterior segment syndrome. **(a)** Diffuse corneal edema with Descemet membrane folds. **(b)** Massive edema and Descemet folds opacify the cornea in an otherwise uninflamed eye.

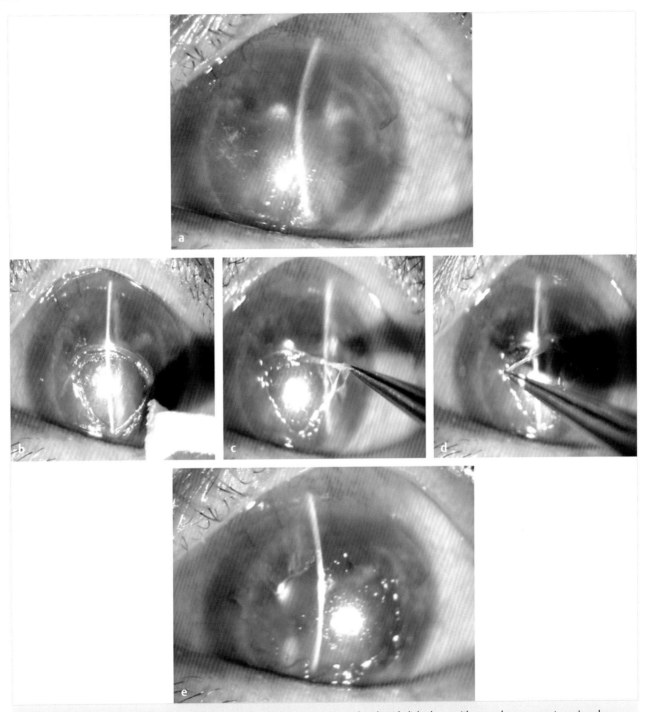

Fig. 4.20 Keratoplasty failure. **(a)** Following keratoplasty rejection, chronic stromal and epithelial edema with secondary recurrent erosions has resulted in thick fibrocellular pannus. **(b–d)** Superficial keratectomy peels loosely adherent fibrocellular pannus from underlying Bowman layer surface. **(e)** Following pannus removal, cornea appears improved but requires repeat keratoplasty to restore anatomical and visual clarity.

shows severe polymegathism, pleomorphism, a markedly decreased cell density, and focal cellular lesions.[36]

Birth Forceps Injury

Breaks in the Descemet membrane can occur from the mechanical stress of forceps-assisted delivery. Initially, the damaged cornea appears profoundly edematous; however, within weeks,

the endothelial defects heal and the stroma clears, leaving typically vertically oriented residual lines (striae) in the Descemet membrane. To the extent that the endothelial cell population has sustained major damage, such corneas may later develop edema (as well as astigmatism with concomitant amblyopia) that can be appropriate for endothelial keratoplasty. ▶ Fig. 4.23 shows the clinical and pathological characteristics of a patient with corneal forceps injury.

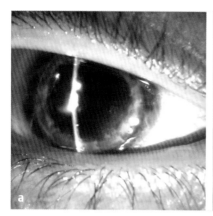
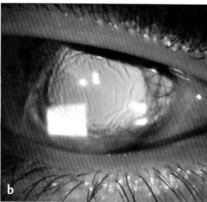

Fig. 4.21 Keratoplasty failure. Following penetrating keratoplasty for aphakic corneal edema, (a) the failed graft is edematous (b) with numerous Descemet membrane folds evident in retroillumination.

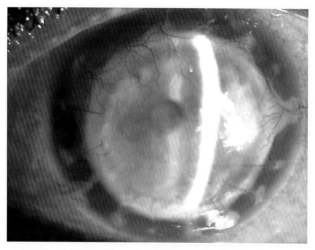

Fig. 4.22 Keratoplasty failure. With long-standing and irreversible corneal graft rejection, the conjunctiva becomes injected and the keratoplasty donor disc is massively edematous with superficial peripheral neovascularization.

Blunt Injury

Following major concussive ocular trauma, among the numerous potential sequelae involving the cornea are lower endothelial cell density with polymegathism and polymorphism. The presence of ocular surface injury or endothelial cell abnormalities is often associated with other anterior and posterior segment comorbidities, collectively impairing visual acuity.[37] A concussive injury can disrupt endothelial cells in an annulus on the perimeter of the impact zone, resulting in transient stromal edema immediately anterior to the injured endothelial cells.[38] A pigmented annulus on the corneal endothelium, the so-called Vossius ring, forms consequent to extreme anterior segment deformation as the compressed cornea impacts the iris. ▶ Fig. 4.24 and ▶ Fig. 4.25 show clinical images of two patients with posttraumatic endothelial injury.

Depending on the extent of injury and postinjury inflammatory consequences, as well as requirement for other anterior segment surgery, such as cataract, iris, or glaucoma procedures, the resultant corneal endothelial compromise may require either endothelial keratoplasty if the stroma remains otherwise intact or PK if extreme scarring and tissue distortion plus other damages requiring anterior segment reconstruction have developed.

Postinflammatory and Postinfectious: Uveitis, Keratitis, Endotheliitis (HSV, VZV, CMV)

Corneal endotheliitis clinically comprises keratic precipitates (KPs), overlying stromal and epithelial edema, and mild iritis. Initially interpreted as an autoimmune process because the linear distribution of KPs resembled the corneal allograft rejection,[39] several viruses have subsequently etiologically implicated including herpes simplex virus (HSV), *Varicella zoster* virus (VZV), and cytomegalovirus (CMV).

Herpes Simplex Virus Endotheliitis

HSV infection incites inflammation in multiple ocular tissues. Its corneal involvement may affect the epithelium, stroma, and/or endothelium.

Etiology

In HSV endotheliitis, either secondary inflammation caused by the virus and/or direct infection of endothelial cells causes endothelial dysfunction with consequent overlying stromal edema. Typically responsive to topical steroid treatment, the so-called disciform keratitis is largely reversible, as is its concomitant stromal edema, and seldom causes intrinsic stromal scarring.

HSV type 1 (HSV-1) causes the majority of the corneal HSV infections, except in neonatal ocular infections, which are usually HSV type 2-related. The herpes viruses not only cause several variants of active ocular infections but also establish latency, largely within the trigeminal ganglion, whereby the viral genome is quietly retained in the absence of virus production. Hence, as the virus is never completely eradicated, various trigger mechanisms may reactivate its infectious and/or immunologic recurrence, frequently at the initial site of infection.

Clinical Features

While both HSV stromal keratitis and endotheliitis can manifest as stromal opacity, they represent distinctly separate pathological processes. The stromal keratitis is driven by inflammation within the stroma that, if persistent, is accompanied by neovascularization. The disciform endotheliitis, in contrast, manifests solely as stromal edema due to HSV-mediated endothelial dysfunction in the absence of stromal inflammation or neovascularization. ▶ Fig. 4.26 shows clinical images of HSV endotheliitis.

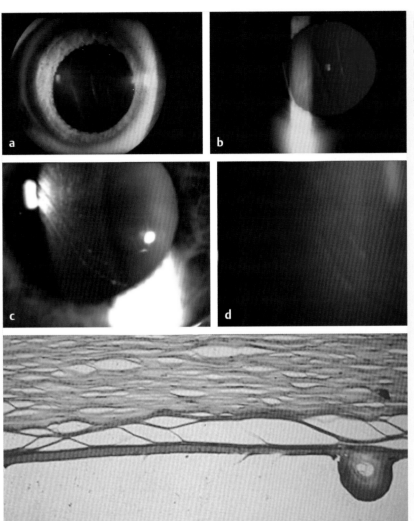

Fig. 4.23 Corneal forceps injury. **(a–d)** Slit lamp photographs with and without retroillumination depict birth forceps injury to the cornea as parallel breaks in the Descemet membrane, which have healed to restore stromal clarity. **(e)** Keratoplasty specimen demonstrates tubular proliferations of the Descemet membrane (far right) in the region of healed breaks (periodic acid-Schiff, ×600).

Often anterior chamber inflammatory reaction and keratin precipitates develop, as well as inflammatory trabeculitis with elevated IOP. Although the diagnosis of HSV endotheliitis is mainly historical and clinical, polymerase chain reaction (PCR) analysis, enzyme-linked assays, and viral culture of the aqueous humor may reveal HSV-1 DNA, protein, or live virus, respectively.

As the disciform reaction is generally sensitive to topical steroids, corneal endothelial function is usually reestablished with stromal clearing and visual improvement. However, given the persistent nature of HSV, multiple recurrences can cause irreversible endothelial damage with resultant chronic edema, thereby requiring keratoplasty. If secondary stromal changes of scarring, thinning, and neovascularization are not advanced, then endothelial keratoplasty is indicated, albeit with vigilant postoperative measures to prevent HSV recurrence as well as immune rejection.

Varicella Zoster Virus Endotheliitis

Etiology

Varicella zoster virus (VZV) can cause severe keratouveitis.[38] Approximately 50% of patients with ophthalmic herpes zoster develop uveitis and/or iritis.[40] Approximately 50% of patients with ophthalmic herpes zoster develop uveitis and/or iritis.[41]

VZV-induced iritis is more common over age 50 years, accounting for approximately 60% of total cases. Most patients are immunocompetent, although inadequate immune development following chickenpox as well as various acquired and pharmacological immunodeficiencies are also implicated. The course of the uveitis is generally uniphasic and of relatively short duration. Secondary glaucoma is common and recalcitrant, as 15% of all patients require surgical intervention. The visual loss associated with VZV is not solely related to uveitis and secondary glaucoma but also to other posterior segment complications.[42]

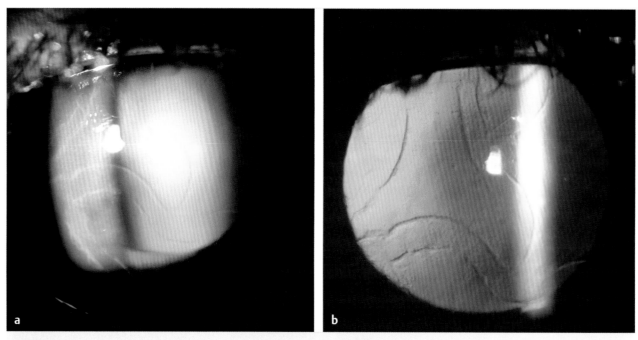

Fig. 4.24 (a) Traumatic rupture of the Descemet membrane. (b) Following blunt trauma, multiple Descemet membrane ruptures have healed to produce a serpiginous pattern most visible by retroillumination. (Courtesy of Gustavo A. Novais, MD, PhD.)

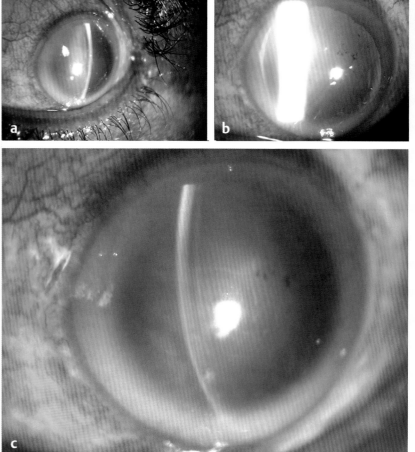

Fig. 4.25 Posttraumatic corneal edema. (a) Following blunt trauma, dislocation of the crystalline lens has caused profound anterior chamber shallowing with localized endothelial contact. (b) Disruption of zonules and Descemet membrane folds are apparent with retroillumination. (c) At higher magnification, diffuse corneal edema, pigment dispersion, and cornea–lenticular contact become evident.

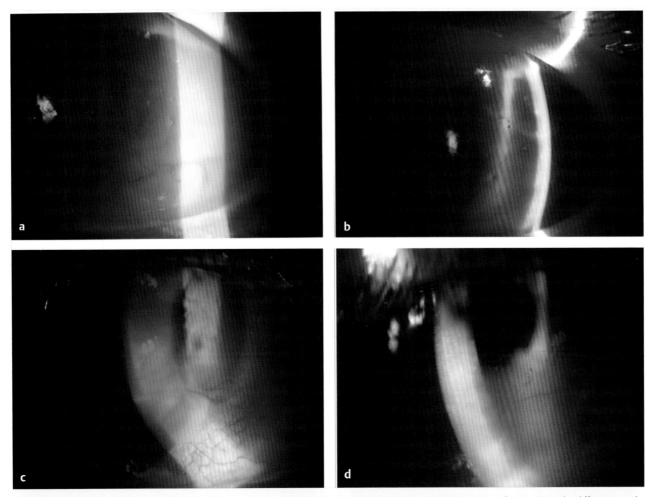

Fig. 4.26 Herpes simplex virus endotheliitis. **(a,b)** Disciform endotheliitis in a patient with previous herpes keratitis infection. Note the diffuse stromal edema. **(c,d)** Linear endotheliitis. Note the keratic precipitates in the endothelial layer in a linear disposition. (Courtesy of Gustavo A. Novais, MD, PhD.)

The significant corneal complications are predominantly consequent to the neurotrophic keratopathy of the virus-induced corneal anesthesia. Most challenging are neurotrophic persistent epithelial defects with potential development of sterile and/or infectious keratolysis. Such defects often heal, with stromal thinning, scarring, and neovascularization. As such, and if the visual axis is involved, penetrating keratoplasty is mandated for tectonic and/or visual rehabilitation. However, in cases retaining stromal integrity and potential visual axis clarity, endothelial dysfunction can potentially be managed by endothelial keratoplasty.

Cytomegalovirus Endotheliitis

Etiology

Human cytomegalovirus (CMV), a ubiquitous lymphotropic herpesvirus, causes various systemic and ocular clinical manifestations, including retinitis in immunocompromised hosts.[43] Recent reports have also demonstrated increasing CMV-associated anterior segment inflammations, including anterior uveitis and/or corneal endotheliitis, in otherwise healthy individuals. Many patients have a past ocular history of recurrent iritis.

Clinical Features

The corneal involvement ranges from small focal areas of corneal edema to diffuse bullous keratopathy in the absence of epithelial and stromal abnormality. In some cases, a distinct horizontal curvilinear demarcation on the endothelium develops and with treatment regresses in a superior-to-inferior direction. KPs of variable thin, filiform, or pigmented appearance occur over the inferior half of the cornea. Anterior chamber inflammation is mild. The iris develops diffuse atrophy without heterochromia, posterior synechiae, or sector atrophy. The IOP is frequently elevated.[44]

The diagnosis of CMV endotheliitis is confirmed by PCR of the aqueous humor.

4.2 Conclusion

The clinicopathologic features of the extensive litany of corneal conditions characterized by either primary or secondary endothelial dysfunction are reviewed. Understanding their fundamental etiologic and morphological aspects thereby affords a basis for determining those specific cases that may be optimally approached and potentially benefited by endothelial keratoplasty.

References

[1] Weiss JS, Møller HU, Aldave AJ, et al. IC3D classification of corneal dystrophies—edition 2. Cornea. 2015; 34(2):117–159

[2] Li YJ, Minear MA, Rimmler J, et al. Replication of TCF4 through association and linkage studies in late-onset Fuchs endothelial corneal dystrophy. PLoS ONE. 2011; 6(4):e18044

[3] Kuot A, Hewitt AW, Griggs K, et al. Association of TCF4 and CLU polymorphisms with Fuchs' endothelial dystrophy and implication of CLU and TGFBI proteins in the disease process. Eur J Hum Genet. 2012; 20(6):632–638

[4] Wieben ED, Aleff RA, Tosakulwong N, et al. A common trinucleotide repeat expansion within the transcription factor 4 (TCF4, E2–2) gene predicts Fuchs corneal dystrophy. PLoS ONE. 2012; 7(11):e49083

[5] Vilas GL, Morgan PE, Loganathan SK, Quon A, Casey JR. A biochemical framework for SLC4A11, the plasma membrane protein defective in corneal dystrophies. Biochemistry. 2011; 50(12):2157–2169

[6] Bucher F, Adler W, Lehmann HC, et al. Corneal nerve alterations in different stages of Fuchs' endothelial corneal dystrophy: an in vivo confocal microscopy study. Graefes Arch Clin Exp Ophthalmol. 2014; 252(7):1119–1126

[7] Amin SR, Baratz KH, McLaren JW, Patel SV. Corneal abnormalities early in the course of Fuchs' endothelial dystrophy. Ophthalmology. 2014; 121(12):2325–2333

[8] Aldave AJ, Han J, Frausto RF. Genetics of the corneal endothelial dystrophies: an evidence-based review. Clin Genet. 2013; 84(2):109–119

[9] Vincent AL. Corneal dystrophies and genetics in the International Committee for Classification of Corneal Dystrophies era: a review. Clin Experiment Ophthalmol. 2014; 42(1):4–12

[10] Klintworth GK. Corneal dystrophies. Orphanet J Rare Dis. 2009; 4:7

[11] Cheng LL, Young AL, Wong AK, Law RW, Lam DS. Confocal microscopy of posterior polymorphous endothelial dystrophy. Cornea. 2005; 24(5):599–602

[12] Grupcheva CN, Chew GS, Edwards M, Craig JP, McGhee CN. Imaging posterior polymorphous corneal dystrophy by in vivo confocal microscopy. Clin Experiment Ophthalmol. 2001; 29(4):256–259

[13] Aldahmesh MA, Khan AO, Meyer BF, Alkuraya FS. Mutational spectrum of SLC4A11 in autosomal recessive CHED in Saudi Arabia. Invest Ophthalmol Vis Sci. 2009; 50(9):4142–4145

[14] Alvarado JA, Underwood JL, Green WR, et al. Detection of herpes simplex viral DNA in the iridocorneal endothelial syndrome. Arch Ophthalmol. 1994; 112(12):1601–1609

[15] Groh MJ, Seitz B, Schumacher S, Naumann GO. Detection of herpes simplex virus in aqueous humor in iridocorneal endothelial (ICE) syndrome. Cornea. 1999; 18(3):359–360

[16] Sacchetti M, Mantelli F, Marenco M, Macchi I, Ambrosio O, Rama P. Diagnosis and Management of Iridocorneal Endothelial Syndrome. Biomed Res Int. 2015; 2015:763093

[17] Levy SG, McCartney AC, Baghai MH, Barrett MC, Moss J. Pathology of the iridocorneal-endothelial syndrome. The ICE-cell. Invest Ophthalmol Vis Sci. 1995; 36(13):2592–2601

[18] Morris RW, Dunbar MT. Atypical presentation and review of the ICE syndrome. Optometry. 2004; 75(1):13–25

[19] Le QH, Xu JJ, Sun XH, Zheng TY. [Morphological changes of cornea in iridocorneal endothelial syndrome under the confocal microscopy]. Zhonghua Yan Ke Za Zhi. 2008; 44(11):987–992

[20] Pezzi PP, Marenco M, Cosimi P, Mannino G, Iannetti L. Progression of essential iris atrophy studied with confocal microscopy and ultrasound biomicroscopy: a 5-year case report. Cornea. 2009; 28(1):99–102

[21] Ljubimov AV, Atilano SR, Garner MH, Maguen E, Nesburn AB, Kenney MC. Extracellular matrix and Na+,K+-ATPase in human corneas following cataract surgery: comparison with bullous keratopathy and Fuchs' dystrophy corneas. Cornea. 2002; 21(1):74–80

[22] Mamalis N, Edelhauser HF, Dawson DG, Chew J, LeBoyer RM, Werner L. Toxic anterior segment syndrome. J Cataract Refract Surg. 2006; 32(2):324–333

[23] Sengupta S, Chang DF, Gandhi R, Kenia H, Venkatesh R. Incidence and long-term outcomes of toxic anterior segment syndrome at Aravind Eye Hospital. J Cataract Refract Surg. 2011; 37(9):1673–1678

[24] Bodnar Z, Clouser S, Mamalis N. Toxic anterior segment syndrome: Update on the most common causes. J Cataract Refract Surg. 2012; 38(11):1902–1910

[25] Avisar R, Weinberger D. Corneal endothelial morphologic features in toxic anterior segment syndrome. Cornea. 2010; 29(3):251–253

[26] Wakefield MJ, Armitage WJ, Jones MN, et al. National Health Service Blood and Transplant Ocular Tissue Advisory Group (OTAG Audit Study 19). The impact of donor age and endothelial cell density on graft survival following penetrating keratoplasty. Br J Ophthalmol. 2015

[27] Mannis MJ, Holland EJ, Gal RL, et al. Writing Committee for the Cornea Donor Study Research Group. The effect of donor age on penetrating keratoplasty for endothelial disease: graft survival after 10 years in the Cornea Donor Study. Ophthalmology. 2013; 120(12):2419–2427

[28] The Collaborative Corneal Transplantation Studies Research Group. The collaborative corneal transplantation studies (CCTS). Effectiveness of histocompatibility matching in high-risk corneal transplantation. Arch Ophthalmol. 1992; 110(10):1392–1403

[29] Kocaba V, Colica C, Rabilloud M, Burillon C. Predicting Corneal Graft Rejection by Confocal Microscopy. Cornea. 2015; 34 Suppl 10:S61–S64

[30] Arnavielle S, Lafontaine PO, Bidot S, Creuzot-Garcher C, D'Athis P, Bron AM. Corneal endothelial cell changes after trabeculectomy and deep sclerectomy. J Glaucoma. 2007; 16(3):324–328

[31] Kim CS, Yim JH, Lee EK, Lee NH. Changes in corneal endothelial cell density and morphology after Ahmed glaucoma valve implantation during the first year of follow up. Clin Experiment Ophthalmol. 2008; 36(2):142–147

[32] Lim KS. Corneal endothelial cell damage from glaucoma drainage device materials. Cornea. 2003; 22(4):352–354

[33] Konowal A, Morrison JC, Brown SV, et al. Irreversible corneal decompensation in patients treated with topical dorzolamide. Am J Ophthalmol. 1999; 127(4):403–406

[34] Giasson CJ, Nguyen TQ, Boisjoly HM, Lesk MR, Amyot M, Charest M. Dorzolamide and corneal recovery from edema in patients with glaucoma or ocular hypertension. Am J Ophthalmol. 2000; 129(2):144–150

[35] Spierer O, Cavuoto KM, Suwannaraj S, Chang TC. Anterior Segment Optical Coherence Tomography Imaging of Haab Striae. J Pediatr Ophthalmol Strabismus. 2015; 52 Online:e55–e58

[36] Mastropasqua L, Carpineto P, Ciancaglini M, Nubile M, Doronzo E. In vivo confocal microscopy in primary congenital glaucoma with megalocornea. J Glaucoma. 2002; 11(2):83–89

[37] Cockerham GC, Lemke S, Rice TA, et al. Closed-globe injuries of the ocular surface associated with combat blast exposure. Ophthalmology. 2014; 121(11):2165–2172

[38] Reid GA, Musa F. OCT imaging of a traumatic endothelial ring. Cornea. 2014; 33(9):952–954

[39] Khodadoust AA, Attarzadeh A. Presumed autoimmune corneal endotheliopathy. Am J Ophthalmol. 1982; 93(6):718–722

[40] Reijo A, Antti V, Jukka M. Endothelial cell loss in herpes zoster keratouveitis. Br J Ophthalmol. 1983; 67(11):751–754

[41] Yawn BP, Wollan PC, St Sauver JL, Butterfield LC. Herpes zoster eye complications: rates and trends. Mayo Clin Proc. 2013; 88(6):562–570

[42] Thean JH, Hall AJ, Stawell RJ. Uveitis in Herpes zoster ophthalmicus. Clin Experiment Ophthalmol. 2001; 29(6):406–410

[43] Suzuki T, Ohashi Y. Corneal endotheliitis. Semin Ophthalmol. 2008; 23(4):235–240

[44] Chee S-P, Bacsal K, Jap A, Se-Thoe S-Y, Cheng CL, Tan BH. Corneal endotheliitis associated with evidence of cytomegalovirus infection. Ophthalmology. 2007; 114(4):798–803

5 Mastering Descemet Stripping Endothelial Keratoplasty

Ashiyana Nariani and Terry Kim

5.1 Background

5.1.1 Evolution

Descemet stripping endothelial keratoplasty (DSEK), or Descemet stripping automated endothelial keratoplasty (DSAEK), is a technique for partial corneal transplantation. It involves removal of the recipient's Descemet membrane and endothelium and replacement with donor posterior stroma, Descemet membrane, and endothelium and is currently the surgical procedure choice for endothelial dysfunction.[1] However, the surgical technique for DSEK has undergone various transformations, thanks to the efforts of expert corneal surgeons who have been fine tuning and perfecting the procedure over the last 2 decades, before it evolved to DSEK as we know today.[2]

Prior to the era of endothelial keratoplasty (EK), corneal transplantation was limited to full-thickness penetrating keratoplasty (PKP). The initial series of the "posterior approach" posterior lamellar keratoplasties (PLKs) included deep lamellar endothelial keratoplasty (DLEK),[2,3,4] stemming from the initial experimental attempts by Ko and colleagues on rabbits in 1993.[5] A similar approach was conceived by Dr. Gerritt Melles of Holland (known as the father of endothelial keratoplasty) and then adopted in the United States by Dr. Francis Price, who termed it Descemet stripping with endothelial keratoplasty, or DSEK.[2,6]

As ongoing experimentation and experience with the procedure continued, improved modifications in surgical technique were conceptualized by Dr. Price, including corneal surface massaging and small paracentral keratotomy vent incisions to help remove graft interface fluid and improve adherence and rebubbling for graft detachments.[2,7] Dr. Mark Gorovoy used an artificial anterior chamber and introduced the variant that became known as Descemet stripping automated endothelial keratoplasty, or DSAEK, which included the use of a blade microkeratome for cutting donor grafts. This transition away from manual lamellar dissection improved postoperative outcomes, resulting from more consistent dissection depths and a smoother donor interface.[1]

The adoption of DSEK in the United States has been rapid. From 2005 to 2014, the Eye Bank Association of America (EBAA) reported an increase in the number of endothelial transplants from 1429 to 28,961, with a simultaneous decrease in the number of full-thickness PK transplants from 45,821 to 38,919.[8,9] In an era where corneal transplantation is at an all-time explosion in innovation, corneal surgeons worldwide are building upon the foundation of DSEK to create new surgical techniques and inventions and to expand on indications for use.

5.1.2 Indications

With the increasing integration of DSEK into ophthalmology practice, the indications and threshold for use have expanded rapidly. In the mid-1980s and -1990s, pseudophakic and aphakic corneal endothelial decompensation due to cataract surgery or from the use of anterior chamber lenses constituted the primary indications. Today, DSEK is being done more commonly for Fuchs endothelial corneal dystrophy, failed EK grafts, under a previously failed PK or in conjunction with cataract surgery for Fuchs, known more commonly as a DSEK-triple. Rarer indications for DSEK include posterior polymorphous corneal dystrophy (PPCD), congenital hereditary endothelial dystrophy (CHED), and iridocorneal endothelial (ICE) syndrome, in the absence of visually significant corneal scarring.[2,9,10,11]

5.1.3 Advantages and Disadvantages

Compared to traditional full-thickness transplantation, EK generally improves vision with lower rates of complication and with a faster visual recovery. This is inherently due to the less invasive nature of EK, allowing for maintenance of the eye and anterior chamber contour throughout the procedure, unlike the "open-sky" approach for PKPs. In maintaining the integrity of the anterior corneal curvature, there is considerably less induced corneal astigmatism, if any. Additionally, EK eliminates the risk of suture-associated complications, notably infection, neovascularization, and rejection.[12]

Given the overall predictability and ease in manipulation of a DSEK corneal donor graft within the anterior chamber, more surgeons continue to perform DSEK over Descemet membrane endothelial keratoplasty (DMEK) as their EK procedure of choice. Though highly controversial and unclear whether graft thickness is clinically important for best corrected visual acuity (BCVA), some corneal surgeons believe that the major disadvantage of DSEK, although less so with ultrathin DSEK, is the limitation in optimal vision due to optical degradation associated with the graft–host lamellar interface or persistent stromal haze. This results from the interface of posterior stromal tissue in a DSEK graft to the recipient stromal tissue.[13,14,15] A retained ophthalmic viscosurgical device (OVD) used during the surgery has also been shown to contribute.[2,16,17,18]

The consideration to switch from DSEK to DMEK and pre-Descemet endothelial keratoplasty (PDEK) stems from this concept that these grafts may yield a more direct optical path and offer better visual and refractive outcomes and a faster visual recovery. Additionally, in minimizing the amount of stromal antigens present, there is also a lower graft rejection rate than with DSEK.[19,20,21,22] Nonetheless, at this point in time in current practice, surgeons performing DMEK will often have a DSEK corneal graft available, should the need for conversion to DSEK occur in cases where the DMEK graft does not behave as desired.[23]

5.1.4 Preoperative Evaluation

The decision as to what type of anesthesia to choose varies among surgeons and cases. In general, for beginning DSEK surgeons or for complicated cases that are predicted to take longer, local anesthesia with peribulbar or retrobulbar block and adjunct intravenous sedation should be considered. Sometimes even general anesthesia may be needed. For more experienced surgeons, acceptable results and patient comfort are obtained with topical anesthesia in conjunction with intravenous sedation and preservative-free intracameral lidocaine.[1,7,24] Be aware that patients generally will experience the most discomfort during a scleral tunnel wound construction, tissue insertion and manipulation in the anterior chamber, air bubble injection (particularly with firm air fill), and wound suturing.

Additional important considerations include the depth of the chamber, severity of endothelial disease, level of corneal scarring and visibility into the anterior chamber, status of the other eye, shape of the pupil, and lens status. If the indication for DSEK is a failed graft, knowing the previous size of the graft will help plan the size for descemetorhexis and graft diameter.

If phakic with a higher-grade cataract, in the setting of endothelial disease, a DSEK triple procedure, involving cataract extraction with intraocular lens (IOL) implantation, may be indicated. With DSEK, the shape of the lenticule may produce a hyperopic shift. Targeting a spherical equivalent of approximately −1.00 when choosing the IOL will generally minimize a hyperopic surprise. The grading of the cataract, endothelial disease, guttae, level of edema, and scarring should be noted and are critical for determining whether to use two procedures—DSEK followed by cataract removal, cataract removal followed by DSEK, or a single DSEK-triple.[25,26] With regard to order, a DSEK followed by cataract extraction and IOL implantation performed as two separate procedures allows for more accurate corneal topography and IOL measurements and optimizes postoperative visual outcomes. Cataract extraction and IOL implantation followed by DSEK is the ideal route for mild endothelial disease, where a DSEK may not be needed.

Generally, a DSEK-triple is elected in the presence of endothelial dysfunction and a cataract and has been shown to be as effective as DSEK alone. Given the ease of carrying out DSEK today, cataract extraction alone is attempted only if endothelial compromise and corneal guttata are minimal, in the setting of Fuchs. Additionally, in cases where there are anesthesia risks or the patient experiences difficulty in remaining in the supine position for prolonged periods, the threshold to proceed with a DSEK-triple is lowered.

5.1.5 Medical Management of Endothelial Disease

Prior to delving into surgical intervention for corneal edema secondary to endothelial corneal disease or decompensation, it is important to recognize that, in clinical practice, a stepwise approach to management includes first attempting medical interventions to treat corneal edema in order to improve visual outcomes. Identifying the etiology for corneal decompensation is critical to effective management. Depending on the etiology, medical interventions for corneal edema include topical sodium chloride 5% dehydrating drops and ointments, intraocular pressure–lowering agents, topical steroids, and evaporative techniques (e.g., use of a hair dryer to dry the cornea), in cases of Fuchs endothelial corneal dystrophy, and supportive treatment for ruptured bullae in the same manner as for a corneal abrasion include topical antibiotics, cycloplegics, and a bandage contact lens. Alternative nonmedical therapies include excimer laser phototherapeutic keratectomy (PTK), amniotic membrane graft, and/or a conjunctival flap, depending on the underlying etiology and degree of condition severity.[27]

5.2 Surgical Technique: DSEK Step by Step

In DSEK, the Descemet membrane and endothelium are stripped in the host eye (descemetorhexis), producing a smooth posterior stream bed in the host.[28]

An automated microkeratome is used to prepare the donor tissue, producing a smoother stream bed and potentially less irregularity in the graft–host interface, carried out either by the surgeon or previously prepared from an eye bank. The order of whether to prepare the host cornea or donor graft first is surgeon dependent. Host preparation first minimizes corneal tissue wastage should the decision be made not to proceed further with the case, while preparing the graft first ensures that the host Descemet membrane and endothelium are removed only once the graft has been confirmed to be present and appropriately prepared for use. The donor tissue is then inserted into the anterior chamber and attached to the host posterior stroma.

5.2.1 Host Preparation

Corneal Marking

Ink an 8–0 corneal marker 360 degrees and center onto the cornea. This will be the landmark for descemetorhexis creation and scoring (▸ Fig. 5.1).

DSEK Instrumentation (Authors' Preference List)

- 8–0 Corneal marker
- Ink marker
- Angle slit laser edge 2.5 mm knife
- 25-gauge 5/8 needle
- 2% Lidocaine + epinephrine
- Healon GV (Abbott Laboratories, Inc., Abbott Park, Illinois) ophthalmic viscoelastic device
- Hemostat
- Paracentesis knife
- 2.4 mm standard I-Knife II (Alcon Laboratories, Inc., Fort Worth, Texas)
- 27-gauge, 4 mm irrigation cannula
- 3 mL syringe
- 23-gauge Gorovoy Irrigating Descemet Stripper (Harvey Instruments, Rotonda West, FL)
- 0.12 mm toothed forceps
- Nontoothed forceps
- Colibri forceps
- Irrigation–aspiration handpiece with Centurion Vision System (Alcon) phaco machine
- 4.1 mm 30 degree angled Satin ShortCut angled knife (Alcon, Forth Worth, Texas)
- Graft spatula
- Ocular Systems Endoserter
- DSEK donor graft tissue (eye bank-prepared)
- Ethilon 10–0 Cutting Suture (Ethicon)
- ReSure Sealant (Ocular Therapeutix, Inc.)
- UltraFit Coronet Donor Punch Set (Angiotech)
- Balanced salt solution (BSS)
- Visitec LASIK Flap Roller (Lindstrom), 14mm sleeve

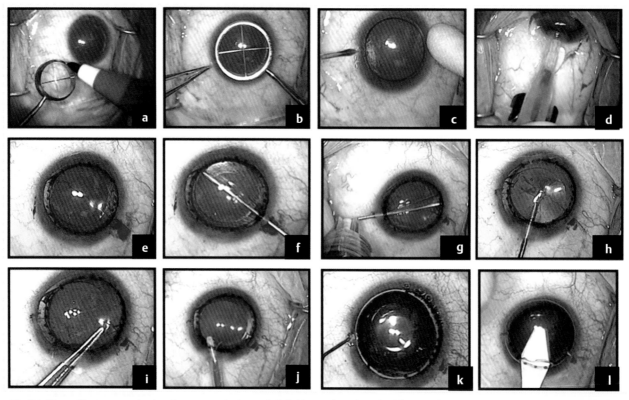

Fig. 5.1 Steps of host preparation in a Descemet stripping endothelial keratoplasty (DSEK)-triple procedure. (a) An 8–0 corneal marker is inked with a marking pen and (b) corneal marker centered and applied on the cornea. (c) Two short, vertically positioned paracenteses are made adjacent to the limbus, approximately 120 to 180 degrees apart. (d,e) Cataract extraction with intraocular lens implant is then carried out. (f,g) The Descemet membrane is scored using a bent 25-gauge needle through each of the paracenteses. (h) A 23-gauge Gorovoy irrigating Descemet stripper cannula is used to remove the host Descemet membrane and endothelium. (i,j) Residual Descemet membrane is removed with forceps followed by irrigation aspiration. (k) Air is injected into the anterior chamber to detect remnants and to test whether the air bubble will hold post–graft placement. (l) The main wound is then enlarged under an air bubble.

Corneal Incisions

Using a super sharp blade or paracentesis blade of choice, make two paracentesis incisions approximately 120 to 180 degrees apart (when positioned temporally, approximately 1 and 5 o'clock positions). The surgeon is positioned temporal to the eye, rather than superiorly, which allows for ease of access without being limited by the nasal bridge. A paracentesis, constructed short and vertical, allows for ease of graft manipulation in the anterior chamber.

The main wound can be made limbal, clear corneal, or scleral, based on surgeon preference, with the length varying between 3 and 6 mm. Several studies using vital dye staining of the endothelium after insertion of the donor corneal tissue have shown that placing tissue through a 3 mm incision causes two to four times more acute damage to the endothelium than does use of a 5 mm incision, regardless of the technique used to place the tissue. However, new methods of tissue insertion may eliminate the trauma associated with the use of a smaller incision size.[29]

Descemet Membrane Scoring

Scoring of the Descemet membrane involves initializing the edges of the Descemet membrane in a circular, continuous manner in preparation for removal of the host Descemet membrane and endothelium (descemetorhexis). Entering through each of the paracenteses, the Descemet membrane can be stripped with a circular pattern using a 25-gauge needle (bent with a hemostat) on a 3 mL cannula. The use of a bent 25-gauge needle provides for the ability to fill the anterior chamber should it shallow while entering and exiting the wounds.

Descemetorhexis

Based on surgeon preference, the Descemet membrane can be stripped using a variety of instruments, including a Sinskey hook (BD Visitec), a specially designed Descemet stripper, and/or an irrigation–aspiration (I-A) handpiece. Aggressive depth while carrying out the descemetorhexis and manipulation while stripping may result in tears in the stromal layer and an irregular interface, interfering with graft attachment and increasing the risk of graft–interface haze.

The stripping can be performed under viscoelastic, air, or irrigation with BSS. Some surgeons feel that it is necessary to strip the Descemet membrane only in cases of Fuchs endothelial dystrophy and not in patients with a failed PK or with pseudophakic bullous keratopathy. Whether the retention of the Descemet membrane in these cases may predispose to dislocation of the graft is controversial. Any retained Descemet membrane fragments can be removed from the anterior chamber with a nontoothed forceps of choice.

Anterior Chamber Aspiration

A thorough aspiration of the anterior chamber, with an I-A tip engaging close to the recipient posterior stromal bed is critical to further ensure removal of any retained Descemet membrane fragments.

Air Injection

An air bubble is injected into the anterior chamber for two major reasons: (1) to identify residual Descemet membrane fragments and (2) to ensure the air bubble injected after graft placement will hold well in the anterior chamber (as it will be critical for graft attachment).

5.2.2 Graft Preparation and Handling

With the advent of the eye bank–prepared DSEK grafts, corneal surgeons have the option of obtaining precut tissue or preparing the tissue in the operating room.

To prepare the corneal donor graft, a microkeratome system, consisting of a blade and an artificial anterior chamber to mount the cornea and fixate the microkeratome is used. The epithelium may be removed prior to the lamellar dissection with a Weck-Cel sponge (Beaver-Visitec). The corneal thickness can be measured using a pachymeter to select the appropriate-size microkeratome head, with the goal of leaving approximately 90 to 120 μm of posterior stroma with Descemet membrane and endothelium, ultrathin DSEK being approximately 60 to 90 μm thick. The donor corneoscleral rim is then pressurized with balanced salt solution (BSS), Optisol storage medium (Bausch), or viscoelastic to ensure a deep and smooth dissection. After the lamellar dissection is performed, the corneal stroma may be marked with an outline of the area of the trephine cut to allow proper centration of the tissue. A central gentian violet mark on the anterior cap is used to center the tissue on the cutting block, and peripheral marks around the circumference of the microkeratome cut are used to center the donor, even if the anterior cap is lost or decentered. Some reports have indicated that gentian violet has produced endothelial toxicity, so its use is limited.[24,30]

The DSEK graft is then ready to be punched using a donor cornea button trephine punch system (e.g., the UltraFit Coronet Donor Punch Set [Angiotech] or the Vacuum Donor Cornea Button Punch [Barron Precision Instruments]) consisting of a cutting block, trephine blade, and seating ring (▶ Fig. 5.2). The graft is then placed on the cutting block and trephined to create a disc-shaped lamella of donor tissue, ensuring the graft is well centered. Decentration of the graft on the cutting block can lead to portions of the donor button outside the area dissected by the microkeratome. Typical DSEK graft diameters generally range from 8 to 9 mm. Ensure a 0.5 mm difference between the graft size desired and the graft bed diameter of the corneal tissue. Once the donor graft has been punched, ensure that the donor is not stuck to the trephine and that no full-thickness edges are on the DSEK graft. These edges can prevent graft attachment. One or two drops of BSS can be placed over the graft and can remain on the cutting block with a cover until ready for use.

Next, the stromal cap with prepared donor graft can be transferred, endothelium side up, to the host, using a graft spatula. While grasping the stromal cap with colibri forceps, a 27-gauge irrigating cannula on a 3 mL syringe is used to identify the lamellar dissection.

5.2.3 Graft Insertion

Initially, the primary method for graft insertion was to fold the donor tissue into a 60/40 "taco" shape that required gently unfolding it within the anterior chamber. However, laboratory studies using vital dye staining, specular microscopy, and scanning electron microscopy have demonstrated a 30 to 40% endothelial cell loss with this technque.[31] Newer methods have been developed that are less traumatic to the endothelium, including the Endoserter (Ocular Systems) (▶ Fig. 5.3), Busin Glide (Moria), Tan EndoGlide (Network Medical), modified lens cartridges using an intraocular lens sheet glide to push or pull the tissue into place, Neusidl Corneal Injector (Fischer Surgical, Inc.), and a suture pull-through technique.[32,33]

The objective is to insert the tissue in a single plane, stromal side up, without having the endothelial cells touch each other, while also maintaining proper orientation of the tissue and reducing the need for intraocular manipulation to unfold it.[34]

While inserting the graft, it is ideal to keep the bottle height and anterior chamber low. If using an inserter, once the tip has been placed into the anterior chamber, irrigation should be on and the anterior chamber deepened. Some corneal surgeons prefer the use of an anterior chamber maintainer to ensure globe stability.

The main wound is then sealed with a 10–0 nylon suture. The "sutureless" DSEK technique can be done by drying the main wound first with a Weck-Cel sponge, followed by preparation and applications of ReSure sealant (▶ Fig. 5.4).

5.2.4 Grafting Attachment

Graft Centration

After tissue placement in the anterior chamber, a 25-gauge bent needle, Sinskey hook, or 27-gauge needle, entered via the paracenteses, can be used to manipulate and center the graft. An "S-stamp" on eye bank–prepared DSEK grafts provides the surgeon a way in which to ensure the correct orientation of the graft.

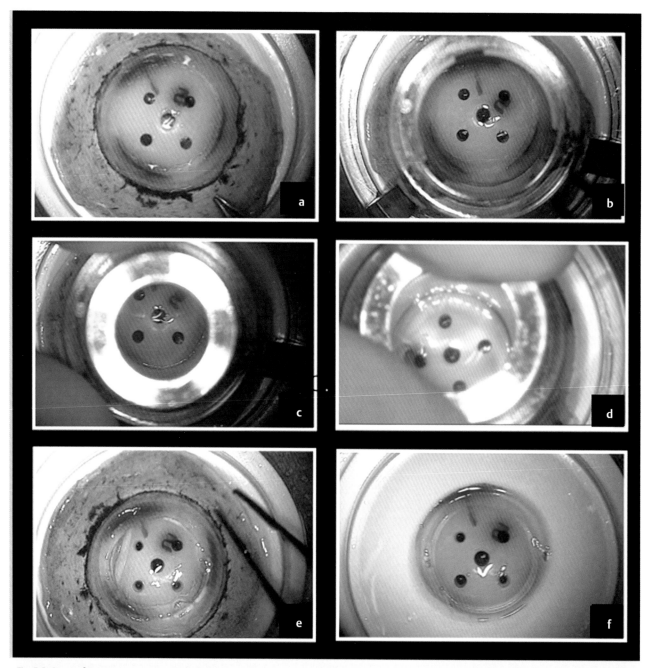

Fig. 5.2 Steps of Descemet stripping endothelial keratoplasty donor graft preparation using an UltraFit Coronet Donor Punch Set. **(a)** After excess storage medium is removed, graft is placed on cutting block. Graft centration is confirmed and graft then trephined. **(b)** Seating ring placed over graft and cutting block. **(c)** Trephine blade diameter confirmed and trephine blade placed into seating ring. **(d)** Graft punched with thumb and scleral rim rotated to ensure complete rotation. **(e)** Scleral rim removed. **(f)** Ensure graft is on cutting block and not adherent to trephine blade and no residual edges on graft.

Air Injection

Once the graft is centered, air, in a 3 mL syringe with 27-gauge cannula, is then injected into the anterior chamber. This is done in order to appose the donor graft against the host stromal bed. A smooth interface both host with good stripping, a graft with proper preparation and no residual edges, increased intraocular pressure and lying flat can optimize graft adherence rates.

Graft Adherence

Intraoperative maneuvers to facilitate adhesion include scraping the peripheral recipient bed, draining fluid from the interface through vertical mid peripheral vent incisions, sweeping the surface of the cornea with a roller, and presoaking the donor tissue in BSS (▶ Fig. 5.5).

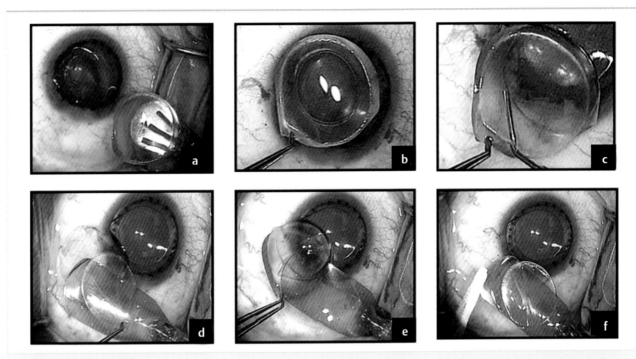

Fig. 5.3 Steps of graft handling with use of an Ocular Systems Endoserter in a Descemet stripping endothelial keratoplasty (DSEK)-triple procedure. **(a)** A graft spatula is used to position the anterior cap with prepared donor graft onto the cornea, endothelial side up. **(b)** Using a Colibri or Maumenee forceps the anterior cap alone is held at its widest point. **(c)** A 27-gauge irrigation cannula on a 3 mL syringe is used to confirm a complete lamellar dissection plane has been made. **(d)** The DSEK graft is brought onto the Endoserter plate, holding only the edge of the graft to minimize endothelial cell loss. **(e)** The anterior cap is removed and **(f)** a Weck-Cel sponge is used to dry the edges of the graft.

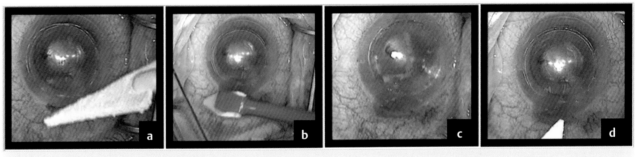

Fig. 5.4 "Sutureless" Descemet stripping endothelial keratoplasty with the use of ReSure Sealant. **(a)** The main incision is dried with a Weck-Cel sponge. **(b)** ReSure Sealant components are mixed and applied with minimal pressure using the applicator. **(c)** Allow for sealant to dry in approximately 20 seconds. **(d)** Test area with Weck-Cel sponge to confirm sealant has dried.

The required duration and pressure of the air fill to ensure adherence of the tissue are controversial. Techniques vary from a full air fill in the operating room for 10 minutes followed by release and replacement with a partial air fill; a full air fill for up to 1 hour, with subsequent partial release at a slit lamp; and a complete air fill overnight, combined with an inferior iridectomy to prevent pupillary block or use of acetazolamide.

5.3 Complications: Prevention and Management

5.3.1 Intraoperative Complications[35]

The following complications can occur during DSEK:

- Poor microkeratome dissection, precluding use of the donor tissue
- Incomplete removal of Descemet tissue
- Poor centration of the donor tissue during trephination, leading to a thick edge and possibly retained epithelial cells that could be implanted into the anterior chamber
- Intraocular hyphema and blood in the interface
- Excessive manipulation of donor tissue, risking endothelial cell loss
- Posterior dislocation of the donor tissue
- Disorientation during placement of donor tissue, leading to placement of the endothelium against the host stream cornea.

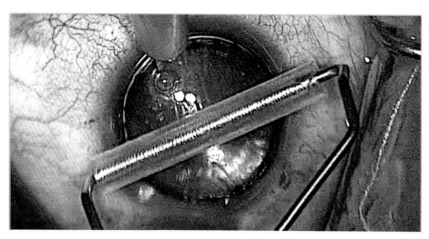

Fig. 5.5 Removal of an air bubble in a Descemet stripping endothelial keratoplasty graft–host interface using a Lindstrom LASIK Flap Roller and a venting incision to release air.

5.3.2 Postoperative Complications

In a typical postoperative follow-up, the patient is seen on postoperative day 1 to ensure that the lenticule is in good position and that no fluid is in the interface. Typically, there is about a 40% air bubble. Over a 3 to 5 day period, the air bubble absorbs and the cornea begins to clear. After 6 months, it is difficult to visualize the interface centrally.

The postoperative medication regimen is similar to that for PK, although some surgeons recommend maintaining the patient on topical corticosteroids for a longer period of time, sometimes on a once-daily dose lifelong.

Inadequate release of the intraoperative air fill may lead to pupillary block from migration of the air behind the iris, thus closing the angle. The acute rise in pressure produces pain and can potentially exacerbate underlying glaucoma. Pupillary dilation beyond the retained air bubble for the first 24 hours may reduce the incidence of this complication. Some corneal surgeons are proponents of performing a prophylactic peripheral iridotomy in the clinic preoperatively using the neodymium: yttrium-aluminum-garnet (Nd:YAG) laser or intraoperatively prior to graft insertion, to avoid risk of pupillary block in DSEK.[36]

The rate of dislocation of the donor graft varies greatly in reported cases, from 4% with experienced surgeons up to 35 to 40% with novice surgeons. Dislocation of the donor graft occurs primarily with the first 24 hours, although occasionally inadvertent trauma from eye rubbing or a sudden blow to the eye has caused the donor disc to be displaced at a later time. Risk factors for graft dislocation include aphakia, complicated IOL placement, or prior aqueous shunt surgery or pars plana vitrectomy.[37,38]

Epithelial ingrowth may first be seen as a white deposit within the interface that can be relatively stable and asymptomatic. In rare cases, epithelial ingrowth may lead to graft failure that is missed on clinical exam but recognized on histological exam of the tissue after a second procedure. The source of the ingrowth may be host surface epithelial cells implanted within the eye during placement of the donor tissue or donor epithelial cells inadvertently left in place and implanted following eccentric trephination beyond the microkeratome dissection.[39]

The primary graft failure rate seen in published reports varies between 3 and 12%, with higher numbers associated with surgeons in the early stages of the learning curve and lower numbers associated with more experienced surgeons, likely due to less endothelial trauma as a consequence of less tissue manipulation and a lower rate of dislocation.[36]

Additional manipulation of tissue risks endothelial cell loss. This may be the result of microkeratome dissection, tissue manipulation, and excess air tamponade. In two different studies, mean endothelial cell loss at 6 months was 34%.[40]

However, in a 6-month to 3-year follow-up by Price and Price, further cell loss was only 8%, which compared favorably with the Cornea Donor Study Investigation Group PK Study that showed 42% cell loss between 6 months and 3 years. The authors attributed these results to the increased diameter of the DSAEK grafts (8.75–9 mm), which provided more surface area and thus more transplanted endothelial cells than traditional PK.[41]

Additional complications associated with DSEK are similar to those seen with PK, including suprachoroidal hemorrhage, retinal detachment, cystoid macular edema, and graft rejection.[42]

5.4 Postoperative Management

If air is removed at the slit lamp within the first hours, it must be released slowly to prevent sudden and dramatic loss of pressure in the eye. Patients are then advised to lie on their back for the first 24 hours to tamponade the donor graft against the posterior stroma with the retained air bubble, whereas others suggest lying flat as much as possible until the bubble resolves. Placement of an inferior anchoring suture may prevent graft dislocation while minimizing the need for the patient to remain supine postoperatively.[28,29,32]

5.5 Conclusion

With the advances in the field of corneal transplantation, DSEK has since gained prominence over PKP as the preferred corneal transplantation technique for numerous indications.[2] Mastering the surgical technique of DSEK, the mainstay endothelial keratoplasty of our time, will allow corneal surgeons to understand variations in technique as well as to delve into newer innovations and corneal transplant procedures that are paving the way of the future, most notably DMEK and PDEK.

References

[1] Gorovoy MS. Descemet-stripping automated endothelial keratoplasty. Cornea. 2006; 25(8):886–889

[2] Price FW, Jr, Price MO. 2009

[3] Fernandez MM, Afshari NA. Endothelial Keratoplasty: From DLEK to DMEK. Middle East Afr J Ophthalmol. 2010; 17(1):5–8

[4] Melles GR. Posterior lamellar keratoplasty: DLEK to DSEK to DMEK. Cornea. 2006; 25(8):879–881

[5] Ko W, Frueh BE, Shields CK, Costello ML, Feldman ST. Experimental posterior corneal transplantation of the rabbit cornea. Invest Ophthalmol Vis Sci. 1993; 34(4):1102 (ARVO Abstract)

[6] Melles GR, Eggink FA, Lander F, et al. A surgical technique for posterior lamellar keratoplasty. Cornea. 1998; 17(6):618–626

[7] Price FW, Jr, Price MO. Descemet's stripping with endothelial keratoplasty in 200 eyes: Early challenges and techniques to enhance donor adherence. J Cataract Refract Surg. 2006; 32(3):411–418

[8] Eye Bank Association of America. http://restoresight.org/

[9] Copeland, R.A. Jr., & Afshari, N. (Eds.). Copeland & Afshari's principles and practice of cornea. New York, NY: JP Medical Publishers. 2013

[10] Price FW, Jr, Price MO. Endothelial keratoplasty to restore clarity to a failed penetrating graft. Cornea. 2006c; 25(8):895–899

[11] Price MO, Price FW, Jr. Descemet stripping with endothelial keratoplasty for treatment of iridocorneal endothelial syndrome. Cornea. 2007; 26(4):493–497

[12] Price MO, Gorovoy M, Price FW, Jr, Benetz BA, Menegay HJ, Lass JH. Descemet's stripping automated endothelial keratoplasty: three-year graft and endothelial cell survival compared with penetrating keratoplasty. Ophthalmology. 2013; 120(2):246–251

[13] Daoud YJ, Munro AD, Delmonte DD, et al. Effect of cornea donor graft thickness on the outcome of Descemet stripping automated endothelial keratoplasty surgery. Am J Ophthalmol. 2013; 156(5):860–866.e1

[14] Wacker K, Bourne WM, Patel SV. Effect of graft thickness on visual acuity after Descemet stripping endothelial keratoplasty: a systematic review and meta-analysis. Am J Ophthalmol. 2016; 163:18–28

[15] Taravella MJ, Shah V, Davidson R. Ultrathin DSAEK. Int Ophthalmol Clin. 2013; 53(2):21–30

[16] Kim K, Alder B, Vora GK, et al. Textural interface opacity after Descemet-stripping automated endothelial keratoplasty. J Cataract Refract Surg. 2014; 40(9):1514–1520

[17] Patel SV, Baratz KH, Hodge DO, Maguire LJ, McLaren JW. The effect of corneal light scatter on vision after descemet stripping with endothelial keratoplasty. Arch Ophthalmol. 2009; 127(2):153–160

[18] Turnbull AM, Tsatsos M, Hossain PN, Anderson DF. Determinants of visual quality after endothelial keratoplasty. Surv Ophthalmol. 2016; 61(3):257–271

[19] Terry MA. Endothelial keratoplasty: why aren't we all doing Descemet membrane endothelial keratoplasty? Cornea. 2012; 31(5):469–471

[20] Tourtas T, Laaser K, Bachmann BO, Cursiefen C, Kruse FE. Descemet membrane endothelial keratoplasty versus descemet stripping automated endothelial keratoplasty. Am J Ophthalmol. 2012; 153(6):1082–90.e2

[21] Price MO, Giebel AW, Fairchild KM, Price FW, Jr. Descemet's membrane endothelial keratoplasty: prospective multicenter study of visual and refractive outcomes and endothelial survival. Ophthalmology. 2009; 116(12):2361–2368

[22] Agarwal A, Agarwal A, Narang P, Kumar DA, Jacob S. Pre-Descemet Endothelial Keratoplasty With Infant Donor Corneas: A Prospective Analysis. Cornea. 2015; 34(8):859–865

[23] Price MO, Fairchild KM, Price DA, Price FW, Jr. Descemet's stripping endothelial keratoplasty five-year graft survival and endothelial cell loss. Ophthalmology. 2011; 118(4):725–729

[24] Price MO, Baig KM, Brubaker JW, Price FW, Jr. Randomized, prospective comparison of precut vs surgeon-dissected grafts for descemet stripping automated endothelial keratoplasty. Am J Ophthalmol. 2008; 146(1):36–41

[25] Jun B, Kuo AN, Afshari NA, Carlson AN, Kim T. Refractive change after descemet stripping automated endothelial keratoplasty surgery and its correlation with graft thickness and diameter. Cornea. 2009; 28(1):19–23

[26] Covert DJ, Koenig SB. New triple procedure: Descemet's stripping and automated endothelial keratoplasty combined with phacoemulsification and intraocular lens implantation. Ophthalmology. 2007; 114(7):1272–1277

[27] Dunn SP, Gal RL, Kollman C, et al. Writing Committee for the Cornea Donor Study Research Group. Corneal graft rejection 10 years after penetrating keratoplasty in the cornea donor study. Cornea. 2014; 33(10):1003–1009

[28] Melles GR, Wijdh RH, Nieuwendaal CP. A technique to excise the descemet membrane from a recipient cornea (descemetorhexis). Cornea. 2004; 23(3):286–288

[29] Terry MA, Saad HA, Shamie N, et al. Endothelial keratoplasty: the influence of insertion techniques and incision size on donor endothelial survival. Cornea. 2009; 28(1):24–31

[30] Chen ES, Terry MA, Shamie N, Hoar KL, Friend DJ. Precut tissue in Descemet's stripping automated endothelial keratoplasty donor characteristics and early postoperative complications. Ophthalmology. 2008; 115(3):497–502

[31] Busin M, Bhatt PR, Scorcia V. A modified technique for descemet membrane stripping automated endothelial keratoplasty to minimize endothelial cell loss. Arch Ophthalmol. 2008; 126(8):1133–1137

[32] Khor WB, Kim T. Descemet-stripping automated endothelial keratoplasty with a donor tissue injector. J Cataract Refract Surg. 2014; 40(11):1768–1772

[33] Mehta JS, Por YM, Poh R, Beuerman RW, Tan D. Comparison of donor insertion techniques for descemet stripping automated endothelial keratoplasty. Arch Ophthalmol. 2008; 126(10):1383–1388

[34] Mehta JS, Por YM, Beuerman RW, Tan DT. Glide insertion technique for donor cornea lenticule during Descemet's stripping automated endothelial keratoplasty. J Cataract Refract Surg. 2007; 33(11):1846–1850

[35] Chen ES, Terry MA, Shamie N, Hoar KL, Friend DJ. Descemet-stripping automated endothelial keratoplasty: six-month results in a prospective study of 100 eyes. Cornea. 2008; 27(5):514–520

[36] Suh LH, Yoo SH, Deobhakta A, et al. Complications of Descemet's stripping with automated endothelial keratoplasty: survey of 118 eyes at One Institute. Ophthalmology. 2008; 115(9):1517–1524

[37] Decroos FC, Delmonte DW, Chow JH, et al. Increased Rates of Descemet's Stripping Automated Endothelial Keratoplasty (DSAEK) Graft Failure and Dislocation in Glaucomatous Eyes with Aqueous Shunts. J Ophthalmic Vis Res. 2012; 7(3):203–213

[38] Afshari NA, Gorovoy MS, Yoo SH, et al. Dislocation of the donor graft to the posterior segment in descemet stripping automated endothelial keratoplasty. Am J Ophthalmol. 2012; 153(4):638–642, 642.e1–642.e2

[39] Koenig SB, Covert DJ. Epithelial ingrowth after Descemet-stripping automated endothelial keratoplasty. Cornea. 2008; 27(6):727–729

[40] Terry MA, Chen ES, Shamie N, Hoar KL, Friend DJ. Endothelial cell loss after Descemet's stripping endothelial keratoplasty in a large prospective series. Ophthalmology. 2008; 115(3):488–496.e3

[41] Price FW, Jr, Price MO. Does endothelial cell survival differ between DSEK and standard PK? Ophthalmology. 2009; 116(3):367–368

[42] Price MO, Jordan CS, Moore G, Price FW, Jr. Graft rejection episodes after Descemet stripping with endothelial keratoplasty: part two: the statistical analysis of probability and risk factors. Br J Ophthalmol. 2009; 93(3):391–395

6 Ultrathin Descemet Stripping Automated Endothelial Keratoplasty

Claudia E. Perez-Straziota

Endothelial keratoplasty (EK) has revolutionized the field of corneal transplantation for focal endothelial disease by providing a safer procedure with more predictable refractive outcomes and less risk for rejection compared to penetrating keratoplasty.[1] Since Tillett's first discussion of posterior lamellar keratoplasty in 1956[2] and Melles's article on endothelial keratoplasty in 1998,[3] several variations have been proposed to improve refractive outcomes and minimize rejection. These include deep lamellar endothelial keratoplasty (DLEK),[4] Descemet stripping endothelial keratoplasty (DSEK),[5] Descemet stripping automated endothelial keratoplasty (DSAEK),[6] Descemet membrane endothelial keratoplasty (DMEK),[7] and ultrathin Descemet stripping automated endothelial keratoplasty (ultrathin DSAEK)[8].[69]

The postoperative outcomes after standard DSAEK typically result in visual acuities better than 20/40[9,10]; however, in some instances, despite a clear graft with no apparent irregularities, the final visual acuity is worse than expected. Two main factors have been proposed to explain this variability in results: graft thickness[11,12,13] (preoperative and postoperative) and the higher-order aberrations (HOAs) induced by irregularities in the donor–host interface and in tissue architecture.[6,14,15,16]

Aside from a thinner lenticule, the double-pass microkeratome technique used for ultrathin DSAEK seems to provide better tissue architecture than a single-pass preparation, with comparable postoperative outcomes to DMEK and without the steep learning curve that DMEK requires to achieve proficiency.[17,18]

In ultrathin DSAEK the lenticule is also significantly thinner than DSAEK, but the surgical technique remains essentially the same. Despite excellent postoperative outcomes with DMEK[19] there is still poor traction for this procedure due to the significant learning curve and technical challenges DMEK presents. The comparative efficacy of DMEK compared to ultrathin DSAEK has yet to be fully elucidated but may be more similar than outcomes for regular-thickness DSEK grafts.

6.1 The Role of Lenticule Thickness in Postoperative Outcomes

In 2011 Neff et al published their findings of thinner lenticules, especially those < 131 µm, achieving better visual acuities than thicker grafts (20/25 in 100% and 20/20 in 71%).[20] There are many reports disputing the association between preoperative lenticule thickness and postoperative outcomes.[21,22,23,24,25] In these reports, preoperative and postoperative donor thicknesses were > 130 µm (> 145 µm in preoperative and >141 µm in postoperative measurements); and when preoperative graft thicknesses < 125 µm were analyzed separately, the percentage of patients with better visual acuities trended toward better visual outcomes.[21,24,26,27] In several publications where only thinner lenticules have been studied the results are still conflicting. Some show a significant improvement in visual

outcomes and rate of detachment and dislocation when lenticules are < 130 µm.[28,29] Others have shown no significant correlation between postoperative graft lenticule thickness and visual outcomes.[30,31] The current evidence associating graft thickness with postoperative visual outcomes is inconclusive, and current available studies do not yet present robust data and statistical analyses to prove or disprove this relationship,[32] specifically with lenticules < 130 µm.

6.2 Interface and Lenticule-Related Higher-Order Aberrations

There is an average hyperopic shift of + 1.0 D after DSAEK.[33,34,35] This seems to be related to tissue architecture and the negative lens effect that lenticules have, which is due to increased peripheral lenticule thickness.[36] In correlation analyses, a thicker lenticule center, a larger lenticule diameter, and negative curvature profiles have all been correlated with a higher refractive shift,[27,34] with stronger correlation when a thicker lenticule and a negative lenticule curvature profile are combined.[27,36]

Despite negligible changes in the anterior corneal topography after all types of endothelial keratoplasty,[15,27,36] there is an increase in posterior corneal HOAs after both DSAEK[13,15,29,35,37] and, to a lower degree, DMEK.[38] No studies are available in regard to HOAs after ultrathin DSAEK.

6.3 The Search for the Thinnest Transplantable Lenticule

In 2006 Melles et al introduced DMEK,[7] limiting the transplanted lenticule to Descemet membrane and endothelium only. DMEK likely represents the thinnest possible tissue routinely amenable to transplantation. However, DMEK poses many technical challenges and a significant learning curve to the surgeon.[17,18] There are some instances in which DMEK lenticule unfolding, which requires specific aqueous dynamics, would be challenging if at all possible, due to complexities from comorbidities or preexisting surgeries. In these patients DSAEK remains the procedure of choice, and a thinner lenticule may be desirable to maximize the postoperative outcomes.

In 2012 Busin et al[8] published their concept of ultrathin DSAEK previously presented at the 2009 European Society of Cataract and Refractive Surgery meeting and proposed the use of a preoperative lenticule thinner than 100 µm by using the "microkeratome double-pass technique" for donor preparation, which would standardize the preparation of grafts, resulting in consistently thinner and more planar lenticules.[39,40]

6.4 Ultrathin DSAEK: Indications

Ultrathin DSAEK is similar to standard DSAEK in terms of the surgical procedure, with the difference being mainly in donor preparation for a lenticule ideally < 100 µm. Even though ultrathin lenticules can still be obtained with a single-pass microkeratome by applying a nomogram for microkeratome head selection,[41,42] the double-pass microkeratome technique yields a more planar surface that offers some advantages in postoperative quality of vision and refractive shift.

Ultrathin DSAEK offers the advantages of minimizing stroma attached to Descemet membrane and endothelium in the donor lenticule while maintaining essentially the same surgical technique that has been used for standard DSAEK, with lenticule thickness measurements as low as 23 µm by 6 months postoperatively.[42]

The concerns for implementation of ultrathin DSAEK lie in tissue manipulation and increased tissue flexibility, which may result in postoperative irregularities in both the stroma interface and the endothelial side that may induce HOAs[21]; however, these concerns could also be applied to the very thin lenticule used in DMEK.

Studies looking at the relationship between DSAEK graft folds and HOAs have shown that thicker grafts actually tend to have more folds and induce more HOAs[43]; however, reports on HOAs after ultrathin DSAEK are not available.

6.5 Donor Tissue Preparation

The main objectives in the donor preparation for endothelial keratoplasty are to achieve a specific target lenticule thickness and to obtain the most planar cut possible in order to minimize postoperative refractive changes while inflicting minimal trauma to the endothelial cells in the graft. Ultrathin DSAEK lenticules can be obtained both with a single-pass and with a double-pass microkeratome technique.

6.6 Single Microkeratome Pass

Different strategies have been suggested in order to consistently obtain thinner cuts with a single microkeratome pass, such as stromal dehydration,[44] development of a nomogram for microkeratome head setting based on central corneal thickness prior to the cut,[42] and adjustment of the translational speed of the microkeratome in thicker donors, since slower translational speeds result in deeper cuts and thinner lenticules.[40] With a single microkeratome cut there is higher variability in thicknesses throughout the lenticule compared to two microkeratome passes.[26,39] This variability results in lenticules that are thinner in the center than in the periphery,[40] which has been related to the postoperative hyperopic shift observed after DSAEK.[36] Additionally, the predictability of the final lenticule thickness decreases as the target thickness decreases, dropping from 78% of cuts within 10 µm when the target is between 90 µm and 120 µm to 48% when the target falls below 91 µm.[41] Nevertheless, with the proper microkeratome head selection based on central corneal thickness, the majority of lenticules fall below 131 µm.[41]

6.7 Double Microkeratome Pass

The double-pass microkeratome technique consists of an initial "debulking" pass of the microkeratome, usually with a head between 300 and 350 µm (▶ Fig. 6.1a), and a second microkeratome pass that is adjusted in order to obtain a lenticule thickness between 100 µm to 130 µm (▶ Fig. 6.1b). The second pass is started 180 degrees away from the first pass and is performed in the opposite direction to obtain a more planar surface.

The head used for this step can be selected according to a nomogram developed by Busin (▶ Table 6.1), targeting a residual bed with a central thickness < 100 µm (▶ Fig. 6.1c); other algorithms have also been suggested to adjust both the first pass in relationship to the initial corneal thickness and the second pass related to stromal bed thickness prior to the cut.[39]

Lenticules created with the double-pass technique tend to be more planar, with a more even distribution of thickness from the center to the periphery after the second pass of the microkeratome.[39]

Pressure in the system must be standardized by raising the infusion bottle to a height of 120 cm above the level of the artificial anterior chamber and then clamping the tubing 50 cm from the entrance. Attention must be given to maintain a uniform, slow movement of the hand-driven microkeratome, requiring 4 to 6 seconds for each dissection, which will produce a planar surface that minimizes interface irregularities and hyperopic shift. ▶ Fig. 6.2 shows the optical coherence tomography images of donor tissue before microkeratome double-pass tissue preparation for ultrathin DSAEK (▶ Fig. 6.2a,b), and before regular single-pass microkeratome for DSAEK preparation (▶ Fig. 6.2c).

With the double-pass microkeratome technique, Busin et al reported 100% of the tissues with a postcut thickness < 151 µm, 95.6% < 131 µm, and 78.3% < 101 µm; and only 2.1% of the tissues were lost due to perforation.[19] Woodward et al[45] obtained 65% of cuts < 100 µm and 92% < 131 µm with the double-pass technique and found no significant difference in rate of perforation when the second pass was done 180 degrees from the first cut (23%) or at the thickest peripheral measurement in the residual bed (29%). Their higher perforation rate compared to the 7% reported by Busin et al[19] can be related to the larger chosen head size for the second cut.

6.8 Femtosecond Laser Ultrathin Lenticule Preparation

The role of the femtosecond laser in donor preparation for DSAEK and ultrathin DSAEK lenticules is still being determined. So far, despite the advantage of more accurate determination of depth of cut, and a faster recovery of visual acuity during the immediate postoperative period, femtosecond laser preparation of DSAEK donors has yielded worse long-term postoperative visual acuities and a higher rate of regrafting when compared to microkeratome grafts.[46] In vitro studies of DSAEK lenticule surfaces after microkeratome and femtosecond cuts have also shown that the surface is much smoother when the microkeratome is used for the cut[47] and that femtosecond cuts have a wavelike or concentric ring configuration of the stromal interface, caused by the applanation of the cornea during the preparation leading to an irregular cut shape due to incomplete cut of the stroma by the femtosecond.[48,49]

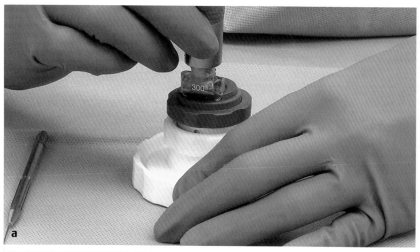

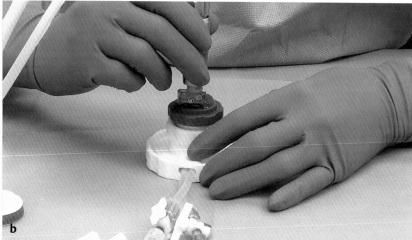

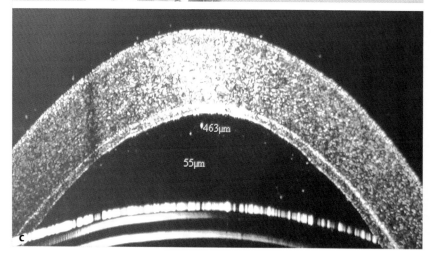

Fig. 6.1 (a) Microkeratome double-pass technique during the first microkeratome pass with a 300 μm head and (b) the second microkeratome pass, in this case with a 90 μm head selected to obtain (c) a final lenticule thickness < 100 μm. (Courtesy of Eric Meineke, Georgia Eye Bank.)

6.9 Surgical Procedure

The surgical procedure for ultrathin DSAEK is essentially the same as that for standard DSAEK. Five-millimeter incisions have been shown to have less endothelial cell loss compared to the 3 mm incisions[50,51]; however, this difference does not appear to be clinically significant postoperatively.[50] The Busin glide and injection devices appear to preserve the endothelium better, compared to manual insertion with forceps,[52,53] yet this difference does not appear to be clinically relevant postoperatively either.[50] The ultrathin DSAEK lenticule slides without difficulties through the 3 mm incision when inserted through a Busin glide; however, this does not necessarily translate into postoperative advantages, and the tissue insertion technique should be selected to maximize the surgeon's performance and minimize iatrogenic tissue trauma through excessive manipulation.

Placing the sutures prior to viscoelastic removal will provide a pressurized eye, which facilitates suture placement to reduce

Table 6.1 Proposed nomogram by Busin et al[19] for microkeratome head selection after the first microkeratome pass in the double-pass technique

Residual stromal bed (µm)	Head selection for second microkeratome pass (µm)
<151	No second cut
151–190	50
191–210	90
211–230	110
>230	130

postoperative astigmatism. It is of equal or greater importance to insert the tissue and then tie the sutures prior to unfolding since not doing so increases the chances of tissue expulsion through the open main incision and through which ultrathin lenticules can be expelled more easily.

Transient interface fluid has been associated with transient interface opacities[54]; therefore, similar precautions need to be taken when performing ultrathin DSAEK in removing all fluid and ocular viscoelastic devices from the donor–host interface. The use of a venting incision has been controversial due to the increased risk of epithelial downgrowth into the interface. The author uses a LASIK Flap Roller (Lindstrom, Visitec®), but any other blunt instrument can be used to "sweep" the corneal surface prior to lenticule adhesion with full air fill in the anterior chamber in order to remove any fluid present in the interface.

6.10 Postoperative Outcomes

After EK there is a degree of corneal deturgescence, mostly during the first postoperative month.[13,25,31,55,56] This causes a decrease in corneal light scatter, especially in subepithelial surface and donor–host interface during the postoperative follow-up, which may be responsible for most of the improvement in visual acuity. Graft thickness has not been directly correlated to the degree of deturgescence; however, the stabilization of postoperative graft thickness is reached earlier with thinner lenticules.[38,56]

The main difference between outcomes in DSAEK and ultrathin DSAEK seems to lie in the proportion of patients achieving distance corrected visual acuity (DCVA) of 20/20 by 1 year.[19,57] By year 2, this gap between both procedures narrows, with visual acuities of 20/20 or better in 34% of DSAEK patients[57] compared to 48.8% after ultrathin DSAEK,[19] with a trend toward better visual acuity after ultrathin DSAEK.

DMEK shows both superior results and faster recovery than DSAEK: by postoperative month 6, 42% of patients have DCVA of 20/20 or better, 72% of patients reach 20/25 or better, and 91% 20/30 or better. By the first year, the proportion of patients that reach DCVA of 20/20 remains stable, and 80% and 98% reach DCVA of 20/25 and 20/30, respectively.[58] To date there have been no direct comparisons between DMEK and ultrathin DSAEK.

The known postoperative hyperopic shift occurs after all cases of EK. In DSAEK cases, this shift averages +1.1 D (range +

0.7 to +1.5D).[33] When ultrathin lenticules are used, this shift decreases to +0.85 D (range −4.50 D to +3.25 D) when a single-microkeratome pass is used for preparation[56] and +0.78 D (range +0 D to +3.25 D) when the double-pass microkeratome technique is used.[19] After DMEK there is still a hyperopic shift, but it is considerably lower at +0.24 D (−1.50 D to +2.25 D).[58]

6.11 Postoperative Complications

Some known complications from DSAEK, such as intraocular pressure elevation (from pupillary block or from steroid response) and interface blood or haze can also occur in ultrathin DSAEK in a comparable rate.[33,56] Endothelial cell loss also seems to be comparable between these two procedures (42% for DSAEK and 35% for ultrathin DSAEK by 12 months),[19,33,59] in contrast with endothelial cell loss after DMEK in the same period of time, which has been reported as 19%.[59] Graft dislocation, detachment, and rejection rates are somewhat different between DSAEK, ultrathin DSAEK, and DMEK.

6.12 Detachment and Dislocation

There seems to be a trend toward higher rates of detachment or dislocation in thicker grafts and older recipients.[28,60] The rates of postoperative graft detachment and dislocation after ultrathin DSAEK[19,56] are lower than those reported in large DSAEK case series[33,60,61] and considerably lower than those reported for DMEK, which is probably related to the surgeon's learning curve[18,59,62,63] and the large proportion of partial detachments in DMEK cases.[59,63,64,65] The vast majority of these detachments resolved after an air reinjection (or "rebubbling") procedure, which is less commonly required after ultrathin DSAEK[19] than after DSAEK[33,66] and DMEK.[58,65,66]

6.13 Primary Graft Failure

There are concerns of increased difficulty in manipulation of ultrathin compared to standard lenticules; however, this has not translated to an increased rate or primary graft failure from excessive tissue manipulation in reported series of ultrathin DSAEK cases[19,56] compared to standard DSAEK.[33,67] The increased rate of 4% after DMEK[64] is likely related to iatrogenic failure due to complexity in tissue manipulation since the main reported cause of primary graft failure in DMEK patients is intraoperative level of difficulty.[68] The histopathological findings in removed DSAEK lenticules show in most primary graft failure cases a significant degree of endothelial cell attenuation, evidence of retained material either on the interface stromal side or in the endothelial side, and retained host Descemet membrane or presence of full-thickness cornea from eccentric trephination,[69,70] and electronic microscopy of DMEK failed grafts most commonly shows a decreased density of endothelial cells and thickened Descemet membrane with diffuse abnormal collagen inclusions. This demonstrates that the main causes of primary graft failure in all EK cases are related to the procedure and tissue manipulation and a possible preexisting endothelial cell dysfunction prior to transplantation.[68]

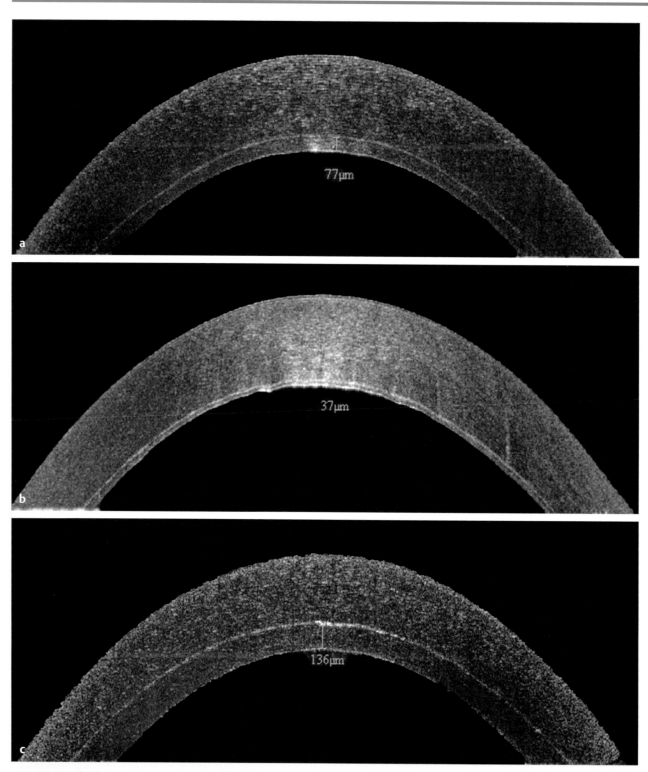

Fig. 6.2 Optical coherence tomography images after lenticule preparation with the **(a,b)** microkeratome double-pass technique and **(c)** after a standard single-microkeratome-pass technique. (Courtesy of Eric Meineke, Georgia Eye Bank.)

6.14 Graft Rejection

The lower rate of immunologic graft rejection with ultrathin DSAEK[19] reported at 1.4% compared to DSAEK reported between 7% and 8%[71,72,73,74] is likely explained be the reduction of transplanted stromal tissue, decreasing the antigenic load associated with the stromal tissue and reducing the chances of immune reaction. This is further demonstrated by the even lower rate of rejection after DMEK,[64] which remains as low as 0.7 to 0.8% after 1 and 2 years, respectively.[66,75]

The Kaplan–Meier predictions of probability of rejection at 12 and 24 months are also lower after ultrathin DSAEK (2.4% and 3.3%, respectively)[19] compared to DSAEK (7.6% and 12%, respectively),[66,74,76] and both are comparable to the projected risk of rejection after penetrating keratoplasty of 5 to 14% and 15 to 29% within the first and second year, respectively.[66,76,77,78,79] In contrast, the projected probabilities of immunologic graft rejection after DMEK are significantly lower at 1% at both the first and second years,[66] providing a significant advantage from the immune reaction standpoint and providing an alternative in patients with a higher risk of immune graft rejection prior to transplantation.

Intensive topical steroid treatment remains the standard treatment for immune graft rejection, and the resolution of graft rejection with any of these strategies has been reported as 73.3 to 94% of cases within 6 months.[74,76]

6.15 Conclusion

Ultrathin DSAEK is an alternative to DSAEK, using lenticules < 100 µm while maintaining the same surgical procedure and indications. Despite the perceived increased difficulty in tissue manipulation, there is no robust evidence proving difficulties in learning curves or changes required in the surgical instrumentation. The rate of immunologic rejection is slightly lower when ultrathin lenticules are used.

The outcomes in terms of visual acuity are also comparable to outcomes with DMEK except for the exceptionally low risk of immunologic rejection that DMEK offers. The role of ultrathin lenticules in substitution of standard DSAEK lenticules has not yet been completely established, and more robust data are required to support or discard it.

References

[1] Price MO, Gorovoy M, Price FW, Jr, Benetz BA, Menegay HJ, Lass JH. Descemet's stripping automated endothelial keratoplasty: three-year graft and endothelial cell survival compared with penetrating keratoplasty. Ophthalmology. 2013; 120(2):246–251

[2] Tillett CW. Posterior lamellar keratoplasty. Am J Ophthalmol. 1956; 41(3):530–533

[3] Melles GR, Eggink FA, Lander F, et al. A surgical technique for posterior lamellar keratoplasty. Cornea. 1998; 17(6):618–626

[4] Terry MA, Ousley PJ. Deep lamellar endothelial keratoplasty in the first United States patients: early clinical results. Cornea. 2001; 20(3):239–243

[5] Melles GR, Wijdh RH, Nieuwendaal CP. A technique to excise the descemet membrane from a recipient cornea (descemetorhexis). Cornea. 2004; 23(3):286–288

[6] Gorovoy MS. Descemet-stripping automated endothelial keratoplasty. Cornea. 2006; 25(8):886–889

[7] Melles GR, Ong TS, Ververs B, van der Wees J. Descemet membrane endothelial keratoplasty (DMEK). Cornea. 2006; 25(8):987–990

[8] Busin M, Patel AK, Scorcia V, Ponzin D. Microkeratome-assisted preparation of ultrathin grafts for descemet stripping automated endothelial keratoplasty. Invest Ophthalmol Vis Sci. 2012; 53(1):521–524

[9] Price FW, Jr, Price MO. Descemet's stripping with endothelial keratoplasty in 50 eyes: a refractive neutral corneal transplant. J Refract Surg. 2005; 21(4):339–345

[10] Ratanasit A, Gorovoy MS. Long-term results of Descemet stripping automated endothelial keratoplasty. Cornea. 2011; 30(12):1414–1418

[11] Chen ES, Shamie N, Terry MA. Descemet-stripping endothelial keratoplasty: improvement in vision following replacement of a healthy endothelial graft. J Cataract Refract Surg. 2008; 34(6):1044–1046

[12] Chen ES, Shamie N, Terry MA, Hoar KL. Endothelial keratoplasty: improvement of vision after healthy donor tissue exchange. Cornea. 2008; 27(3):279–282

[13] Hindman HB, Huxlin KR, Pantanelli SM, et al. Post-DSAEK optical changes: a comprehensive prospective analysis on the role of ocular wavefront aberrations, haze, and corneal thickness. Cornea. 2013; 32(12):1567–1577

[14] Koenig SB, Covert DJ, Dupps WJ, Jr, Meisler DM. Visual acuity, refractive error, and endothelial cell density six months after Descemet stripping and automated endothelial keratoplasty (DSAEK). Cornea. 2007; 26(6):670–674

[15] Rudolph M, Laaser K, Bachmann BO, Cursiefen C, Epstein D, Kruse FE. Corneal higher-order aberrations after Descemet's membrane endothelial keratoplasty. Ophthalmology. 2012; 119(3):528–535

[16] Muftuoglu O, Prasher P, Bowman RW, McCulley JP, Mootha VV. Corneal higher-order aberrations after Descemet's stripping automated endothelial keratoplasty. Ophthalmology. 2010; 117(5):878–884.e6

[17] Terry MA. Endothelial keratoplasty: why aren't we all doing Descemet membrane endothelial keratoplasty? Cornea. 2012; 31(5):469–471

[18] Dapena I, Ham L, Droutsas K, van Dijk K, Moutsouris K, Melles GR. Learning Curve in Descemet's Membrane Endothelial Keratoplasty: First Series of 135 Consecutive Cases. Ophthalmology. 2011; 118(11):2147–2154

[19] Busin M, Madi S, Santorum P, Scorcia V, Beltz J. Ultrathin descemet's stripping automated endothelial keratoplasty with the microkeratome double-pass technique: two-year outcomes. Ophthalmology. 2013; 120(6):1186–1194

[20] Neff KD, Biber JM, Holland EJ. Comparison of central corneal graft thickness to visual acuity outcomes in endothelial keratoplasty. Cornea. 2011; 30(4):388–391

[21] Terry MA, Straiko MD, Goshe JM, Li JY, Davis-Boozer D. Descemet's automated endothelial keratoplasty: the tenuous relationship between donor thickness and postoperative vision. Ophthalmology. 2012; 119(10):1988–1996

[22] Woodward MA, Raoof-Daneshvar D, Mian S, Shtein RM. Relationship of visual acuity and lamellar thickness in descemet stripping automated endothelial keratoplasty. Cornea. 2013; 32(5):e69–e73

[23] Van Cleynenbreugel H, Remeijer L, Hillenaar T. Descemet stripping automated endothelial keratoplasty: effect of intraoperative lenticule thickness on visual outcome and endothelial cell density. Cornea. 2011; 30(11):1195–1200

[24] Phillips PM, Phillips LJ, Maloney CM. Preoperative graft thickness measurements do not influence final BSCVA or speed of vision recovery after descemet stripping automated endothelial keratoplasty. Cornea. 2013; 32(11):1423–1427

[25] Ahmed KA, McLaren JW, Baratz KH, Maguire LJ, Kittleson KM, Patel SV. Host and graft thickness after Descemet stripping endothelial keratoplasty for Fuchs endothelial dystrophy. Am J Ophthalmol. 2010; 150(4):490–497.e2

[26] Nieuwendaal CP, van Velthoven ME, Biallosterski C, et al. Thickness measurements of donor posterior disks after descemet stripping endothelial keratoplasty with anterior segment optical coherence tomography. Cornea. 2009; 28(3):298–303

[27] Lombardo M, Terry MA, Lombardo G, Boozer DD, Serrao S, Ducoli P. Analysis of posterior donor corneal parameters 1 year after Descemet stripping automated endothelial keratoplasty (DSAEK) triple procedure. Graefes Arch Clin Exp Ophthalmol. 2010; 248(3):421–427

[28] Acar BT, Akdemir MO, Acar S. Visual acuity and endothelial cell density with respect to the graft thickness in Descemet's stripping automated endothelial keratoplasty: one year results. Int J Ophthalmol. 2014; 7(6):974–979

[29] Dickman MM, Cheng YY, Berendschot TT, van den Biggelaar FJ, Nuijts RM. Effects of graft thickness and asymmetry on visual gain and aberrations after descemet stripping automated endothelial keratoplasty. JAMA Ophthalmol. 2013; 131(6):737–744

[30] Daoud YJ, Munro AD, Delmonte DD, et al. Effect of cornea donor graft thickness on the outcome of Descemet stripping automated endothelial keratoplasty surgery. Am J Ophthalmol. 2013; 156(5):860–866.e1

[31] Shinton AJ, Tsatsos M, Konstantopoulos A, et al. Impact of graft thickness on visual acuity after Descemet's stripping endothelial keratoplasty. Br J Ophthalmol. 2012; 96(2):246–249

[32] Wacker K, Bourne WM, Patel SV. Effect of Graft Thickness on Visual Acuity After Descemet Stripping Endothelial Keratoplasty: A Systematic Review and Meta-Analysis. Am J Ophthalmol. 2016; 163:18–28

[33] Lee WB, Jacobs DS, Musch DC, Kaufman SC, Reinhart WJ, Shtein RM. Descemet's stripping endothelial keratoplasty: safety and outcomes: a report by the American Academy of Ophthalmology. Ophthalmology. 2009; 116 (9):1818–1830

[34] Esquenazi S, Rand W. Effect of the shape of the endothelial graft on the refractive results after Descemet's stripping with automated endothelial keratoplasty. Can J Ophthalmol. 2009; 44(5):557–561

[35] Clemmensen K, Ivarsen A, Hjortdal J. Changes in Corneal Power After Descemet Stripping Automated Endothelial Keratoplasty. J Refract Surg. 2015; 31 (12):807–812

[36] Dupps WJ, Jr, Qian Y, Meisler DM. Multivariate model of refractive shift in Descemet-stripping automated endothelial keratoplasty. J Cataract Refract Surg. 2008; 34(4):578–584

[37] Newman LR, Rosenwasser GO, Dubovy SR, Matthews JL. Clinicopathologic correlation of textural interface opacities in descemet stripping automated endothelial keratoplasty: a case study. Cornea. 2014; 33(3):306–309

[38] van Dijk K, Droutsas K, Hou J, Sangsari S, Liarakos VS, Melles GR. Optical quality of the cornea after Descemet membrane endothelial keratoplasty. Am J Ophthalmol. 2014; 158(1):71–79.e1

[39] Sikder S, Nordgren RN, Neravetla SR, Moshirfar M. Ultra-thin donor tissue preparation for endothelial keratoplasty with a double-pass microkeratome. Am J Ophthalmol. 2011; 152(2):202–208.e2

[40] Villarrubia A, Cano-Ortiz A. Development of a nomogram to achieve ultrathin donor corneal disks for Descemet-stripping automated endothelial keratoplasty. J Cataract Refract Surg. 2015; 41(1):146–151

[41] Choulakian MY, Li JY, Ramos S, Mannis MJ. Single-Pass Microkeratome System for Eye Bank DSAEK Tissue Preparation: Is Stromal Bed Thickness Predictable and Reproducible? Cornea. 2016; 35(1):95–99

[42] Nahum Y, Leon P, Busin M. Postoperative Graft Thickness Obtained With Single-Pass Microkeratome-Assisted Ultrathin Descemet Stripping Automated Endothelial Keratoplasty. Cornea. 2015; 34(11):1362–1364

[43] Seery LS, Nau CB, McLaren JW, Baratz KH, Patel SV. Graft thickness, graft folds, and aberrations after descemet stripping endothelial keratoplasty for fuchs dystrophy. Am J Ophthalmol. 2011; 152(6):910–916

[44] Thomas PB, Mukherjee AN, O'Donovan D, Rajan MS. Preconditioned donor corneal thickness for microthin endothelial keratoplasty. Cornea. 2013; 32 (7):e173–e178

[45] Woodward MA, Titus MS, Shtein RM. Effect of microkeratome pass on tissue processing for Descemet stripping automated endothelial keratoplasty. Cornea. 2014; 33(5):507–509

[46] Heinzelmann S, Maier P, Böhringer D, Auw-Hädrich C, Reinhard T. Visual outcome and histological findings following femtosecond laser-assisted versus microkeratome-assisted DSAEK. Graefes Arch Clin Exp Ophthalmol. 2013; 251(8):1979–1985

[47] Jones YJ, Goins KM, Sutphin JE, Mullins R, Skeie JM. Comparison of the femtosecond laser (IntraLase) versus manual microkeratome (Moria ALTK) in dissection of the donor in endothelial keratoplasty: initial study in eye bank eyes. Cornea. 2008; 27(1):88–93

[48] Soong HK, Mian S, Abbasi O, Juhasz T. Femtosecond laser-assisted posterior lamellar keratoplasty: initial studies of surgical technique in eye bank eyes. Ophthalmology. 2005; 112(1):44–49

[49] Phillips PM, Phillips LJ, Saad HA, et al. "Ultrathin" DSAEK tissue prepared with a low-pulse energy, high-frequency femtosecond laser. Cornea. 2013; 32 (1):81–86

[50] Price MO, Bidros M, Gorovoy M, et al. Effect of incision width on graft survival and endothelial cell loss after Descemet stripping automated endothelial keratoplasty. Cornea. 2010; 29(5):523–527

[51] Terry MA, Saad HA, Shamie N, et al. Endothelial keratoplasty: the influence of insertion techniques and incision size on donor endothelial survival. Cornea. 2009; 28(1):24–31

[52] Bahar I, Kaiserman I, Sansanayudh W, Levinger E, Rootman DS. Busin Guide vs Forceps for the Insertion of the Donor Lenticule in Descemet Stripping Automated Endothelial Keratoplasty. Am J Ophthalmol. 2009; 147(2):220–226.e1

[53] Foster JB, Swan KR, Vasan RA, Greven MA, Walter KA. Small-incision Descemet stripping automated endothelial keratoplasty: a comparison of small-incision tissue injector and forceps techniques. Cornea. 2012; 31(1):42–47

[54] Juthani VV, Goshe JM, Srivastava SK, Ehlers JP. Association between transient interface fluid on intraoperative OCT and textural interface opacity after DSAEK surgery in the PIONEER study. Cornea. 2014; 33(9):887–892

[55] Di Pascuale MA, Prasher P, Schlecte C, et al. Corneal deturgescence after Descemet stripping automated endothelial keratoplasty evaluated by Visante anterior segment optical coherence tomography. Am J Ophthalmol. 2009; 148(1):32–7.e1

[56] Roberts HW, Mukherjee A, Aichner H, Rajan MS. Visual Outcomes and Graft Thickness in Microthin DSAEK—One-Year Results. Cornea. 2015; 34 (11):1345–1350

[57] Li JY, Terry MA, Goshe J, Davis-Boozer D, Shamie N. Three-year visual acuity outcomes after Descemet's stripping automated endothelial keratoplasty. Ophthalmology. 2012; 119(6):1126–1129

[58] Guerra FP, Anshu A, Price MO, Giebel AW, Price FW. Descemet's membrane endothelial keratoplasty: prospective study of 1-year visual outcomes, graft survival, and endothelial cell loss. Ophthalmology. 2011; 118(12):2368–2373

[59] Gorovoy IR, Gorovoy MS. Descemet membrane endothelial keratoplasty postoperative year 1 endothelial cell counts. Am J Ophthalmol. 2015; 159(3):597–600.e2

[60] Hood CT, Woodward MA, Bullard ML, Shtein RM. Influence of preoperative donor tissue characteristics on graft dislocation rate after Descemet stripping automated endothelial keratoplasty. Cornea. 2013; 32(12):1527–1530

[61] Suh LH, Yoo SH, Deobhakta A, et al. Complications of Descemet's stripping with automated endothelial keratoplasty: survey of 118 eyes at One Institute. Ophthalmology. 2008; 115(9):1517–1524

[62] Brockmann T, Brockmann C, Maier AK, et al. Clinicopathology of graft detachment after Descemet's membrane endothelial keratoplasty. Acta Ophthalmol (Copenh). 2014; 92(7):e556–e561

[63] Green M, Wilkins MR. Comparison of Early Surgical Experience and Visual Outcomes of DSAEK and DMEK. Cornea. 2015; 34(11):1341–1344

[64] Hamzaoglu EC, Straiko MD, Mayko ZM, Sáles CS, Terry MA. The First 100 Eyes of Standardized Descemet Stripping Automated Endothelial Keratoplasty versus Standardized Descemet Membrane Endothelial Keratoplasty. Ophthalmology. 2015; 122(11):2193–2199

[65] Price MO, Giebel AW, Fairchild KM, Price FW, Jr. Descemet's membrane endothelial keratoplasty: prospective multicenter study of visual and refractive outcomes and endothelial survival. Ophthalmology. 2009; 116(12):2361–2368

[66] Anshu A, Price MO, Price FW, Jr. Risk of corneal transplant rejection significantly reduced with Descemet's membrane endothelial keratoplasty. Ophthalmology. 2012; 119(3):536–540

[67] Letko E, Price DA, Lindoso EM, Price MO, Price FW, Jr. Secondary graft failure and repeat endothelial keratoplasty after Descemet's stripping automated endothelial keratoplasty. Ophthalmology. 2011; 118(2):310–314

[68] Ćirković A, Schlötzer-Schrehardt U, Weller JM, Kruse FE, Tourtas T. Clinical and ultrastructural characteristics of graft failure in DMEK: 1-year results after repeat DMEK. Cornea. 2015; 34(1):11–17

[69] Suh LH, Dawson DG, Mutapcic L, et al. Histopathologic examination of failed grafts in descemet's stripping with automated endothelial keratoplasty. Ophthalmology. 2009; 116(4):603–608

[70] Oster SF, Ebrahimi KB, Eberhart CG, Schein OD, Stark WJ, Jun AS. A clinicopathologic series of primary graft failure after Descemet's stripping and automated endothelial keratoplasty. Ophthalmology. 2009; 116(4):609–614

[71] Jordan CS, Price MO, Trespalacios R, Price FW, Jr. Graft rejection episodes after Descemet stripping with endothelial keratoplasty: part one: clinical signs and symptoms. Br J Ophthalmol. 2009; 93(3):387–390

[72] Bruce AD, Terry MA, Price FW, Price MO, Griffin NB, Claesson M. Corneal Transplant Rejection Rate and Severity after Endothelial Keratoplasty. Cornea 2007;26:1039-1042

[73] Li JY, Terry MA, Goshe J, Shamie N, Davis-Booker D. Graft Rejection After Descemet's Stripping Automated Endothelial Keratoplasty. Ophthalmology 2012;119:90-94

[74] Wu EI, Ritterband DC, Yu G, Shields RA, Seedor JA. Graft rejection following descemet stripping automated endothelial keratoplasty: features, risk factors, and outcomes. Am J Ophthalmol. 2012; 153(5):949–957.e1

[75] Dapena I, Ham L, Netuková M, van der Wees J, Melles GR. Incidence of early allograft rejection after Descemet membrane endothelial keratoplasty. Cornea. 2011; 30(12):1341–1345

[76] Price MO, Jordan CS, Moore G, Price FW, Jr. Graft rejection episodes after Descemet stripping with endothelial keratoplasty: part two: the statistical analysis of probability and risk factors. Br J Ophthalmol. 2009; 93(3):391–395

[77] Alldredge OC, Krachmer JH. Clinical types of corneal transplant rejection. Their manifestations, frequency, preoperative correlates, and treatment. Arch Ophthalmol. 1981; 99(4):599–604

[78] Claesson M, Armitage WJ, Fagerholm P, Stenevi U. Visual outcome in corneal grafts: a preliminary analysis of the Swedish Corneal Transplant Register. Br J Ophthalmol. 2002; 86(2):174–180

[79] Price MO, Gorovoy M, Benetz BA, et al. Descemet's stripping automated endothelial keratoplasty outcomes compared with penetrating keratoplasty from the Cornea Donor Study. Ophthalmology. 2010; 117(3):438–444

7 Descemet Membrane Endothelial Keratoplasty Surgical Technique

Christopher S. Sáles and Mark A. Terry

7.1 Introduction

Our collective efforts have advanced endothelial keratoplasty to the point where we can now attain a very nearly perfect anatomical replacement of the diseased endothelium and Descemet membrane with healthy donor tissue.[1] To our patients, this means that we can deliver visual outcomes and rejection rates that are far superior to penetrating keratoplasty (PK) and even better than Descemet stripping automated endothelial keratoplasty (DSAEK). To the corneal transplant surgeon, it means that we have the opportunity to learn a new surgical skill set that is very different from that for DSAEK.

The procedure for Descemet membrane endothelial keratoplasty (DMEK) has many nuances that can be important for success. This chapter's goal is to ease the learning curve of the novice DMEK surgeon by introducing the most critical details of our standardized surgical technique. It should not be considered an adequate substitute for a "hands-on" DMEK course, where one can assist an experienced DMEK surgeon at the operating microscope and gain experience in the DMEK in vitro wet lab.

7.2 Case Selection

7.2.1 Relative Contraindications for DMEK

Case selection plays a decisive role in the success of DMEK surgery, especially in the early days of one's learning curve. We routinely use DMEK for cases of Fuchs dystrophy and pseudophakic bullous keratopathy (PBK) in the absence of any other complicating issues. Although others have achieved success in a number of these scenarios, we opt for DSAEK instead of DMEK if any of the following are present: anterior chamber intraocular lens (IOL), filtering tube, trabeculectomy, aphakia, extensive peripheral anterior synechiae, and a history of posterior vitrectomy. We also perform DMEK in eyes with a prior failed DSAEK or PK, but in the latter scenario the procedure can be more difficult than in eyes with a virgin cornea (▶ Table 7.1).

7.2.2 The Ideal First Case for DMEK

Two key components that make DMEK surgery easier during the manipulation of the graft are the presence of a small pupil (1–2 mm) and an easily shallowed anterior chamber. The ideal surgical candidate for the new DMEK surgeon is a nontriple case because it does not require dilation agents, which can prevent a complete and brisk response to Miochol (Bausch & Lomb). The ideal candidate also has an eye with a normal or small anterior chamber and minimal vitreous syneresis of the posterior segment.

All of these traits are most often found in younger patients between the ages of 30 and 50, who are frequently phakic. However, the novice DMEK surgeon must also take into account the additional stress of damaging the crystalline lens during anterior segment maneuvers when the chamber is shallow, which is why *a young pseudophakic patient with a small- to average-sized anterior chamber is probably the best first case.*

In addition, although we prefer to place a surgical inferior iridotomy at the time of DMEK surgery, it always presents a small risk of iris vessel bleeding. Thus, for the first few cases of DMEK, the novice DMEK surgeon should also consider placing a *generous* inferior iridotomy by laser applications 1 or 2 weeks prior to the scheduled DMEK surgery (▶ Table 7.2).

7.3 Ordering DMEK Tissue

7.3.1 Prestripped and S-Stamped Tissue

As was the case with their introduction of precut DSAEK tissue, eye banks have made DMEK more feasible to adopt by minimizing the risk of tissue loss. The introduction of prestripped tissue by eye banks has eliminated the risk of failed donor preparation by the surgeon. The "S" stamp has further eliminated iatrogenic primary graft failure caused by inadvertently implanting the graft upside-down.

We obtain all of our prestripped and S-stamped tissue from the Lions Vision Gift (LVG) Eye Bank in Portland, Oregon, a leading eye bank in the Eye Bank Association of America (EBAA). An increasing number of eye banks have begun offering DMEK tissue, but should your local eye bank not provide this service, their tissue can be shipped to LVG in Portland for prestripping the day before scheduled DMEK surgery. LVG has shipped DMEK tissue as far as Asia and Europe.

Table 7.1 Conditions to consider Descemet stripping automated endothelial keratoplasty (DSAEK) instead of Descemet membrane endothelial keratoplasty (DMEK)

Relative contraindications to DMEK	Rationale
Posterior vitrectomy	• Inability to shallow the anterior chamber
Anterior chamber intraocular lens	• Trauma to the graft from the intraocular lens • Frequent coincidence of posterior vitrectomy
Aphakia	• Risk of tissue loss into the posterior segment • Frequent coincidence of posterior vitrectomy
Glaucoma with a filtering tube	• Trauma to the graft from the tube • Risk of graft separation due to postoperative hypotony and/or bubble migration
Glaucoma with a trabeculectomy	• Risk of tissue loss into the sclerotomy • Risk of graft separation due to postoperative hypotony and/or bubble migration
Peripheral anterior synechiae	• If extensive (e.g., in iridocorneal endothelial syndrome), difficulty unscrolling the graft without a smooth iris plane

Prestripped DMEK tissue is 90% stripped by a skilled eye bank technician, leaving a hinge of attachment of Descemet membrane to the peripheral posterior stroma. This allows

the donor tissue to remain attached and still be shipped in Optisol GS (Bausch & Lomb) in the same plastic viewing chamber as standard tissue. A "notch" that is cut from the scleral rim designates the location of the hinge. Tissue is evaluated by slit lamp after prestripping, and specular microscopy is performed prior to and after preparation of the DMEK tissue (▶ Fig. 7.1).

Table 7.2 The ideal first case for the novice Descemet membrane endothelial keratoplasty (DMEK) surgeon

Key factors to consider	Small pupil	Easily shallowed anterior chamber	Minimal risk of intraoperative hemorrhage
Desirable traits	Nontriple procedure	Short or average axial length	Preplaced laser peripheral iridotomy
		Minimal vitreous syneresis (30–50 years of age)	
		Phakic[a]	
Ideal first case for the novice DMEK surgeon	Young pseudophakic[a] patient with a small- to average-sized anterior chamber and a preplaced inferior laser peripheral iridotomy		

[a] Phakic eyes are generally easier to shallow than pseudophakic eyes, but the additional stress of potentially damaging the crystalline lens during anterior chamber maneuvers must be weighed against the potential benefits. In general, it may be better to choose a pseudophakic eye for one's first case.

7.3.2 Donor Age

Younger donor age correlates with more tightly scrolled DMEK tissue, which can be more difficult to unscroll intraoperatively, especially if the anterior chamber cannot be easily shallowed. Donor age is therefore a very important factor to consider during one's initial cases, although in our experience it becomes less of a consideration as the surgeon becomes more adept at the procedure. As of 2016, we routinely implant tissue from donors that are 50 years of age or older using a tapping technique, and we suspect that this age may continue to decrease as new techniques emerge. One such example is the specialized Fogla DMEK Cannula (Storz Bausch & Lomb Surgical), which has horizontally oriented orifices on each side of a closed-ended cannula to "jet" the leaflets of a tight scroll into a double-scroll configuration (▶ Fig. 7.2).

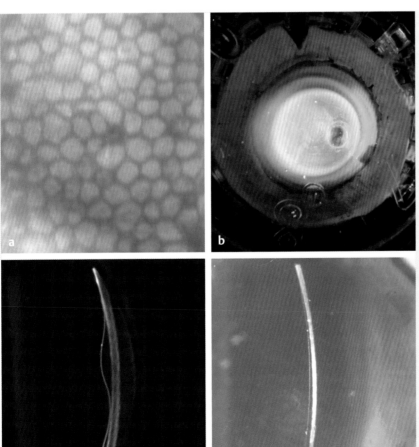

Fig. 7.1 (a) Specular microscopy. **(b)** View of the prestripped and S-stamped tissue in the viewing chamber, with a notch in the scleral rim to designate the location of the hinge. **(c,d)** Slit lamp biomicroscopy of the Descemet membrane endothelial keratoplasty tissue in the viewing chamber. Figure courtesy of Philip Dye, Lions VissionGift, Portland OR.

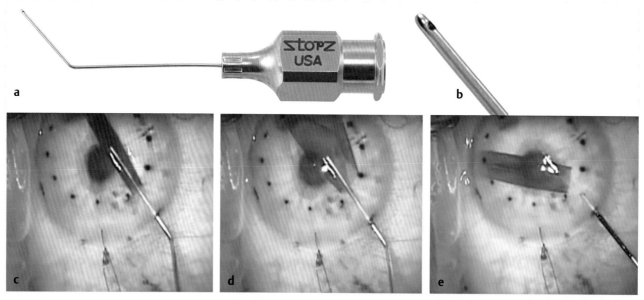

Fig. 7.2 (a) Fogla DMEK Cannula (Storz Bausch & Lomb Surgical) for reconfiguring tighter, younger scrolls into double scrolls using horizontally directed jets of fluid. **(b)** The Fogla Cannula features a closed-ended cannula tip with two horizontally directed orifices that are opposite each other. **(c)** The Fogla DMEK Cannula is positioned in the lumen of a tight DMEK scroll. **(d)** Horizontally directed jets of balanced salt solution force the leaflets of the scroll open. **(e)** The leaflets of the scroll curl back toward each other, thus reconfiguring the graft into a "double scroll." Surgical photos courtesy of Michael Straiko, Devers Eye Institute, Portland, OR.

7.4 Preoperative Medications

It is very important that the pupil is as small as possible for the insertion and unscrolling of the DMEK tissue; therefore we prefer not to use any cycloplegic drops preoperatively, even when concurrent cataract surgery is planned. In "triple" procedures, we use 1 to 3 drops of phenylephrine 2.5% to augment the dilation attained from a well-placed retrobulbar block, and we avoid the use of nonsteroidal drops to prevent persistent dilation. If the eye already has a posterior chamber IOL, we do not routinely use pilocarpine to constrict the pupil preoperatively because it may cause longer-term miosis that can either lead to posterior synechiae in the presence of a gas bubble or interfere with pupil dilation postoperatively should it be needed.

Nonsteroidal drops in DMEK cases that are performed without cataract surgery do not interfere with the miotic effects of Miochol, and can be given based on the surgeon's preference. Other preoperative drops such as antibiotics can also be given according to the surgeon's preference.

Discontinuation of systemic anticoagulants is ideal but not mandatory if a surgical peripheral iridotomy is planned.

7.5 Anesthesia

DMEK surgery is easiest in the first few cases with the patient under general anesthesia, as the stress and frustration level of the novice DMEK surgeon can be high, and it is always better when the patient does not hear the surgeon curse! Otherwise, DMEK can be performed under retrobulbar/peribulbar anesthesia quite easily and comfortably. Well-placed blocks can cause temporary mydriasis, which can help with some parts of the case (e.g., cataract surgery, stripping of Descemet membrane), but must be reversed with Miochol prior to injecting the tissue.

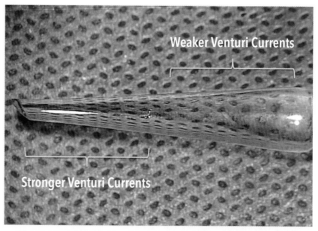

Fig. 7.3 The shape of the Straiko injector creates a Venturi effect that slows the tissue as it is aspirated from the tube's narrower, high-flow orifice into its wider, low-flow base–this makes the injector safer. A fully assembled injector consists of a 3 ml BD syringe (BD Worldwide), 14 French tubing, and a modified Jones tube (Gunther Weiss Scientific Glass Blowing) used off-label for Descemet membrane endothelial keratoplasty surgery.

7.6 Preparing the Injector

The Straiko injector consists primarily of a modified glass Jones tube that has been reshaped and polished by the Gunther Weiss Scientific Glass Blowing Company to resemble the profile of a medicine dropper—tapered distally, and bulb shaped in its midsection (▶ Fig. 7.3). Dr. Mike Straiko chose this design because it creates a venturi effect that slows the tissue as it is aspirated from the tube's narrower, high-flow orifice into its wider, low-flow base. The risk of inadvertently damaging the tissue by sucking it into the syringe is therefore reduced. The modified

Jones tube is coupled to a 3 mL syringe with a short piece of 14 French single-lumen suction tubing, and used off-label for DMEK surgery. Dr. Straiko designed the injector to be a closed system, which makes injection of the tissue highly controlled by ensuring that there is absolutely no reflux of fluid from the anterior chamber into the injector once its tip fully occludes the main incision (▶ Fig. 7.4).

The Straiko injector is constructed in the operating room by cutting a 14 French single-lumen suction tube anywhere along its length with heavy scissors, wetting the cut end with balanced salt solution (BSS), and twisting it onto a 3 mL Luer-lock syringe until it is firmly seated. The tubing is then trimmed to approximately 15 mm in length at a 45-degree angle, and this end is twisted onto the proximal end of the modified Jones tube. A well-constructed Straiko injector should require very little movement of the plunger to move the tissue into and out of the Jones tube. Care should be taken to minimize the gap between the syringe's orifice and the proximal end of the Jones tube, which ensures that the injector responds predictably to inputs made with the plunger. The injector must also be watertight and purged of all air, both of which can make the injector less responsive to actions on the plunger.

A modified Jones tube can be obtained from Gunther Weiss Scientific Glassblowing Company, Inc., in Portland, Oregon

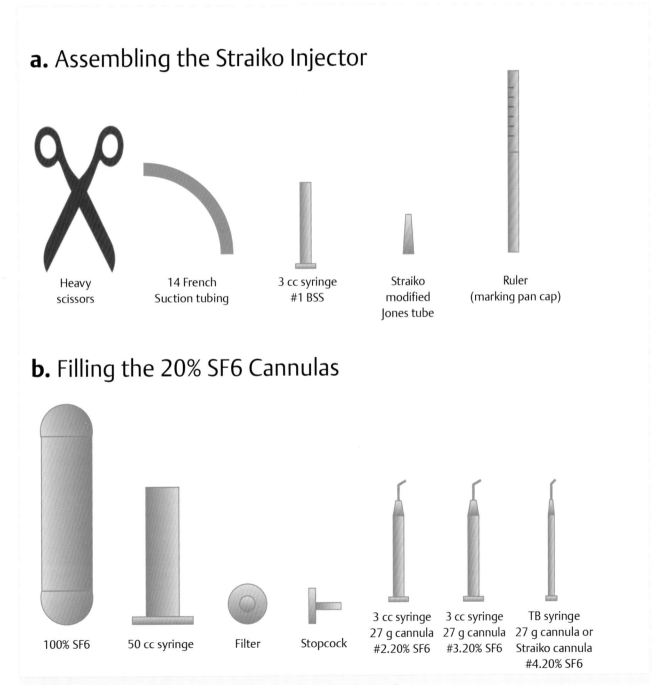

a. Assembling the Straiko Injector

Heavy
scissors

14 French
Suction tubing

3 cc syringe
#1 BSS

Straiko
modified
Jones tube

Ruler
(marking pan cap)

b. Filling the 20% SF6 Cannulas

100% SF6

50 cc syringe

Filter

Stopcock

3 cc syringe
27 g cannula
#2.20% SF6

3 cc syringe
27 g cannula
#3.20% SF6

TB syringe
27 g cannula or
Straiko cannula
#4.20% SF6

Fig. 7.4 (a) Assembling the Straiko injector. (b) Filling the 20% SF6 cannulas. *(continued)*

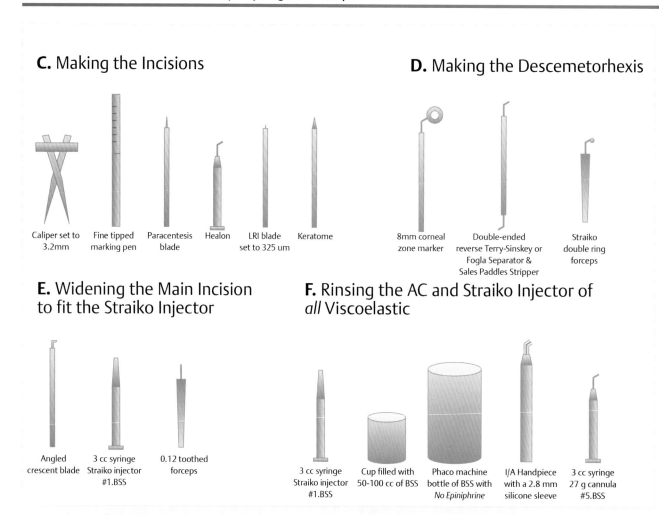

C. Making the Incisions

Caliper set to 3.2mm

Fine tipped marking pen

Paracentesis blade

Healon

LRI blade set to 325 um

Keratome

D. Making the Descemetorhexis

8mm corneal zone marker

Double-ended reverse Terry-Sinskey or Fogla Separator & Sales Paddles Stripper

Straiko double ring forceps

E. Widening the Main Incision to fit the Straiko Injector

Angled crescent blade

3 cc syringe Straiko injector #1.BSS

0.12 toothed forceps

F. Rinsing the AC and Straiko Injector of *all* Viscoelastic

3 cc syringe Straiko injector #1.BSS

Cup filled with 50-100 cc of BSS

Phaco machine bottle of BSS with *No Epiniphrine*

I/A Handpiece with a 2.8 mm silicone sleeve

3 cc syringe 27 g cannula #5.BSS

Fig. 7.4 *(continued)* **(c)** Making the incisions. **(d)** Making the descemetorhexis. **(e)** Widening the main incision to fit the Straiko injector. **(f)** Rinsing the anterior chamber and Straiko injector of all viscoelastic.

(503–644–4056, info@guntherweiss.com). Although these glass injectors may be labeled for single use due to local regulatory requirements, they are easily sterilized with standard methods and can be used multiple times as long as the tip remains smooth and unchipped.

7.7 Preparing the Recipient

The description of our surgical technique is from the perspective of the surgeon sitting temporally.

7.7.1 Paracentesis Sites

Calipers set at 3.2 mm are used to mark the clear corneal limbus at the 180-degree meridian for the main wound, and this is embellished with a surgical marking pen on the epithelium. Two additional ink marks are made in the superior and the inferior temporal limbal cornea to mark the locations of the paracentesis sites. Square-shaped, self-sealing stab incisions are then made at the two sites with a 1 mm keratome. The anterior chamber is filled with cohesive viscoelastic (Healon, Abbott Medical Optics, Inc.).

7.7.2 Descemetorhexis

The central surface of the cornea is marked with an 8 mm circle indentation, and this is embellished with multiple spots of marking pen ink to establish a template for the descemetorhexis. Care is taken to ensure that the surface template does not overlap the paracentesis or the main wound openings into the anterior chamber (▶ Fig. 7.5). With the chamber filled with cohesive viscoelastic, a reverse Terry-Sinskey hook is used to strip Descemet membrane, making sure to score exactly along the circular mark so that a full 8 mm area of stroma is bared. The goal is to attain a recipient stromal bed that is 0.5 mm larger than the donor DMEK tissue so that there is minimal, and ideally no, overlap between the donor and recipient Descemet membranes because any overlap can increase the risk of graft edge separation. Kruse and colleagues have termed this technique overstripping.

More so than in DSAEK surgery, extra care is taken during the descemetorhexis to ensure that the overlying stromal fibers are not disrupted because a rough stromal bed can increase the risk of graft separation in DMEK. Specialized instruments designed to protect the stroma during this step of the procedure are available, including the Sáles Paddle Stripper (▶ Fig. 7.6) and

G. Preparing the Donor at the Back Table

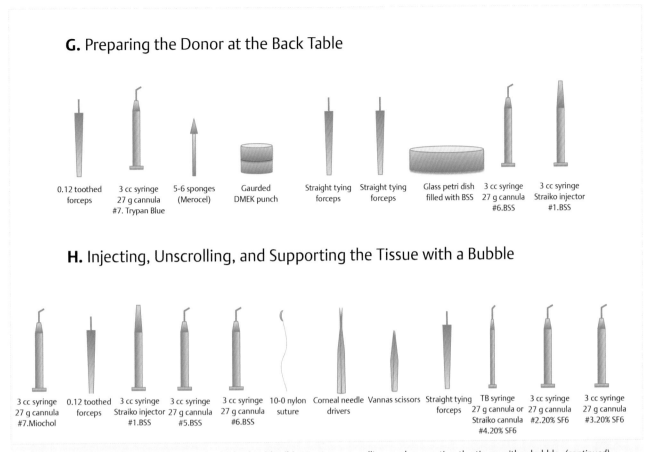

| 0.12 toothed forceps | 3 cc syringe 27 g cannula #7. Trypan Blue | 5-6 sponges (Merocel) | Gaurded DMEK punch | Straight tying forceps | Straight tying forceps | Glass petri dish filled with BSS | 3 cc syringe 27 g cannula #6.BSS | 3 cc syringe Straiko injector #1.BSS |

H. Injecting, Unscrolling, and Supporting the Tissue with a Bubble

| 3 cc syringe 27 g cannula #7.Miochol | 0.12 toothed forceps | 3 cc syringe Straiko injector #1.BSS | 3 cc syringe 27 g cannula #5.BSS | 3 cc syringe 27 g cannula #6.BSS | 10-0 nylon suture | Corneal needle drivers | Vannas scissors | Straight tying forceps | TB syringe 27 g cannula or Straiko cannula #4.20% SF6 | 3 cc syringe 27 g cannula #2.20% SF6 | 3 cc syringe 27 g cannula #3.20% SF6 |

Fig. 7.4 *(continued)* **(g)** Preparing the donor at the back table. **(h)** Injecting, unscrolling, and supporting the tissue with a bubble. *(continued)*

the Fogla Separator (▶ Fig. 7.7) (Storz Bausch & Lomb Surgical). Unlike DSAEK surgery, *scraping the stroma is not performed in the DMEK procedure.*

The chamber is filled again with Healon to pressurize the eye, and the main wound is created. A guarded diamond knife is set for 325 µm and a vertical 3.2 mm incision is made at the temporal limbus where previously marked. A 2.8 mm diamond or steel microkeratome is placed through the vertical incision edge to create a beveled entrance wound about 1.5 mm in length. The stripped Descemet membrane is then removed with forceps, or if available, Straiko Twin Ring Forceps (Storz Bausch & Lomb Surgical), which have been designed to grasp the tissue without engaging the stroma (▶ Fig. 7.8).

7.7.3 Inferior Peripheral Iridotomy

The inferior peripheral iridotomy is then performed if it has not already been made preoperatively with a laser. To make the iridotomy as peripheral as possible, a few microliters of Miochol are placed directly onto the iris surface beneath the Healon to constrict the pupil. In phakic eyes, we perform the iridotomy by excising iris that has been externalized from the eye through an overlying vertical paracentesis with forceps. In pseudophakic eyes, Healon is then injected into the anterior chamber and also placed between the iris pigment epithelium and the anterior capsule inferiorly. A needle driver is used to make two bends in a half-inch 30-gauge needle, one at the beveled tip and one at the hub, to fashion an ergonomic reversed hook that has a

sharp cutting edge. The bent needle tip is placed through the superior paracentesis site, passed through the pupil, walked along the posterior iris inferiorly, and then pressed upward against the far peripheral iris pigment epithelium. At the same time, a straight Sinskey hook is placed through the inferior paracentesis or the main incision and onto the iris stroma. The hook is then used to scrape down onto the location of the needle tip that is tenting up the iris tissue in the inferior periphery. Once the tip of the needle perforates the iris from behind, this creates a hole where the tip of the Sinskey hook can then be placed. Using the needle and the hook, the small iridotomy can be stretched to open it further. Intraocular MST Scissors (Micro-Surgical Technology) are then used to excise a full-thickness wedge of iris from the inferior periphery to ensure that the peripheral iridotomy remains patent (▶ Fig. 7.9). *When making the peripheral iridotomy, care should be taken to place it as peripheral and as close to 6 o'clock as possible to allow for a large bubble, and to avoid lacerating iris stromal vessels and pulling radially on the iris root, which can result in hemorrhage. In addition, the surgeon must be absolutely certain that iris pigment is excised (and not just iris stroma) to ensure patency of the peripheral iridotomy.*

7.7.4 Main Incision

The 2.8 mm main incision is then widened and custom-fit to the injector tip. A crescent blade is used to widen the incision incrementally to approximately 3.2 mm, or until the injector tip

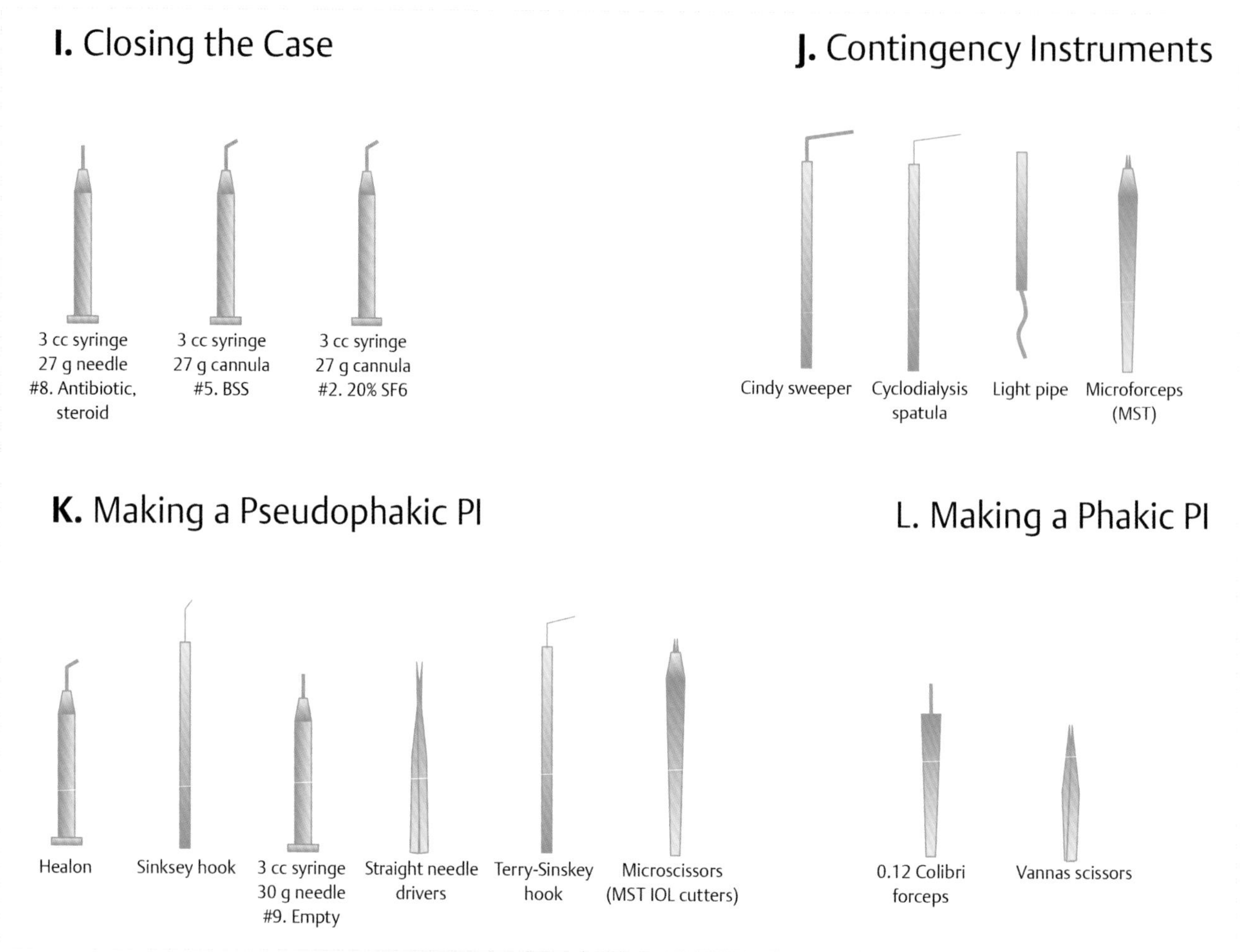

I. Closing the Case

3 cc syringe 27 g needle #8. Antibiotic, steroid	3 cc syringe 27 g cannula #5. BSS	3 cc syringe 27 g cannula #2. 20% SF6

J. Contingency Instruments

Cindy sweeper	Cyclodialysis spatula	Light pipe	Microforceps (MST)

K. Making a Pseudophakic PI

Healon	Sinskey hook	3 cc syringe 30 g needle #9. Empty	Straight needle drivers	Terry-Sinskey hook	Microscissors (MST IOL cutters)

L. Making a Phakic PI

0.12 Colibri forceps	Vannas scissors

Fig. 7.4 *(continued)* **(i)** Closing the case. **(j)** Contingency instruments. **(k)** Making a pseudophakic peripheral iridotomy (PI). **(l)** Making a phakic PI.

fits snugly into the incision. One or two test-fits with the injector may be necessary. *When widening the main incision, care should be taken to make its shape trapezoidal such that the injector's tapered midsection completely occludes the internal and external wounds.* A watertight main incision is imperative to safe injection of DMEK tissue into the anterior chamber. Care must also be taken not to widen the incision excessively, which can make it more difficult to disengage the tissue because the injector must be inserted further into the anterior chamber to maintain a watertight seal, thereby reducing the space available between the angle and the distal tip.

7.7.5 Evacuation of Viscoelastic

The anterior chamber is then evacuated with an irrigation/aspiration tip, preferably with a silicone sleeve to help to occlude the enlarged main incision and prevent iris prolapse. *The Straiko injector is also flushed at least three times with BSS to ensure that there is absolutely no viscoelastic in the injector system.*

7.7.6 Final Check

The eye is brought to a normal to slightly hypertensive pressure with BSS to prevent any bleeding from the iridotomy or from

episcleral reflux. *As a systemic measure to prevent mishaps in the operating room, we review the following checklist before moving to the donor table: (1) completion of the descemetorhexis, (2) completion of the inferior peripheral iridotomy, (3) widening of the main incision, and (4) evacuation of the anterior chamber* and *the Straiko injector of viscoelastic.*

7.8 Preparing the Donor

Our methods of handling the donor tissue ensure that the DMEK graft is touched only once at its far periphery during the entire transplant surgery. All preparation of the donor and loading of the injector is performed under an operating microscope.

The donor corneoscleral rim is removed from the viewing chamber with forceps by grasping the scleral notch placed by the eye bank. The tissue is then placed endothelial side up onto the donor table, where trypan blue is dripped onto the endothelium and left to stain for 1 minute. The trypan blue is wicked away using a polyvinyl-alcohol (Merocel) sponge placed at the edge of the donor Descemet flap opposite its hinge, while raising the hinged side of the corneoscleral rim with forceps. *Care should be taken to seat the prestripped Descemet membrane flat against the underlying posterior stroma when draining the fluid.*

M. Accounting of All of the Syringes opened for a DMEK case

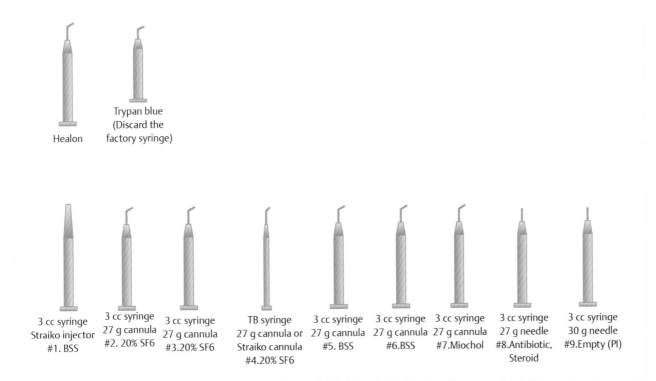

Fig. 7.4 (continued) (m) Accounting of all of the syringes opened for a Descemet membrane endothelial keratoplasty case.

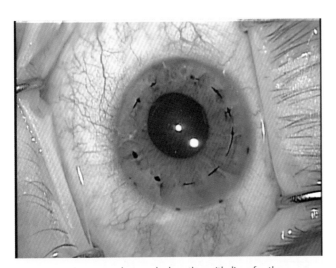

Fig. 7.5 An 8 mm template marked on the epithelium for the descemetorhexis, two 1 mm paracentesis sites, and a 3.2 mm biplanar incision.

If the membrane does not lie flat, especially along any of its edges, refloat it with BSS and wick the fluid again until the folds are gone.

The corneoscleral rim is placed on a 7.5 mm Moria punch block, which has been specially designed for partial-thickness trephination of DMEK tissue (▶ Fig. 7.10). The tissue is then positioned on the block to comfortably incorporate the S-stamp into the punch while simultaneously excluding as much damaged endothelium as possible, which can be visualized as punctate trypan blue staining of the endothelium. The trephine punch is then lowered very slowly onto the block until the blade meets the endothelium. A partial-thickness punch is made by pressing firmly on the trephine and allowing the preset depth guard to make contact with the corneoscleral rim. The trephine is then carefully removed. If alternative trephines are used, then forceful tapping by the surgeon of the trephine surface will render a partial-thickness trephination of Descemet membrane without creating a full-thickness stromal cut.

Tying forceps are used to remove the peripheral ring of Descemet membrane. Great care must be taken not to pull this tissue away too quickly because even the sharpest trephine will sometimes fail to make a full 360-degree cut. After tearing the ring opposite the hinge with two smooth forceps, each free end can be reflected onto itself much like a capsulorhexis flap in cataract surgery. *Should there be an area of incomplete trephination, the tissue can be torn along the intended contour of the cut without risking radial extension using this technique* (▶ Fig. 7.11). Two peripheral segments of Descemet membrane are placed into a petri dish filled with BSS for later use in testing the injector.

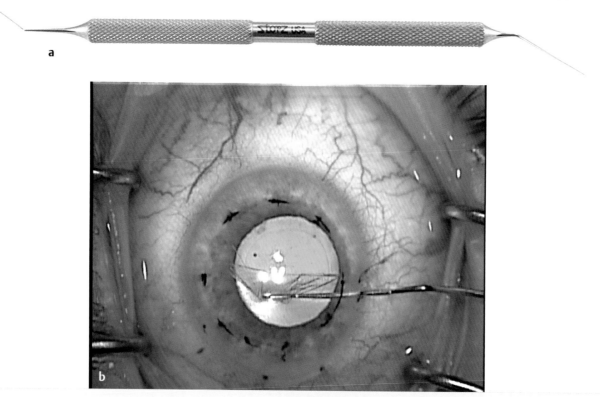

Fig. 7.6 **(a)** Combined Sáles Paddle Stripper and reverse Terry-Sinskey hook; the paddle is also available with a Fogla Separator (Storz Bausch & Lomb Surgical). **(b)** The Sáles Paddle Stripper provides a broad point of contact that protects the overlying stroma from damage; it is used in a "windshield wiper" sweeping action to efficiently strip the diseased endothelial Descemet membrane complex from the recipient.

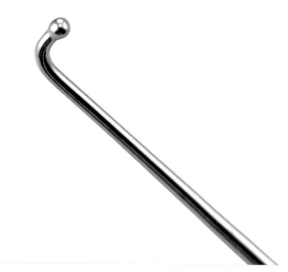

Fig. 7.7 The Fogla Separator (Storz Bausch & Lomb Surgical) features a dull ball-point tip to protect the overlying stroma from damage.

To facilitate grasping the tissue with forceps, the edge opposite the scleral notch is floated with gentle jets of BSS until it is no longer incarcerated in the stromal incision made by the trephine. With the trephined tissue now fully covered in BSS, the smallest peripheral area of tissue possible is grasped with tying forceps. The graft is then lifted from the stroma and completely

peeled off of the corneoscleral rim. *Care should be taken not to drag the endothelium on the donor stroma by bringing the forceps toward the notch and simultaneously elevating them.* Once the tissue is freely dangling in the air as a scroll, it is dropped back into the pool of BSS, which is then slowly drained from the corneoscleral rim with a premoistened Merocel sponge. The graft is then completely covered in trypan blue to stain for 3 to 4 minutes. Longer staining times do not damage the endothelium (▶ Fig. 7.12).

7.9 Testing the Straiko Injector

Remember the NASA space program in its early days? Before we sent an astronaut to the moon, we first sent a monkey into space to confirm that all systems were "go" without any glitches. We like to do the same with DMEK surgery. Our spaceship is the Straiko injector. Our "space monkeys" are the discarded peripheral pieces of donor Descemet membrane. "To infinity and beyond!" (▶ Fig. 7.13).

The Straiko injector is primed with 2 mL of BSS and all air bubbles are purged from the system. The distal tip of the Jones tube is then submerged into a petri dish filled with BSS, where the space monkeys were previously placed. With the tip bevel up, one of the space monkeys is engaged and suctioned far enough into the Jones tube to allow it to float in the distal portion of the tube's wider midsection. The tissue is then injected back into the petri dish, and the routine is practiced until the surgeon feels comfortable that the system is foolproof. During

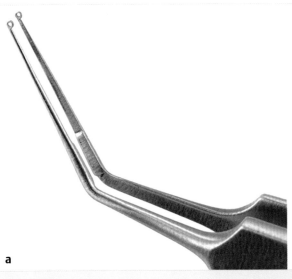
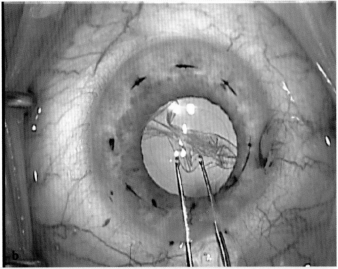

Fig. 7.8 **(a)** The Straiko Twin Ring Forceps (Storz Bausch & Lomb Surgical) feature smooth tips that are shaped like "rings" and are directed up toward the cornea to facilitate grasping of the stripped endothelial Descemet membrane complex without damaging the overlying stroma. **(b)** The Straiko Twin Ring Forceps are used to remove the stripped endothelial Descemet membrane complex and any remaining tags of membrane from the overlying stroma.

these trial runs, one should confirm that the plunger is positioned *in the middle of its travel* and that it moves freely. If the action of the injector feels sluggish, check for leaks, air bubbles, and a large gap between the proximal orifice of the Jones tube and the syringe.

Very short, staccato pulses on the plunger should translate into direct movement of the tissue out of a well-constructed injector. Long, slow depressions on the plunger will be much less effective at propelling the tissue and will raise the risk of overpressurizing the anterior chamber by overfilling it. By committing to memory what these inputs feel like, the surgeon knows when the upper limits of normal have been exceeded and too much volume is being injected into the eye. This awareness is paramount to preventing the dreaded complication of tissue ejection.

7.10 Loading the Straiko Injector

Before loading the injector, the space monkeys are first discarded from the petri dish, which will serve as a rescue pool for the DMEK graft should any unforeseen complications occur.

We prefer to load the injector directly from the corneoscleral rim so as to minimize touching and damaging the donor tissue. However, our DMEK graft is like a "shark" in "ink water"—the endothelium is on the *outside* surface of the scroll and ready to "bite" the surgeon under the dark cover of trypan blue stain if the trypan blue fluid is drained too quickly. To drain the trypan blue safely, it is first diluted with a few drops of BSS to better visualize the scroll. Premoistened Merocel sponges are then used to slowly wick fluid out of the corneoscleral rim by dabbing the peripheral meniscus so that fluid flows through the lumen of the scroll. This process is repeated until the tissue is easily seen as a dark blue scroll floating in nearly clear BSS in the corneoscleral rim (▶ Fig. 7.14).

The tip of the injector is placed bevel up into the corneoscleral rim and positioned so that the tip of the bevel is beneath one end of the DMEK scroll. The graft is then gently aspirated into the modified Jones tube until it is in the tube's distal flared midsection. *Again, very short, staccato pulls on the plunger are best; long, slow withdrawals on the plunger are much less effective and will tend to drain the corneoscleral rim of BSS rather than aspirate the tissue* (▶ Fig. 7.15).

7.11 Determining DMEK Scroll Orientation in the Injector: The Veldman Venn

We use the Veldman Venn to maximize our chances of injecting the tissue right side up. Prior to injecting the tissue, the very distal tip of the scroll is inspected in the modified Jones tube under the operating microscope while rolling the syringe between one's fingers. The "V" is defined by the overlapping edges of the scroll. This can be illustrated to oneself in a scale model by cutting a large circle out of tightly wound wrapping paper. When the V moves in the same direction as the rotation, the surgeon is looking at the graft right side up. When the V moves in the opposite direction, the graft is upside-down. Where the bevel is pointed when the scroll is right side up is mentally noted (e.g., bevel left), so that after the modified Jones tube is inserted bevel down, it can be rotated to the appropriate direction (e.g., left) prior to injecting the tissue. This method is not foolproof because the scroll can roll out of position at any point during the injection and withdrawal of the injector, but in our experience it delivers the tissue in the right side up orientation fairly consistently (▶ Fig. 7.16).

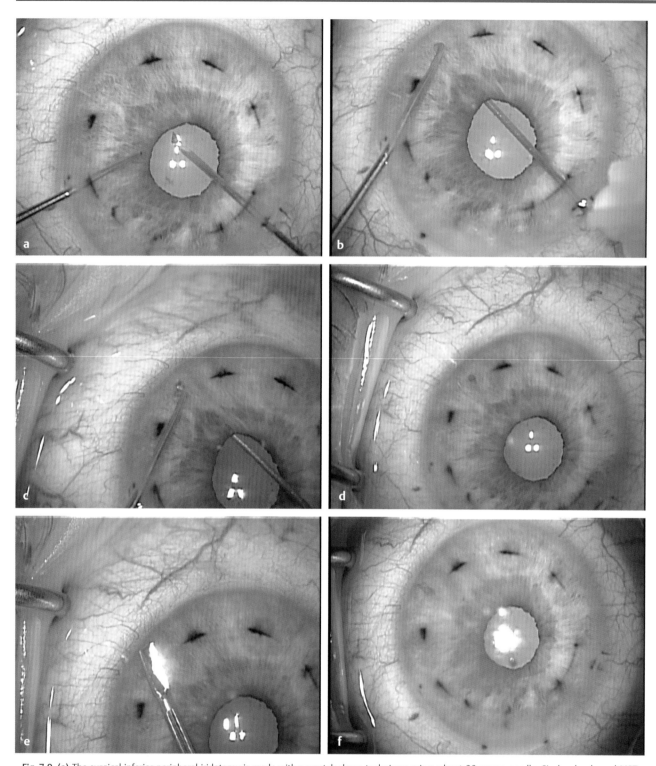

Fig. 7.9 **(a)** The surgical inferior peripheral iridotomy is made with a scratch-down technique using a bent 30-gauge needle, Sinskey hook, and MST IOL Cutters (MicroSurgical Technology). **(b)** The bent needle tip is placed through the superior paracentesis site, passed through the pupil, walked along the posterior iris inferiorly, and then pressed upward against the far peripheral iris pigment epithelium. At the same time, a straight Sinskey hook is placed through the inferior paracentesis or the main incision and onto the iris stroma. **(c)** The Sinskey hook is then used to scrape down on the location of the needle tip that is tenting up the iris tissue in the inferior periphery. **(d)** Once the tip of the needle perforates the iris from behind, this creates a hole where the tip of the Sinskey hook can then be placed. Using the needle and the Sinskey hook, the small iridotomy can be stretched to open it further. **(e)** Intraocular MST Scissors (IOL Cutters, MicroSurgical Technology) are then used to excise a full-thickness wedge of iris from the inferior periphery to ensure that the peripheral iridotomy remains patent. **(f)** Completed surgical inferior peripheral iridotomy.

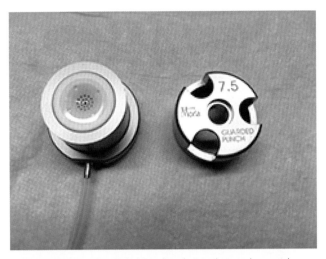

Fig. 7.10 The Moria Guarded Punch is designed to render partial-thickness trephinations of Descemet membrane without making a full-thickness cut through the stroma.

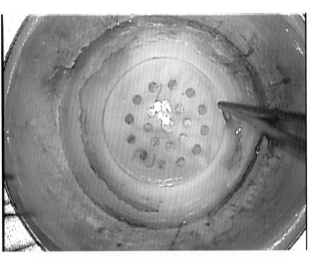

Fig. 7.11 When removing excess Descemet membrane, radial tears in the graft are prevented by reflecting the tissue onto itself, like the flap of a capsulorhexis.

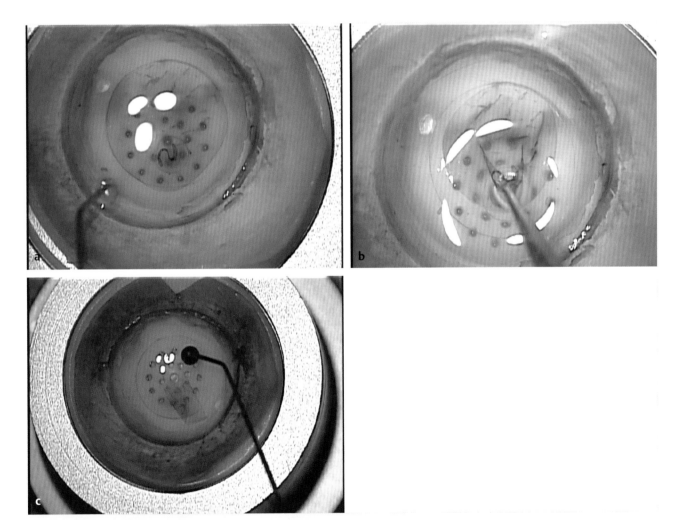

Fig. 7.12 (a) The incarcerated edge of the graft is freed from the stroma with jets of balanced salt solution. (b) The graft is lifted from the corneoscleral rim with tying forceps. This is the only time that the tissue is ever directly touched during the procedure. (c) The graft is stained with trypan blue for 3 to 4 minutes.

7.12 Injecting the DMEK Graft into the Anterior Chamber

7.12.1 Final Preparation of the Recipient

A small pupil reduces the risk of trauma to the endothelium when the DMEK graft is injected and opened. Miochol, which is short acting and therefore less apt to cause posterior synechiae, is injected into the anterior chamber to constrict the pupil to at least 3 mm, preferably 1 to 2 mm. If needed, the iris stroma can be gently stroked with a cannula to coax the sphincter into

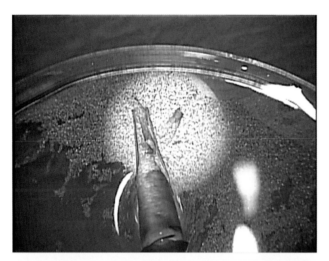

Fig. 7.13 Testing the Straiko injector in a glass petri dish with "space monkeys" consisting of discarded Descemet membrane from the peripheral corneoscleral rim.

constricting further. Once the pupil is sufficiently small, the anterior chamber is rinsed free of Miochol and any remaining debris with BSS. If fibrin strands are suspected or small bubbles are extensive, an irrigation/aspiration tip can be used to evacuate the anterior chamber before injection of the tissue.

In addition to the pupil being as small as possible, the recipient eye should be titrated with BSS to a normotensive pressure and a normal anterior chamber depth. For the novice DMEK surgeon, the starting point of the anterior chamber is important to preventing chamber collapse when inserting the injector. A chamber that is too shallow prior to inserting the injector can collapse if the surgeon is too tentative with the insertion of the injector tip. Chamber collapse, while beneficial to unscrolling the tissue, can be a major hindrance to injecting the DMEK scroll if it causes the iris and the IOL to obstruct the injector's tip. The more controllable scenario for a novice DMEK surgeon is to have a well-formed chamber that is more forgiving of a slower insertion. *The key, however, is to decompress the chamber if needed before injecting the tissue to prevent overpressurization.*

Final Checklist before Injecting DMEK Tissue into the Anterior Chamber

1. Descemetorhexis with no loose tags of Descemet membrane or stroma
2. Patent inferior peripheral iridotomy
3. Main incision widened to accommodate the Straiko injector and form a watertight seal
4. Evacuation of all viscoelastic from the anterior chamber *and* the injector
5. Pupil smaller than 3 mm, constricted with Miochol *not* Miostat

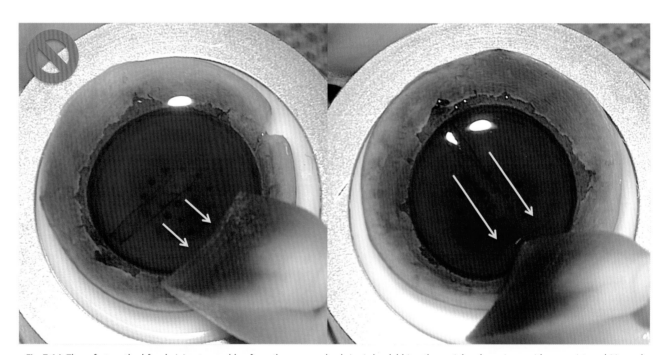

Fig. 7.14 The safest method for draining trypan blue from the corneoscleral rim is by dabbing the peripheral meniscus with premoistened Merocel sponges so that fluid flows through the lumen of the scroll. This prevents the scroll from rolling onto the sponge.

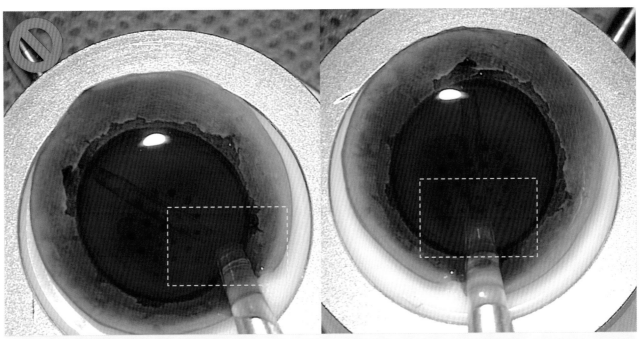

Fig. 7.15 The most effective method for aspirating the Descemet membrane endothelial keratoplasty (DMEK) scroll with the Straiko injector is placing it bevel up into the corneoscleral rim so that the tip of the bevel is beneath one end of the DMEK scroll.

6. Evacuation of any pigment debris, fibrin debris, and small bubbles from the anterior chamber immediately prior to injecting the tissue
7. Normotensive and normal anterior chamber depth immediately prior to insertion of the injector to prevent occlusion of the injector from chamber collapse

7.12.2 Tissue Injection

The tip of the modified Jones tube is *briskly* inserted into the main incision bevel down with the aid of forceps for countertraction until it is snugly seated against the walls of the wound. *At no point during tissue injection should this watertight seal ever be broken.* The tube is then rotated as needed to orient the tissue right side up. After visually confirming that the anterior chamber is normal to slightly shallow in depth, the tissue is moved into the anterior chamber with several short staccato bursts of BSS, all the while observing the depth of the anterior chamber. Regardless of the tissue's position, when the chamber becomes too deep (and the pressure in the eye is therefore high), a cannula is used to decompress the chamber through one of the paracentesis sites. *Decompression is repeated as many times as needed during the process of tissue injection. The surgeon should* never *proceed unless the chamber is normal or slightly shallow in depth and the eye pressure is normal to soft.*

Once the tissue is in the chamber, it is sometimes helpful to give a few additional short bursts of fluid while pivoting the

injector ever so slightly in the main incision (without breaking the watertight seal) to spin the scroll like a propeller so that it is oriented perpendicularly to the injector tip. Alternatively, the tissue can be tapped into this position with a cannula. Orienting the tissue in this manner is not mandatory, but it can increase the margin of safety when withdrawing the injector by making it more difficult for the tissue to reenter the injector tip or exit the main incision (▶ Fig. 7.17).

7.12.3 Injector Withdrawal

Prior to removing the injector tip, the anterior chamber is evacuated of fluid via one of the paracentesis sites until it is nearly collapsed and the eye is very soft. Failure to sufficiently decompress the chamber to this extent will almost certainly end in partial or complete tissue ejection.

A cannula is used to depress the anterior corneal surface just distal to the tip of the injector so that the incision is sealed as the injector exits. *To aid in sealing the incision during withdrawal, the injector tip should be simultaneously pointed downward as it is pulled out of the eye to allow the anterior and posterior surfaces of the incision to progressively close.* Even if the chamber is collapsed, gaping of the main incision with an uncontrolled withdrawal of the injector can also lead to tissue ejection (▶ Fig. 7.18).

Once the tip is removed, immediately place one interrupted 10–0 nylon suture in the wound to close it. Suture tension should not be too tight or it will create a horizontal crease in the cornea that can hinder unscrolling the graft by making the chamber depth uneven. Now the "DMEK dance" begins!

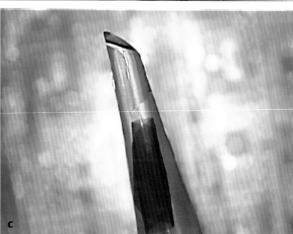

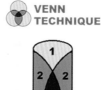

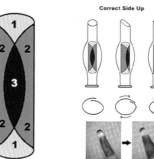

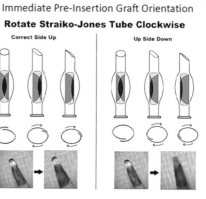

Fig. 7.16 (a) The "V" is defined by the overlapping edges of the scroll. (b) The Veldman Venn technique for determining graft orientation: When the V moves in the same direction as the rotation, the surgeon is looking at the graft right side up. When the V moves in the opposite direction, the graft is upside-down. (c) Where the bevel is pointed when the scroll is right side up is mentally noted (e.g., bevel right), so that after the modified Jones tube is inserted bevel down, it can be rotated to the appropriate direction (e.g., right) prior to injecting the tissue. Schematic diagram courtesy of Peter Veldman, Massachusetts Eye and Ear Infirmary, Boston, MA.

7.13 The DMEK Dance—Unscrolling and Centering the DMEK Graft

7.13.1 Graft Orientation

Introduction of the S-stamp has completely eliminated the incidence of upside-down DMEK grafts in our practice. It has also changed our approach to unscrolling the tissue, which no longer hinges on determining the graft's orientation at every step of the DMEK dance. Whereas we once began the dance with a careful inspection of the leaflets to determine whether they were scrolling toward or away from us, we now employ the Veldman Venn and begin opening the scroll as soon as it is safely in the anterior chamber.

When using both the Venn and the S-stamp, there is less of a need to inspect which direction the leaflets are scrolling because the surgeon can proceed under the reasonable assumption that the scroll is right side up, which is *usually but not always* true. In most cases, the graft is tapped open and the S-stamp reveals itself right side up. If, however, it becomes evident that the S-stamp is upside-down, the tissue is rolled over with short bursts of BSS from the paracentesis sites so that it is

right side up, and tapped open again until the S-stamp can be visualized. Once the S-stamp confirms the correct orientation, the surgeon can complete unscrolling and centering of the graft without further concern about it being upside down.

7.13.2 Unscrolling the Tissue

The key to unscrolling DMEK tissue is to make the anterior chamber shallow enough to prevent the scroll from reforming as it is opened. Once the chamber has been titrated to the right depth, staccato taps on the corneal epithelium generate fluid waves inside the scroll's leaflets that "push" them open. The posterior stroma then "catches" the unfurling edges of the leaflets to keep the tissue from scrolling up again. This tapping technique was well described by Dr. Yoeruek in his original articled published in the journal *Cornea* in 2013.[2] Alternatively, fluid currents that "pull" the leaflets open can be generated with a cannula inserted into a paracentesis site by "flicking" the incision open while quickly removing the cannula. The same can be done with the main incision, but this can be fraught with a very high risk of tissue ejection in inexperienced hands (▶ Fig. 7.19).

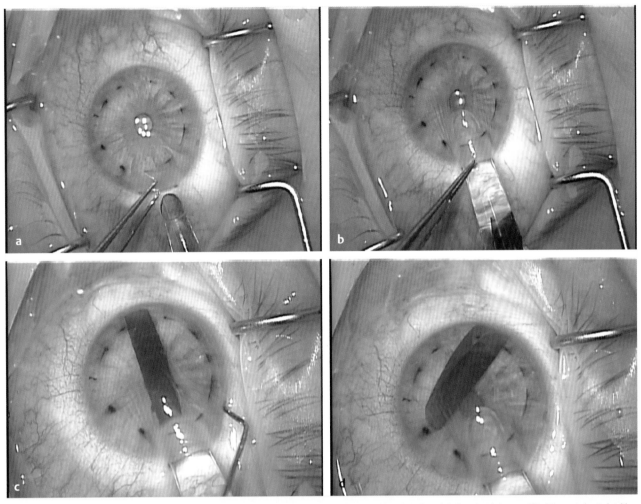

Fig. 7.17 Injecting the Descemet membrane endothelial keratoplasty scroll into the anterior chamber. **(a)** The tip of the modified Jones tube is *briskly* inserted into the main incision bevel down with the aid of forceps for countertraction until it is snugly seated against the walls of the wound. **(b)** *At no point during tissue injection should this watertight seal ever be broken.* **(c)** After visually confirming that the anterior chamber is normal to slightly shallow in depth, the tissue is moved into the anterior chamber with several short staccato bursts of balanced salt solution, all the while observing the depth of the anterior chamber. **(d)** Once the tissue is in the chamber, it is sometimes helpful to give a few additional short bursts of fluid while pivoting the injector ever so slightly in the main incision (without breaking the watertight seal) to spin the scroll like a propeller so that it is oriented perpendicularly to the injector tip.

7.13.3 Rolling the Tissue Over

In the event that the S-stamp is upside down, the tissue can be rolled over after it has been partially reconfigured back into a scroll. First, the chamber is deepened with BSS to provide sufficient space for the maneuver. A cannula is then inserted through one of the paracentesis sites and advanced until the tip of the cannula is in close proximity to the tissue. *Being closer to the tissue makes it possible to use only a small volume of BSS to make the graft roll.* Gentle jets of BSS are then directed along either the iris or the corneal plane to create swirling currents that cause the scroll to roll over. If the anterior chamber ever becomes overfilled, fluid must be evacuated before proceeding with further attempts.

7.13.4 Moving the Tissue

DMEK tissue can be moved with either fast or slow dance moves (▶ Table 7.3). When the graft is very nearly centered,

we either leave it alone or attempt to move it with slow, but preferably not fast, dance moves. Especially for the novice DMEK surgeon, fast moves are more apt to overshoot the mark or cause the graft to behave unpredictably in these sensitive situations. Patience can be a virtue in DMEK surgery.[3]

Fast moves can be performed by either "pushing" the tissue with rapid "golf stroke" taps to the limbus, or "pulling" the tissue by either "flicking" one of the incisions open or executing a "touch and release" maneuver by depressing the cornea and quickly lifting the cannula in the direction of desired movement. Pushing the tissue with golf strokes can sometimes result in a yo-yo movement of the scroll because it tends to rebound from the initial stroke. One method for reducing this phenomenon is to interconnect a series of back-to-back smaller golf strokes created by alternating both hands, like playing a snare drum. This shuffling technique, which we call the "cha cha," can sometimes be slower and more predictable.

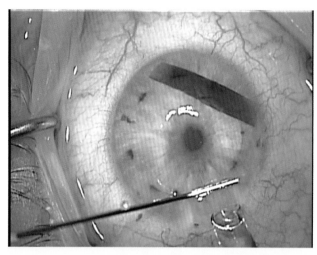

Fig. 7.18 Withdrawal of the injector: A cannula is used to depress the anterior corneal surface just distal to the tip of the injector so that the incision is sealed as the injector exits. To aid in sealing the incision during withdrawal, the injector tip should be simultaneously pointed downward as it is pulled out of the eye to allow the anterior and posterior surfaces of the incision to progressively close.

Table 7.3 Dance moves to center the tissue in Descemet membrane endothelial keratoplasty (DMEK) surgery

	Faster, bigger, less predictable movement	Slower, smaller, more predictable movement
"Push"	"Golf-stroke" the limbus	"Walk" the tissue
		"Shuffle" the tissue by executing back-to-back golf-strokes and slowly releasing the final stroke
"Pull"	"Flick" fluid out of the paracentesis sites	
	"Touch and release" the cornea	
When to Dance Fast and When to Dance Slow	Tissue is far from centered → Tissue is nearly centered	

The best way to slowly move the tissue is to "push" it into a relatively deeper portion of the anterior chamber by shallowing the chamber behind it. To execute this move, the cornea is depressed just behind the tissue, which causes it to nudge ever so slightly away from the cannula. Without moving this cannula, a second cannula is depressed between the first one and the trailing end of the tissue to nudge it forward. Repeating this cannula-over-cannula maneuver "walks" the tissue across the chamber. Once the tissue is in the desired position, the cannula closest to the tissue is *slowly* released to prevent the creation of a fluid wave that might cause the tissue to rebound backward. When moving a partially unscrolled graft with this method, if the leading edge of the tissue is unscrolled it will tend to rescroll as it is dragged along the posterior corneal stroma. Intermittently tapping the leading edge of the leaflet as the tissue is walked across the chamber can prevent this from happening.

7.14 Injecting 20% SF6 Gas

With the S-Stamp confirmed to be right side up, the graft fully unscrolled, and a very shallow (but not flat) anterior chamber, 20% SF6 gas is used to *slowly* elevate the tissue against the recipient stromal bed and reform the chamber. The Straiko cannula on a *1 mL* Luer-lock tuberculin syringe is inserted with the surgeon's "finger off the trigger" into the paracentesis site that is furthest from the graft's edge and advanced along the iris stroma until the tip is under the corneal apex. With the eye looking straight at the ceiling in primary position, a bubble of gas is *slowly* injected and expanded until it is almost the size of the graft, while simultaneously withdrawing the cannula from the eye. *Care should be taken not to inject the gas prematurely or rotate the eye out of primary position during this delicate part of the procedure because either action may cause the graft to decenter.* If there is insufficient space between the iris and the graft

after unscrolling it, a very small volume of BSS can be slowly injected into the paracentesis site to ever so slightly deepen the chamber and make advancing the cannula safer (▶ Fig. 7.20).

All of the graft's edges must be completely unfurled before the bubble is enlarged to its full extent. Any "flat edge" of the circular tissue must be investigated for the graft folding onto itself and corrected to reduce the risk of graft detachment. It is relatively easy to unfold a graft edge that is folded onto itself. With the bubble about the diameter of the tissue, the eye is rotated *toward* the folded edge, which in turn drives the bubble away from the problem and leaves the edge with only fluid beneath it. With the eye in this position, a few taps with a cannula on the surface of the cornea will unfold the problematic edge. When this is accomplished, the eye is then righted and the bubble is allowed to resume its central position. This technique was first described by Melles et al and termed bubble bumping. A final check of the graft should show clean round edges with no folds and good centration within the over-stripped stromal bed.

With the bubble now protecting the tissue from being inadvertently decentered or rescrolled, a very *slow* injection of BSS is directed *away* from the graft into the pupil to fill the anterior and posterior chambers until the eye is fully formed and no longer hypotonous, but still soft. *Although this will shrink the bubble, it will reduce the chances of injecting gas behind the iris during final bubble titration.* Using a 3 mL syringe, 20% SF6 gas is then injected until the bubble occupies 80 to 90% of the anterior chamber, or until the bubble's peripheral meniscus is within 0.5 to 1 mm of the limbus. Final bubble titration is performed by alternately injecting either gas or BSS from *the surface of the paracentesis* as needed. This allows the gas or BSS to travel into the anterior chamber while permitting the incision to self-seal immediately to prevent egress. Bigger bubbles that do not occlude the inferior peripheral iridotomy are best because they reduce the risk of rebubble.

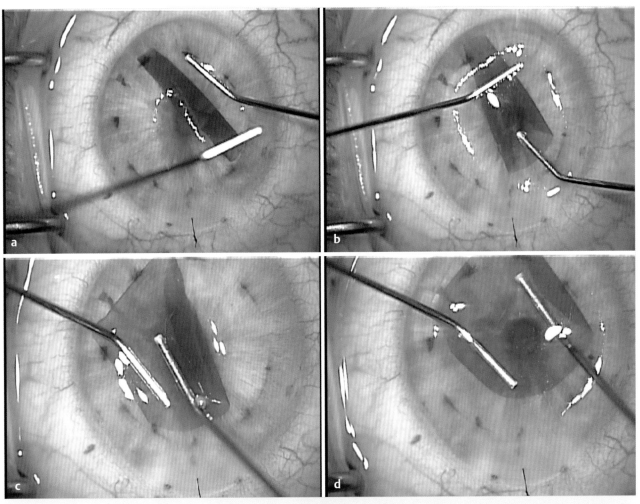

Fig. 7.19 Unscrolling the tissue in the anterior chamber. **(a)** One end of the scroll is tapped with a cannula oriented perpendicularly to the long axis of the scroll. **(b)** Once one end of the scroll begins to open, further taps with the cannula oriented parallel to the long axis of the scroll are used to open the leaflets further. **(c)** A Dirisamer technique is executed by using one cannula to shallow one side of the anterior chamber and another cannula to tap open the scrolled leaflet into the deeper side of the chamber. **(d)** The graft has been nearly completely unscrolled using the Dirisamer technique.

7.15 Closing the Case

At the conclusion of the case, the iris plateau should be flat, the chamber deep, and the intraocular pressure normal. If general anesthesia was used for the case, only a Fox shield is placed on the eye, and the patient is immediately started on antibiotic and steroid drops every 2 hours while awake. If retrobulbar or peribulbar anesthesia is used, the eye is dressed with a dissolving collagen shield that has been soaked in antibiotic and steroid, and the lid is closed and lightly patched until the first postoperative visit the next day. As an alternative to the collagen shield delivery system, the surgeon can inject antibiotics and steroids into the subconjunctival or sub-Tenon space.

A 3 mL syringe of 20% SF6 gas and a 3 mL syringe of BSS are set aside in a sterile baggy if the surgeon wishes to examine the patient at a slit lamp for signs of impending pupillary block about 1 hour after the conclusion of the case. The anterior chamber is examined for uniform depth, approximate tactile pressure is obtained with a cannula, and if needed, the bubble size is titrated with BSS and 20% SF6 gas.

7.16 Postoperative Care

7.16.1 Positioning

The patient is instructed to lie supine ("with your nose facing the ceiling") as much as possible the day of surgery, allowing 20 minutes for bathroom or meal breaks and 2 to 3 minutes every hour to ease any back pain. The patient can sleep in whatever position is comfortable the night of surgery, *but absolutely not prone* to prevent the bubble from moving posterior to the iris and causing iris bombe. For the first 2 days after surgery, the patient follows a simplified positioning routine: "Two-by-two for two days." What this means is the patient spends 2 consecutive hours lying supine followed by 2 consecutive hours sitting up or standing. Starting on postoperative day 3, there are no further positioning requirements (▶ Table 7.4).

7.16.2 Medications

Prednisolone 1% is prescribed every 2 hours for the first week and then tapered to 4 times daily until the 3-month visit, when it is replaced with fluorometholone 0.1%. At the 3-month visit, fluorometholone 0.1% is prescribed 3 times daily for 2 months, 2 times daily for 1 month, and then once daily. Ketorolac or an equivalent nonsteroidal anti-inflammatory drug is prescribed 3 times daily until the bottle is empty or 1 month, and ofloxacin is prescribed 4 times daily until the bottle is empty. Lubricating ointment is prescribed for use at bedtime for the first month. Glaucoma drops, if taken by the patient preoperatively, are resumed immediately after surgery (▶ Table 7.4).

7.16.3 Postoperative Visits

The patient is seen on postoperative day 1, 6, and 14, and then seen at postoperative months 1, 3, 6, and 12. The single "safety suture" of the main wound is removed usually at the 1-week postoperative visit. Patients whose graft edges are progressively

detaching or who have persistent central corneal edema are seen more frequently. An anterior segment optical coherence tomography (OCT) scan that can image the entire diameter of the graft is invaluable in assessing the graft's overall function, edge position, and improvement or worsening of graft separation. For routine cases of DMEK, an anterior segment OCT scan is obtained preoperatively and postoperatively on day 1, week 1, month 1, and month 6. Specular microscopy is obtained at postoperative month 6 and then annually.

7.16.4 Rebubbling

Our practice is to rebubble grafts for any of three reasons: (1) > 30% area of separation of the graft, (2) progressive separation of the graft or diffuse corneal edema, and (3) patient request for faster clearing of the area of graft separation.

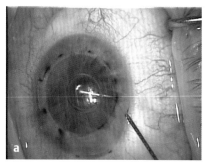
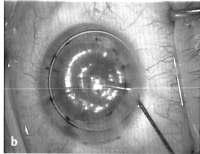
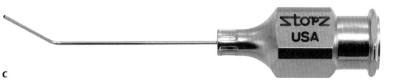

Fig. 7.20 (a) A bubble of 20% SF6 gas is *slowly* injected under the corneal apex using a 1 mL syringe and a standard 27-gauge cannula; alternatively, a Straiko cannula can be used for easier positioning of the cannula in the center of the chamber. (b) A bubble of gas is expanded until it is almost the size of the graft, while simultaneously withdrawing the cannula from the eye. (c) The Straiko DMEK Cannula (Storz Bausch & Lomb Surgical) features a longer segment after the cannula's "elbow" to make positioning the tip of the cannula in the center of the chamber easier.

Table 7.4 Postoperative care of Descemet membrane endothelial keratoplasty (DMEK) patients

	Positioning	Medications
Day of surgery	Supine as much as possible, with 2- to 3-minute breaks every hour and 20 minutes permitted for bathroom and meal breaks. Sleep in a position of comfort, supine if possible, but *absolutely no sleeping in the prone position.*	None—light eye patch and shield are in place
Days 1–2	2 hours supine followed by 2 hours sitting or standing. Sleep in a position of comfort, supine if possible, but *absolutely no sleeping in the prone position.*	• Prednisolone acetate 1% every 2 hours • Fourth-generation quinolone 4 times per day • NSAID of choice according to standard dosing
Days 3–7	• None • If the graft is rebubbled, it is usually by weeks 2–3. Repeat the positioning schedule from the day of surgery and days 1–2 after a rebubble.	
Weeks 2–4	None	• Prednisolone acetate 1% 4 times per day • Fourth-generation quinolone 4 times per day • NSAID of choice according to standard dosing
Months 2–3	None	• Prednisolone acetate 1% 4 times per day
Months 4–5	None	• Fluorometholone 0.1% 3 times per day
Month 5	None	• Fluorometholone 0.1% 2 times per day
Months 6–12	None	• Fluorometholone 0.1% 1 time per day

Abbreviation: NSAID, nonsteroidal anti-inflammatory drug.

Criteria for Rebubbling a DMEK Graft

1. Greater than 30% area of separation of the graft
2. Progressive separation of the graft or diffuse corneal edema
3. Patient request for faster clearing of the area of graft separation

Rebubbling is performed in the clinic at the slit lamp in the vast majority of cases. A disposable 27-gauge cannula is attached to standard 43-inch intravenous (IV) extension tubing, which is then coupled to a 5 mL syringe. After breaking through the epithelium of the inferior paracentesis site with jeweler's forceps at the slit lamp, the tip of the blunt cannula is inserted and advanced to the pupil, the shaft of the cannula is depressed against the posterior edge of the wound to release fluid from the anterior chamber for a count of three, and the plunger is depressed by the other hand to fill the anterior chamber with a

bubble of air. Since the syringe is attached to the cannula via 43 inches of IV tubing, it can be held in the hand that is simultaneously manipulating the slit lamp's joystick to maintain focus. This technique was well described by our team in 2015 and published in the journal *Cornea* in 2016 (▶ Fig. 7.21).[4]

7.17 Conclusion

The following are the most important components of our standardized technique[1]:

- The Straiko injector[5,6]
- Prestripped and S-stamped tissue with post-processing tissue validation[5,6,7]
- Overstripping the recipient descemetorhexis[8]
- Unscrolling the graft by shallowing the anterior chamber and tapping on the corneal epithelium[2,5,6]
- Supporting the graft with a 20% SF6 gas bubble tamponade[9]

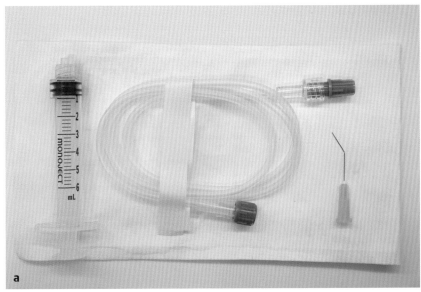

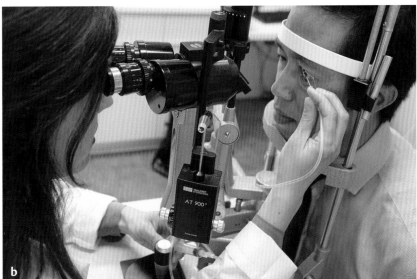

Fig. 7.21 (a) The materials needed for rebubbling a Descemet membrane endothelial keratoplasty (DMEK) graft at the slit lamp are a 27-gauge cannula, 5 mL syringe, and standard 43-inch intravenous extension tubing. **(b)** Method for rebubbling a DMEK graft at the slit lamp.

Summary of the Devers Standardized DMEK Technique

1. Straiko injector
2. Prestripped and S-stamped tissue with post-processing tissue validation
3. Overstripping the recipient descemetorhexis
4. Unscrolling the graft by shallowing the anterior chamber and tapping on the corneal epithelium
5. Supporting the graft with a 20% SF6 gas bubble tamponade

We have achieved equivalent or better outcomes using our standardized DMEK technique compared to our standardized DSAEK technique. In comparison to the first 100 DSAEK cases performed at our center, the first 100 DMEK cases achieved superior visual acuity at 6 months by nearly one line on an Early Treatment Diabetic Retinopathy Study (ETDRS) chart (DSAEK vs. DMEK: 0.20 ± 0.13 vs. 0.11 ± 0.13, $P < 0.001$) with equivalent endothelial cell loss ($25.9 \pm 14\%$ vs. $27.9 \pm 16\%$, $P = 0.38$) and frequency of rebubble (2% vs. 6%, $P = 0.28$). There were no iatrogenic primary graft failures in the DSAEK group and four in the DMEK group ($P = 0.12$), but these cases were before incorporating the S-stamp into our standardized technique. Since the introduction of the S-stamp, we have had no further cases of iatrogenic primary graft failure from upside-down grafts.

Others[2,8,9,10,11,12,13,14] have achieved similar success using techniques that differ to varying degrees from ours, and to be sure, new techniques are always emerging. Whether or not the novice surgeon adopts our technique, the best approach to confronting DMEK's steep learning curve is studying the *nuances* that can be lost in the high points of any technique's bulleted summary. This chapter provides a good foundation for learning DMEK's important details, but nothing can replace hands-on training in the DMEK in vitro wet lab and assisting an experienced DMEK surgeon at the operating microscope.

References

[1] Terry MA. Endothelial keratoplasty: why aren't we all doing Descemet membrane endothelial keratoplasty? Cornea. 2012; 31(5):469–471

[2] Yoeruek E, Bayyoud T, Hofmann J, Bartz-Schmidt KU. Novel maneuver facilitating Descemet membrane unfolding in the anterior chamber. Cornea. 2013; 32(3):370–373

[3] Sáles CS, Terry MA, Veldman PB, Mayko ZM, Straiko MD. The relationship between tissue unscrolling time and endothelial cell loss. Cornea. 2016; 35(4):471–476

[4] Sáles CS, Straiko MD, Terry MA. Novel technique for rebubbling DMEK grafts at the slit lamp using intravenous extension tubing. Cornea. 2016; 35(4):582–585

[5] Terry MA, Straiko MD, Veldman PB, et al. Standardized DMEK Technique: Reducing Complications Using Prestripped Tissue, Novel Glass Injector, and Sulfur Hexafluoride (SF6) Gas. Cornea. 2015; 34(8):845–852

[6] Hamzaoglu EC, Straiko MD, Mayko ZM, Sáles CS, Terry MA. The first 100 eyes of standardized Descemet stripping automated endothelial keratoplasty versus standardized Descemet membrane endothelial keratoplasty. Ophthalmology. 2015; 122(11):2193–2199

[7] Veldman PB, Dye PK, Holiman JD, et al. The S-stamp in Descemet Membrane Endothelial Keratoplasty Safely Eliminates Upside-down Graft Implantation. Ophthalmology. 2016; 123(1):161–164

[8] Kruse FE, Laaser K, Cursiefen C, et al. A stepwise approach to donor preparation and insertion increases safety and outcome of Descemet membrane endothelial keratoplasty. Cornea. 2011; 30(5):580–587

[9] Güell JL, Morral M, Gris O, Elies D, Manero F. Comparison of Sulfur Hexafluoride 20% versus Air Tamponade in Descemet Membrane Endothelial Keratoplasty. Ophthalmology. 2015; 122(9):1757–1764

[10] Dapena I, Moutsouris K, Droutsas K, Ham L, van Dijk K, Melles GR. Standardized "no-touch" technique for descemet membrane endothelial keratoplasty. Arch Ophthalmol. 2011; 129(1):88–94

[11] Droutsas K, Giallouros E, Melles GR, Chatzistefanou K, Sekundo W. Descemet membrane endothelial keratoplasty: learning curve of a single surgeon. Cornea. 2013; 32(8):1075–1079

[12] Price MO, Giebel AW, Fairchild KM, Price FW, Jr. Descemet's membrane endothelial keratoplasty: prospective multicenter study of visual and refractive outcomes and endothelial survival. Ophthalmology. 2009; 116(12):2361–2368

[13] Busin M, Leon P, Scorcia V, Ponzin D. Contact Lens-Assisted Pull-Through Technique for Delivery of Tri-Folded (Endothelium in) DMEK Grafts Minimizes Surgical Time and Cell Loss. Ophthalmology. 2016; 123(3):476–483

[14] Gorovoy MS. DMEK Complications. Cornea. 2014; 33(1):101–104

8 Techniques to Unroll the DMEK Graft in Difficult Situations

Brandon Daniel Ayres

8.1 Introduction

Posterior lamellar keratoplasty is full of complexity from graft preparation, donor insertion, and donor graft unfolding. Unfolding of the donor graft can be particularly difficult in the case of Descemet membrane endothelial keratoplasty (DMEK) for several reasons. The first challenge is visualization of the DMEK graft tissue and orientation in the anterior chamber, second is the very fragile nature of the DMEK graft. Finally, unrolling a graft that would prefer to scroll up on itself, instead of taking a planar configuration as in DSEK surgery, is difficult as well. These are just a few of the factors that make DMEK surgically challenging in a routine case and even more so in a complex case.

8.2 Visualization of DMEK Graft

As a general surgical principle, any improper technique early in a case will amplify difficulty in a later step of the surgery. This rule certainly holds true with DMEK surgery. Making sure the endothelial graft can be visualized in the anterior chamber is essential. Staining the donor graft in a mixture of balanced salt solution (BSS) and trypan blue is critical to visualizing the graft in the anterior chamber. Over time the blue color will dilute out of the graft so timely unfolding is beneficial. Once the graft has lost all color it is exceedingly difficult to see it in the anterior chamber, and unfolding becomes much more difficult, though not impossible. Staining the graft in a 50/50 mixture of trypan blue and BSS for 5 minutes or so should impart enough color to the graft to allow adequate visualization. Good visualization will help with unfolding of the graft in any situation.

Similar to Descemet stripping endothelial keratoplasty (DSEK), the endothelial graft in DMEK must open and be in the correct orientation, with endothelial cells posterior and membrane anterior. Visualizing the orientation of the DMEK graft can be very difficult under the operating microscope but is essential in graft survival and patient satisfaction. Several techniques can be employed to ensure proper graft orientation.

8.2.1 Stromal Marking

Marking of the stroma has been employed in DSEK surgery for many years. Many eyebanks and surgeons are now able to put a stromal orientation mark on the membrane side of DMEK tissue. The mark is typically stamped with gentian violet ink, minimizing loss of the endothelial cells under the mark. Stromal marking can be associated with very minimal cell loss, but greatly facilitates proper graft orientation and prevents graft failure. No long-term cell loss is caused by the orientation stamp (▶ Fig. 8.1).[1] Most surgeons agree that the stromal mark helps in graft orientation and decreases overall surgical time with no need for special instrumentation or technique needed to visualize the graft. The small amount of cell loss associated with the stromal mark is far less damaging than unfolding and attaching a graft upside down.

8.2.2 Indirect Lighting

The visualization of the DMEK graft is difficult even with adequate trypan blue staining under the operating microscope. The use of a light pipe or endoilluminator has been described to assist with visualization of the graft.[2] The use of indirect lighting enhances the surgeon's understanding of graft position and dynamics. This can be especially beneficial when the view into the anterior chamber is reduced due to corneal edema or scarring. In a similar fashion some surgeons have advocated the use of a handheld slit lamp to help with visualization of the graft.[3] In these cases the slit lamp is used to help confirm graft orientation in the anterior chamber.

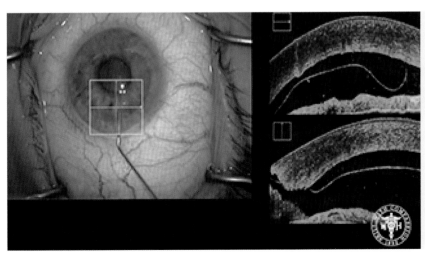

Fig. 8.1 Photo of intraoperative optical coherence tomography being used to confirm correct orientation of the Descemet membrane endothelial keratoplasty graft. Note how the edges of the graft scroll toward the posterior stroma of the host cornea, confirming orientation. In this case a stromal S-stamp is also visible on the graft, further confirming correct graft orientation.

8.2.3 Intraoperative Optical Coherence Tomography

Anterior segment optical coherence tomography (OCT) is commonly used to visualize the DMEK graft postoperatively to ensure proper attachment and orientation. Over the past few years intraoperative OCT has become available to assist with anterior segment surgery.[4] The add-on to the surgical microscope allows the OCT image to be overlayed in the surgeon's view. This allows visualization of the DMEK tissue in real time without the use of any additional instrumentation or stains. Using the OCT helps the surgeon to confirm proper graft orientation and better understand the dynamics of the endothelial graft. As the use of intraoperative OCT increases we will see if it helps novice surgeons transition to DMEK surgery and assists experienced surgeons in more difficult cases.

8.2.4 Direct Visualization

Many surgeons do not have access to intraoperative OCT, light pipes, or portable slit lamps for use in the operating room. As long as you are able to stain the cornea with trypan blue, graft orientation can be determined using what has been called the Moutsouris sign. Using this technique, a cannula is placed over the double scroll of the graft. The cannula is then slid to the right or left. If the cannula turns blue once over the scrolled portion of the graft you can be sure the DMEK tissue is in the correct orientation. If the cannula does not turn blue the graft is upside down and needs to be rotated in the anterior chamber.

8.2.5 Rotation "Flipping" of Graft Tissue

Regardless of the technique used to place a DMEK tissue graft into the anterior chamber the situation will arise when the graft ends up in the incorrect orientation. This may be determined on OCT, by seeing the orientation mark upside down, or with the Moutsouris sign. Once you have confirmed that the graft is upside-down in the anterior chamber it must be flipped. Although it may seem difficult at first, the technique to flip a graft is quite easy as long as the graft can be visualized. In this situation a deep anterior chamber is needed. By deepening the anterior chamber, the DMEK graft will scroll up on itself. After making sure the main incision is closed with a suture, aggressive irrigation through a paracentesis will cause fluid waves in the anterior chamber, allowing the DMEK graft to tumble on itself.

Once the graft tumbles 180 degrees the anterior chamber can be shallowed to hold the graft in place. With some luck the tissue will still be in a double scroll, which will facilitate unfolding. Using a variety of techniques, the graft can then be unfolded in the correct orientation (▸ Fig. 8.2). If the graft rolls up into a single scroll the jets of fluid will eventually allow a leaflet to unscroll. Once a small part of the Descemet graft begins to open, the remainder of the graft can be unscrolled using the Dirisamer technique (▸ Fig. 8.3). The anterior chamber over the open end of the DMEK graft is shallowed using a cannula; this holds the open portion against the iris and deepens the anterior chamber over the scroll. While one is holding the first cannula a second is used to "tap" on the cornea over the scroll to selectively open the remaining graft.

8.2.6 Unfolding DMEK Graft Tissue

Many techniques have been described to help unfold a scroll of DMEK tissue. For the most part the technique(s) used will depend on the ability to maintain a soft eye, a shallow anterior chamber, and how the graft presents itself in the anterior chamber. In many cases more than one technique will need to be employed to open and position the graft. As a general rule, tissue from older donors will open more easily as it tends to form a looser scroll, leading to shorter unfolding times.[5] The more challenging the case the more important it is to be selective as to donor age.

The easiest situation is the **lazy** graft (▸ Fig. 8.4). In this case the Descemet graft presents itself in the anterior chamber in a very loose scroll. The lazy graft is one of the easiest to open. In many cases by keeping the eye soft and the anterior chamber shallow just a few taps on the cornea directly over the DMEK graft will allow the graft to open. Once open, air of 20% sulfur hexaflouride gas (SF6) can be used to attach the graft to the overlying host stroma.

Most of the time the DMEK graft is not lazy and tends to scroll endothelium outward in the anterior chamber. The graft may take the configuration of a single scroll or a double scroll. These shapes are more challenging configurations to unfold, but as long as the eye remains soft and the anterior chamber can remain shallow unfolding is relatively straightforward. The first step is to make sure the graft is in the correct orientation (endothelium down). Knowing the orientation may not be possible until the graft is partially unfolded to allow visualization of an orientation mark or evaluate for the Moutsouris sign. Before unfolding make sure to close the primary incision to ensure the graft will not be expelled from the anterior chamber. Always shallow the chamber through a peripheral paracentesis (though I have seen grafts even go through small peripheral incisions). A no-touch technique may be employed to help with initial graft unfolding. In many instances this will allow one half of the graft to unfold, leaving the other scrolled up on itself. With this configuration the open portion of the graft is held in position by shallowing the anterior chamber with a cannula. Using a second cannula with a sweeping motion the scrolled portion of the graft is opened. Once open, the graft is centered in the anterior chamber and then gas or air is used to affix the graft to the overlying host stroma.

In most cases a no-touch and the Dirisamer technique are all that will be necessary to efficiently open the endothelial graft.[6] As comfort with DMEK grows, more challenging cases may be attempted. Performing DMEK in eyes with glaucoma tube shunts[7] or eyes that have had vitrectomy is possible but may be more challenging and have a higher complication rate.[8,9] As long as the anterior chamber can be shallowed, the technique is no different than that in standard eyes. In some situations (in the author's opinion this is especially true in postvitrectomy eyes) the anterior chamber cannot be shallowed or will not remain shallow. If the anterior chamber will not shallow, the graft will continue to curl on itself, making unfolding almost impossible. In these cases, an air bubble may be employed to assist with unfolding. The use of a bubble to assist with unfolding is named after Isabel Dapena. In the Dapena maneuver an air bubble is injected between the DMEK graft and the overlying host corneal stroma. Manipulation of the air bubble on the

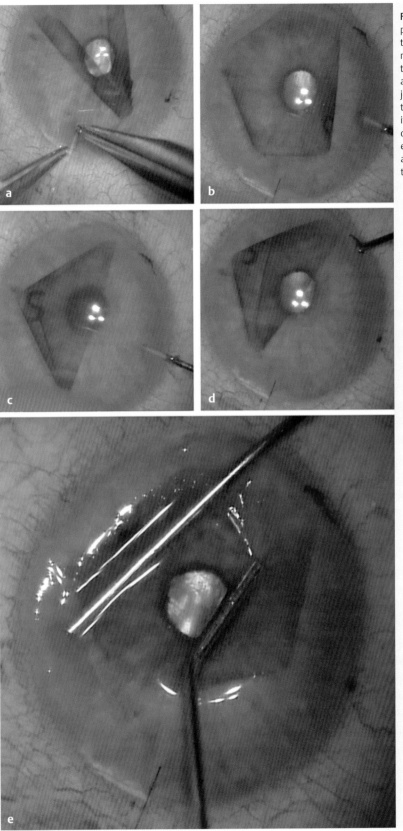

Fig. 8.2 (a) Descemet membrane endothelial keratoplasty (DMEK) graft unfolding upside-down (notice the S-stamp on left side of image). Place suture to make sure the wound cannot open when deepening the anterior chamber. **(b)** The chamber is deep, allowing the DMEK graft to scroll on itself. **(c)** Using jets of balanced salt solution the DMEK tissue is tumbled in the anterior chamber until it everts on itself. **(d)** The DMEK graft is now in the correct orientation in a shallow chamber through paracentesis to hold the graft in position. **(e)** The DMEK now in a good position, being unfolded using the Dirisamer technique.

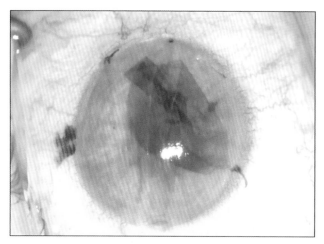

Fig. 8.3 With the Dirisamer technique one cannula shallows the anterior chamber over the open portion of the DMEK graft and a second cannula is used to tap and sweep the cornea opening the second portion of the graft.

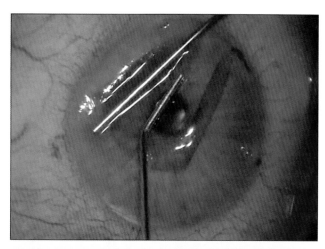

Fig. 8.4 Clinical photo of a "lazy" Descemet membrane endothelial keratoplasty graft. Notice how the graft is not in a tight scroll in the anterior chamber, making it easier to unfold the tissue.

external cornea allows the small bubble to act as a tool to unfold the graft. Once the graft is unfolded the air bubble is removed and air is placed under the graft for final attachment. Though the technique sounds quite simple, it can be very challenging to know exactly where you are in the anterior chamber and what is the position of the cannula over the graft. Care must be taken to make sure that the air is injected in the correct place or it will make unfolding the graft even more difficult.

DMEK can be a challenging surgical procedure, even when operating conditions and the clinical scenario are optimized. In many cases with tubes, trabeculectomies, and postvitrectomized eyes DSEK may be a simpler choice for visual rehabilitation. If DMEK is to be attempted multiple techniques may need to be employed to help with unfolding the graft. With patience and surgical skill cases with anterior segment complications beyond corneal edema can safely and effectively be treated with the DMEK procedure.

References

[1] Veldman PB, Dye PK, Holiman JD, et al. The S-stamp in Descemet Membrane Endothelial Keratoplasty Safely Eliminates Upside-down Graft Implantation. Ophthalmology. 2016; 123(1):161–164

[2] Jacob S, Agarwal A, Agarwal A, Narasimhan S, Kumar DA, Sivagnanam S. Endoilluminator-assisted transcorneal illumination for Descemet membrane endothelial keratoplasty: enhanced intraoperative visualization of the graft in corneal decompensation secondary to pseudophakic bullous keratopathy. J Cataract Refract Surg. 2014; 40(8):1332–1336

[3] Burkhart ZN, Feng MT, Price MO, Price FW. Handheld slit beam techniques to facilitate DMEK and DALK. Cornea. 2013; 32(5):722–724

[4] Cost B, Goshe JM, Srivastava S, Ehlers JP. Intraoperative optical coherence tomography-assisted descemet membrane endothelial keratoplasty in the DISCOVER study. Am J Ophthalmol. 2015; 160(3):430–437

[5] Heinzelmann S, Hüther S, Böhringer D, Eberwein P, Reinhard T, Maier P. Influence of donor characteristics on descemet membrane endothelial keratoplasty. Cornea. 2014; 33(6):644–648

[6] Liarakos VS, Dapena I, Ham L, van Dijk K, Melles GR. Intraocular graft unfolding techniques in descemet membrane endothelial keratoplasty. JAMA Ophthalmol. 2013; 131(1):29–35

[7] Bersudsky V, Treviño A, Rumelt S. Management of endothelial decompensation because of glaucoma shunt tube touch by Descemet membrane endothelial keratoplasty and tube revision. Cornea. 2011; 30(6):709–711

[8] Yoeruek E, Rubino G, Bayyoud T, Bartz-Schmidt KU. Descemet membrane endothelial keratoplasty in vitrectomized eyes: clinical results. Cornea. 2015; 34(1):1–5

[9] Weller JM, Tourtas T, Kruse FE. Feasibility and Outcome of Descemet Membrane Endothelial Keratoplasty in Complex Anterior Segment and Vitreous Disease. Cornea. 2015; 34(11):1351–1357

9 Pre-Descemet Endothelial Keratoplasty

Priya Narang and Amar Agarwal

9.1 Introduction

Endothelial keratoplasty (EK) consists of Descemet membrane endothelial keratoplasty (DMEK) and Descemet stripping endothelial keratoplasty (DSEK) as the major variants, whereas many surgeons worldwide have also employed their automated version of Descemet membrane automated endothelial keratoplasty (DMAEK) and Descemet stripping automated endothelial keratoplasty (DSAEK). In terms of visual output, DMEK as an EK procedure has always been successful in spite of it being technically challenging as compared to other subtypes. Melles et al described DMEK that represents the perfect anatomical replacement of the diseased Descemet membrane (DM)–endothelium complex with a healthy donor DM–endothelium complex.[1,2]

Pre-Descemet endothelial keratoplasty (PDEK),[3] being a new variant in the field of EK, further extends the lexicon of EK, which mainly consists of the separation of the pre-Descemet layer (PDL) along with the DM–endothelium complex from the residual donor stroma by the formation of a type 1 bubble (bb).[4] The feasibility of the PDEK procedure with both adult and infant donor tissue[3,5] makes it highly acceptable in the era of donor tissue shortage.

9.2 Importance of Air Dissection and Types of Bubbles

Air dissection is a well-established entity that relegates the use of microforceps or a microkeratome for dissection of the corneal stroma. An air-filled syringe is used to inject air into the stroma with the endothelial side up and is advanced under direct observation at a required depth beneath the endothelium. The advantage with air dissection is that it is cost-effective because it is done manually by the surgeon. The major drawback is that it requires a certain amount of surgical skill on behalf of the surgeon because the needle that is employed to inject air must be introduced at the correct depth below the DM–endothelium complex.

9.2.1 Type 1 Bubble

This is the kind of bb that is essential to obtain for performing a PDEK procedure. This bb typically spreads from the center to the periphery and is dome shaped. The diameter of the bb usually varies from 7.5 to 8.5 mm; this bb never extends to the extreme periphery due to adhesions between the PDL and the residual stroma. Injection of air leads to separation of the PDL–DM–endothelium complex in toto from the residual stromal bed (▶ Fig. 9.1). This type 1 bb is created using a 30-gauge needle connected to a 5 mL syringe with the bevel up (▶ Fig. 9.2).

9.2.2 Type 2 Bubble

This type of bb is typically formed when the air enters the plane between the PDL and the DM–endothelium complex. A type 2 bb typically spreads from the periphery to the center and is around 10 to 11 mm in diameter. It extends up to the extreme periphery because there are no adhesions between the PDL and the DM (▶ Fig. 9.3). With the formation of this bb, it becomes essential to perform a DMEK instead of a PDEK procedure. Immense care should be taken when a type 2 bb is formed because it has a thin wall, and if it is subjected to excessive air push the bb can rupture leading to perforation of the graft and eventually transcending into donor tissue wastage.

9.2.3 Type 3—Mixed Bubble

When both type 1 and type 2 bbs are formed and they coexist, a mixed bubble is said to have been achieved. This is a type 3 big bb (▶ Fig. 9.4). These types of bbs pose a surgical challenge to the surgeon because they require delicate handling and manipulation to avoid bb rupture.

9.3 Surgical Technique

9.3.1 Donor Graft Preparation

Bubble Creation

The donor button with the corneoscleral rim is dissected from the whole cornea and is placed with the endothelial side up. For the process of bb creation, a 30-gauge needle is used that is attached to an air-filled 5 mL syringe. The needle is introduced with a bevel-up position from the periphery up to the midperipheral area at a considerable depth from the DM so as to create a plane of separation between the PDL and the residual stroma (▶ Fig. 9.5a). If one does not get a bb after repeated attempts (more than 10 at least) with air one can try with fluid using the McCarey Kaufman (MK) medium or Optisol (Chiron Ophthalmics) or balanced salt solution (BSS). If a bb still does not form then the surgeon can use visocoelastic. Air is injected and a dome-shaped type 1 bb is formed that is approximately 8 mm in diameter.

Graft Staining

The graft is stained with trypan blue that allows a considerable clear visualization of the graft. The bb is penetrated with a side-port blade at the extreme periphery (▶ Fig. 9.5b), and trypan blue is injected inside (▶ Fig. 9.5c). The bb is then cut all across the periphery with corneoscleral scissors (▶ Fig. 9.5d) and is placed in the storage media. The donor graft is loaded onto the injector when ready for insertion (▶ Fig. 9.6).

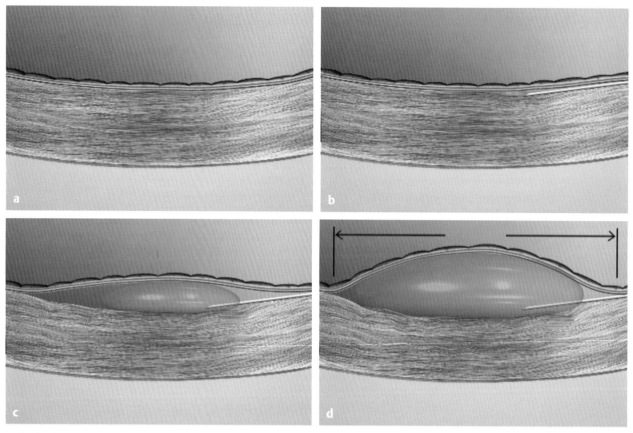

Fig. 9.1 Graphical display of the creation of a type 1 bubble (bb). **(a)** The image demonstrates all the layers of cornea with the graft placed endothelial side up. **(b)** An air-filled 30-gauge needle is introduced from the periphery beneath the pre-Descemet layer (PDL). The PDL–Descemet membrane (DM)–endothelium complex is seen lying above the bevel of the needle. **(c)** Further injection of air lifts the entire PDL–DM–endothelium complex that consists of a pre-Descemet endothelial keratoplasty graft above the residual stroma. **(d)** A fully formed type 1 bb is shown.

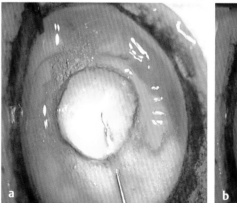

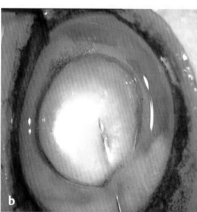

Fig. 9.2 Type 1 big bubble–donor graft preparation. **(a)** A small type 1 bubble is formed. **(b)** The type 1 bubble is enhanced with air.

9.3.2 Recipient Bed Preparation

The procedure is performed under local anesthesia with supplemental anesthesia administered as necessary.

In cases of bullous keratopathy, the initial step consists of scrapping and debridement of the epithelium. This facilitates an enhanced intraoperative view during the surgical procedure. An anterior chamber maintainer (ACM) or a trocar anterior chamber maintainer (TACM)[6] is introduced in to the eye that is connected to the air pump. This helps to maintain adequate anterior chamber depth at all times, and it also ensures the appropriate shift between air and fluid infusion as and when required (▶ Fig. 9.7). A 2.8 mm corneal tunnel is made and two side port incisions are framed. With the anterior chamber completely inflated with air, the DM is scored and stripped using a reverse Sinskey hook. Inferior iridectomy is performed with a vitrectomy probe introduced from the corneal incision. This maneuver ensures prevention of pupillary block at a later stage.

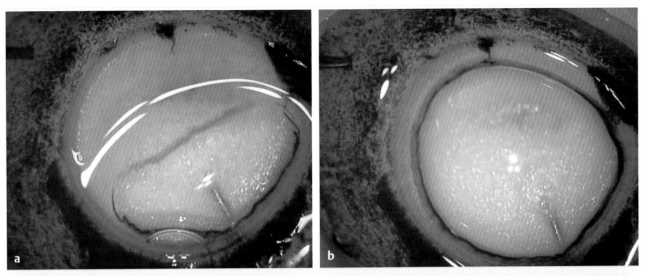

Fig. 9.3 Type 2 big bubble. **(a)** Type 2 bubble being formed after air injection. The bubble spreads from periphery to center. **(b)** Type 2 bubble fully formed.

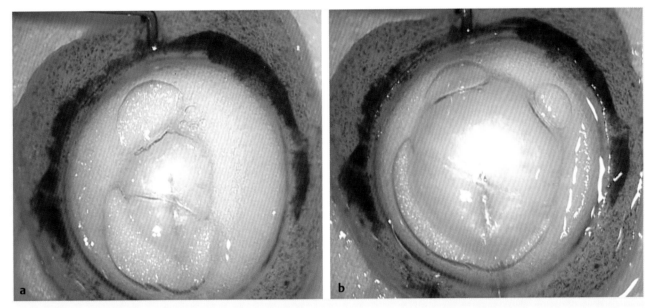

Fig. 9.4 Type 3 big bubble. Both type **(a)** 1 and type **(b)** 2 bubbles are formed.

9.3.3 Donor Graft Insertion

The graft is held gently with a nontoothed forceps and is placed into the cartridge of a foldable intraocular lens that is filled with BSS (▶ Fig. 9.7).[7] Air infusion is stopped and the graft is gently injected into the anterior chamber through a clear corneal incision, avoiding wound-assisted implantation. Graft orientation is verified and the graft is gently unfolded using air and fluidics. Corneal indentation and massaging are also performed to facilitate the graft unrolling. Once the graft has partly unrolled, a small air bb is injected beneath the graft, which helps it to adhere to the corneal surface. The peripheral edges of the graft can be unrolled by gently manipulating it with a reverse Sinskey hook. Once the graft has fully unrolled, air infusion is started, which facilitates total adherence of the graft to the recipient bed. Corneal sutures are taken and there is complete closure of all wounds to achieve a well-formed anterior chamber in the postoperative period (▶ Fig. 9.8 and ▶ Fig. 9.9).

9.3.4 Postoperative Care

In the immediate postoperative period, the patient is advised to lie in a supine position for approximately 3 hours and to continue doing so for most of the day. Slit lamp examination confirms the graft centration and location. On the second postoperative day, intraocular pressure is checked and the patency of the inferior iridectomy is confirmed. Topical antibiotics and steroids are prescribed, which are slowly tapered over a period of 4 months.

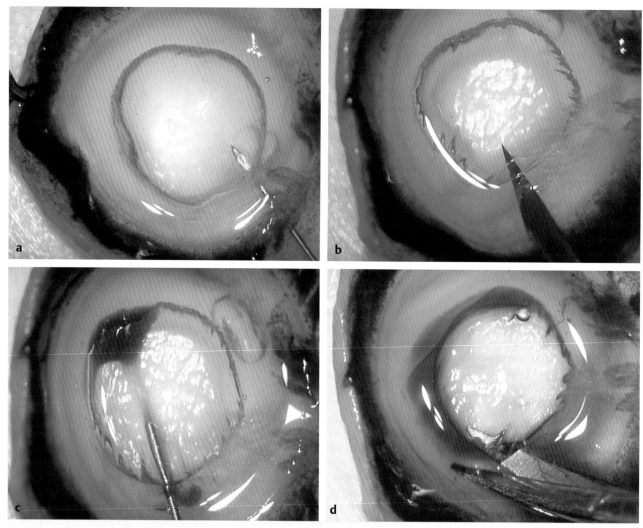

Fig. 9.5 Donor graft preparation. **(a)** An air-filled 30-gauge needle is introduced from the corneoscleral rim up to the midperiphery and air is injected to create a type 1 bubble (bb). **(b)** The bb is punctured at the extreme periphery with the help of a side port blade. **(c)** Trypan blue is injected to stain the bb. **(d)** The graft is cut along the peripheral edge of the bb with the corneoscleral scissor.

9.3.5 PDEK

EK as a technique has evolved from deep lamellar endothelial keratoplasty (DLEK) and transitioned to DSEK/DSAEK and further to DMEK. PDEK, being the latest entry in this list, is expected to have broad acceptance due to its similar characteristics of rapid visual recovery, predictable wound strength, and a significant greater optical predictability similar to a DMEK procedure. There is also less likelihood of donor tissue loss due to the DM tearing away as well as improved graft maneuverability due to extra strength and the splinting effect of the PDL on the DM–endothelium complex. Differences between DSEK, DMEK, and PDEK are shown in ▶ Table 9.1. Like DMEK, preparation of a PDEK graft does not require large investment in addition to all the other benefits of a DMEK procedure. PDEK involves the addition of the PDL in the donor graft, which increases the thickness of the graft to approximately 30 to 35 μm as measured with optical coherence tomography (OCT). The graft is comparatively thicker than that of the DMEK but is thinner as compared to DSEK/DSAEK or an ultrathin DSAEK (UT-DSAEK). Visual rehabilitation after PDEK is comparatively

faster as compared to other EK techniques, except DMEK, which involves pure DM transplantation.

Clinically, in our series we have observed that the incidences of graft dislocation and rebubbling rate are comparatively lower in PDEK as compared to DMEK, which can probably be attributed to the addition of the PDL to the donor graft, which enhances the graft sustainability. Validation of the PDEK procedure by other surgeons would enhance the acceptability of the technique before it is widely emulated and performed worldwide, taking into consideration the complications and feasibility of the technique. The risk of donor tissue loss can be minimized by the eye banks if they supply premade, ready-to-use donor graft tissue.

9.4 Infant Donor Cornea for PDEK

There is a substantial shortage of donor tissue for EK worldwide. The feasibility of using infant donor graft for PDEK has been highlighted in the past and could potentially increase the pool of suitable donor tissue for PDEK.[5]

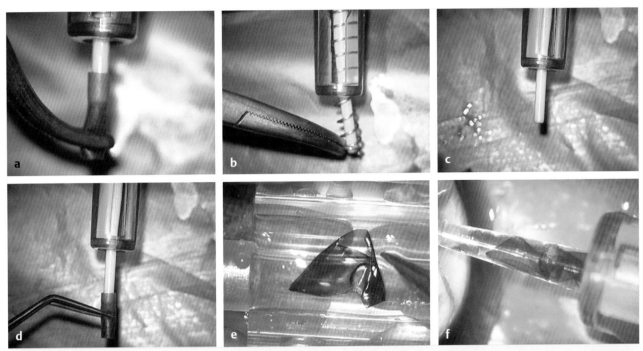

Fig. 9.6 Loading the graft. (a) The sponge tip from the injector is removed. (b) The spring of the injector is grasped and pulled out. (c) The injector tip with the spring removed is illustrated. (d) The sponge tip is refixed onto the injector. (e) The graft is placed on the cartridge. (f) The cartridge is loaded onto the injector and the graft is ready to be injected into the anterior chamber.

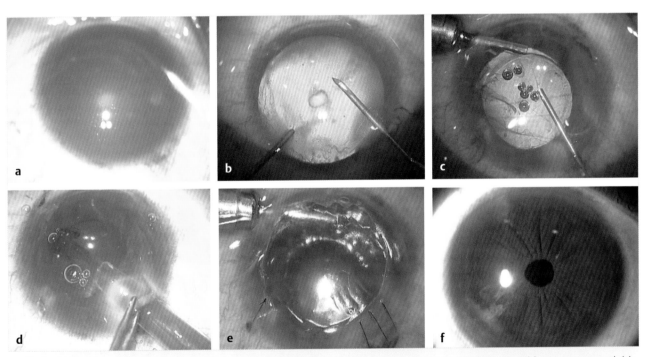

Fig. 9.7 Pre-Descemet endothelial keratoplasty with cataract. (a) Preoperative status of the recipient eye. (b) Rhexis started for cataract removal. (c) Side port incision made to introduce an anterior chamber maintainer (ACM). Notice the intraocular lens in the eye. Now descemetorhexis will be started. (d) Donor graft is inserted into the anterior chamber. Wound-assisted graft insertion is avoided. (e) Graft unrolling is attempted with air and fluidics. Endoilluminator is used to enhance the graft visualization and also to check the correct orientation. (f) One month postoperative image.

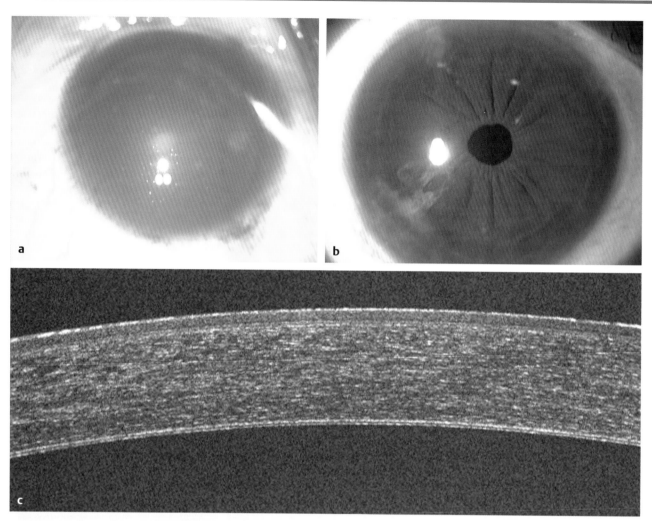

Fig. 9.8 Preoperative and postoperative images. **(a)** Preoperative image of the eye. **(b)** One month postoperative image of the eye after cataract extraction by phacoemulsification and pre-Descemet endothelial keratoplasty. **(c)** Anterior segment optical coherence tomography shows attached graft.

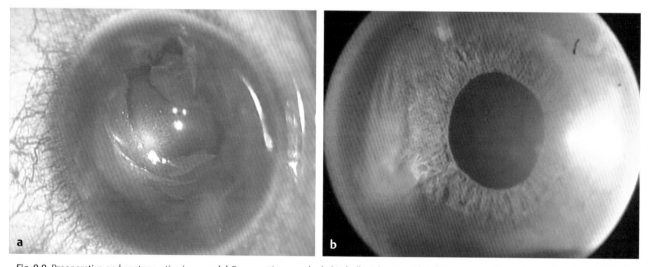

Fig. 9.9 Preoperative and postoperative images. **(a)** Preoperative pseudophakic bullous keratopathy. **(b)** Three months postoperative vision is 20/20.

Table 9.1 Comparison of the different endothelial keratoplasty techniques

	DSEK	DMEK	PDEK
Surgical layers	Stroma + DM + endo	DM + endo	Pre-Descemet + DM + endo
Technical difficulty	Easy	Difficult	Moderate
Type of procedure	Tissue additive	Tissue neutral	Minimal tissue additive
Artificial anterior chamber	Required	NR	NR
Microkeratome	Required (DSAEK)	NR	NR
Induced hyperopia	Yes	NO	No
Corneal thickness	Increased	Normal	Minimal
Intrastromal interface	Yes	No	Minimal
Cost	Costly	Cost-effective	Cost-effective
Eye bank prepared donor tissue	Available	No	Can be made available
Graft unrolling	Easy	Difficult	Moderate
Tissue handling	Good	Difficult	Good
Visual recovery	Slow	Fast	Fast

Abbreviations: DM, Descemet membrane; endo, endothelium; DMEK, Descemet membrane endothelial keratoplasty; DSAEK, Descemet stripping automated endothelial keratoplasty; DSEK, Descemet stripping endothelial keratoplasty; NR, not required; PDEK, pre-Descemet endothelial keratoplasty.

The upper age limit for donor tissue usage is considered to be around 75 years, but there is still not a clear-cut consensus on the lower age limit of donor tissue usage. Under such circumstances, most centers accept tissue from pediatric donors over 6 months of age. Infant donor tissue has not been used in the past due to various reasons involved with the concerns surrounding implanting immature tissue, although it runs high on endothelial cell density (ECD) count, along with the technical reason for implanting tissue with a greater corneal curvature and increased antigenicity, which would increase the risk of immune reaction. Increased steepness, elasticity, and flexibility of the infant donor tissue have limited its application for graft replacement, especially for a penetrating keratoplasty (PK). The same criteria also apply for EK, where difficulty in unrolling the graft is observed more so in a DMEK. Harvesting a donor tissue for DMEK with young donors below 40 years of age is considered to be difficult and should be avoided due to presumed strong adhesions between the DM and stroma that can lead to tearing of the DM during harvesting of donor tissue.

Use of young donor tissue with favorable outcomes has been reported for DSEK[8] and of infant donor tissue for DSAEK.[9] Sun et al have reported conflicting results with neonate corneas in DSEK procedure[10] whereas in our study, we reported the feasibility of an infant donor tissue in PDEK[5] (▶ Fig. 9.10, ▶ Fig. 9.11, ▶ Fig. 9.12, ▶ Fig. 9.13, ▶ Fig. 9.14).

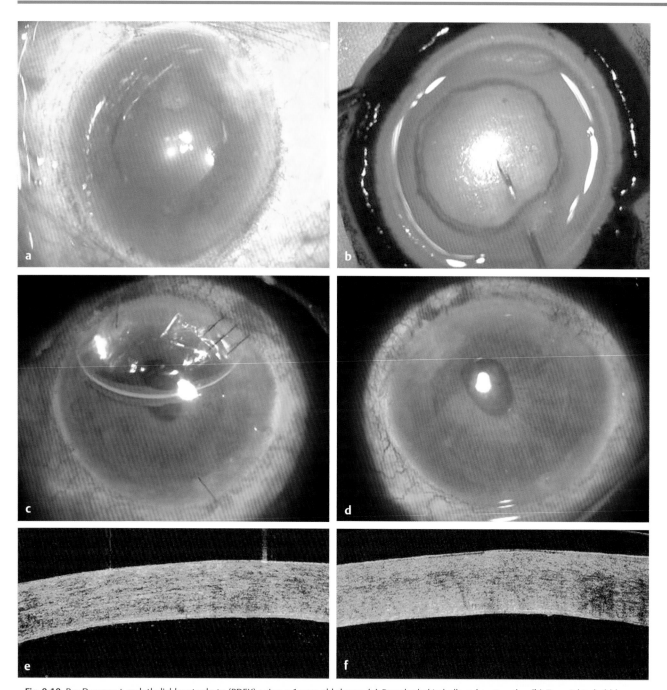

Fig. 9.10 Pre-Descemet endothelial keratoplasty (PDEK) using a 1-year-old donor. (a) Pseudophakic bullous keratopathy. (b) Type 1 big bubble prepared for PDEK graft. (c) Postoperative day 1 after PDEK. (d) Postoperative 1 week after PDEK. (e) Anterior segment optical coherence tomography (OCT) postoperative day 1. (f) Anterior segment OCT 1 week postoperative.

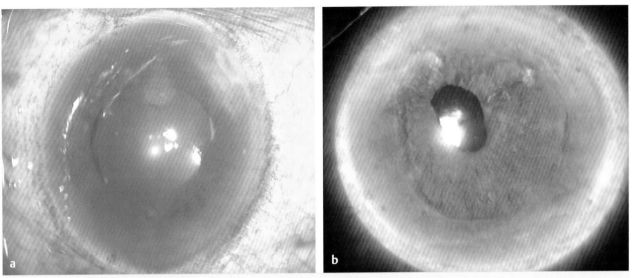

Fig. 9.11 Preoperative and postoperative follow-up images of pre-Descemet endothelial keratoplasty using a 1-year-old donor. (a) Preoperative clinical photograph showing the corneal decompensation. (b) Postoperative image of the same case at 15-month follow-up with vision being 20/20.

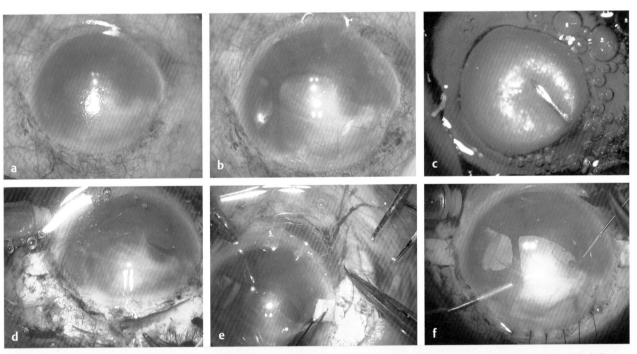

Fig. 9.12 Surgical procedure of pre-Descemet endothelial keratoplasty (PDEK) with a 9-month-old infant donor cornea, step 1. (a) Pseudophakic bullous keratopathy with decentered intraocular lens (IOL). (b) Epithelium removed. Note corneal vascularization and corneal haze. (c) Type 1 big bubble prepared for PDEK graft. (d) IOL explanted. (e) Glued IOL. (f) Pupilloplasty.

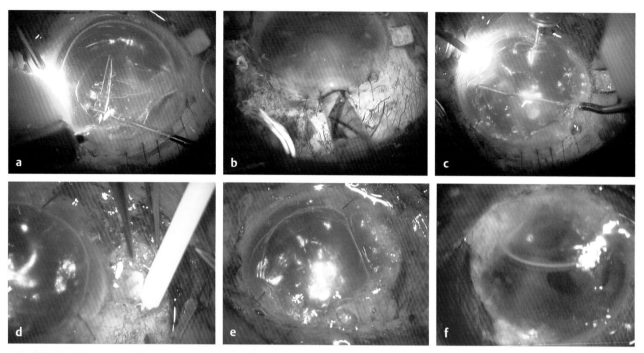

Fig. 9.13 Surgical procedure of pre-Descemet endothelial keratoplasty (PDEK) with a 9-month-old infant donor cornea, step 2. **(a)** Descemetorhexis being performed under air. The endoilluminator helps to enhance the visualization. **(b)** The infant donor graft is loaded onto the cartridge of a foldable intraocular lens (IOL) injector (the spring is removed to prevent any damage to the graft), and is slowly injected into the eye. **(c)** The donor graft is unrolled, and the endoilluminator helps to identify the correct graft orientation. **(d)** Fibrin glue is being applied beneath the scleral flaps. **(e)** Corneal incisions are closed with 10–0 nylon suture and the anterior chamber is filled with air. **(f)** Postoperative image of the case on postoperative day 4.

9.5 Discussion

Posterior lamellar keratoplasty has the benefit of transferring the healthy endothelium from the donor with or without the addition of the stromal tissue.

Surgeons have performed DSEK with neonate corneas where they have reported achieving the maximum size of lenticule as 8 mm along with the thinner central lenticule as compared to a thicker peripheral rim of the lenticule. This can be attributed to the increased corneal curvature in newborns as compared to that in adults. They also observed that, due to increased flexibility of the cornea, the unrolling of the graft was a bit difficult and as a result there were increased chances of graft dislocation and lenticule contraction in the postoperative period.[10]

Another group of surgeons has performed DSEK with pediatric donor tissue and has reported good outcomes. The employment of young donor tissue for EK has a theoretical advantage of transferring a donor lenticule with high ECD, which could compensate for ECD loss that eventually occurs postsurgery. In EK, a frequent concern among surgeons is potential tissue loss as a result of DM graft preparation failure, which is minimized with the PDEK procedure, because failure to get a type 1 bb may be associated with the formation of a type 2 bb. Under such a scenario the surgeon can perform a DMEK instead of a PDEK procedure.

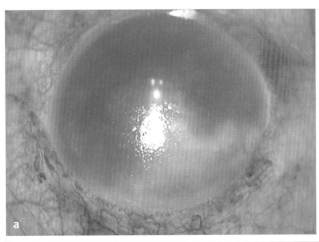
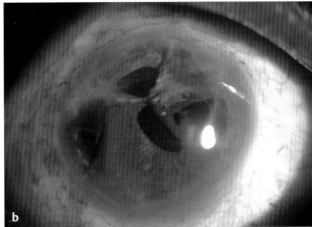
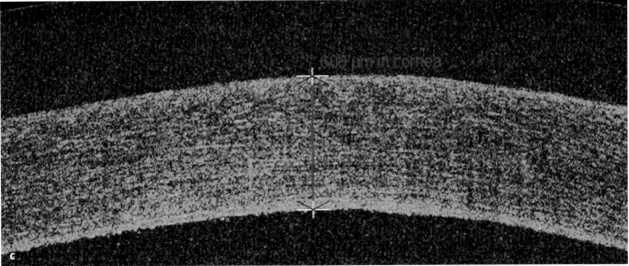

Fig. 9.14 Preoperative and postoperative follow-up images using a 9-month-old donor. **(a)** Preoperative image of decentered intraocular lens with bullous keratopathy with anterior stromal haze. **(b)** Postoperative image at 6-month follow-up. Vision is 20/30. **(c)** Anterior segment optical coherence tomography showing the attached graft.

In conclusion, a stepwise approach to donor preparation and donor insertion makes PDEK a standardized and reproducible procedure with a successful outcome with usage of young donor corneas with high ECD. The procedure of PDEK also involves a surgical skill set to create a type 1 bb, but this limitation is circumvented by the fact that PDEK does not require the employment of a costly microkeratome as in a DSAEK, DMAEK, or UT-DSEK, thereby cutting the cost of the surgical procedure and also inculcating the use of infant donor cornea with a graft thickness of around 35 µm, which is eventually less as compared to DSAEK or UT-DSEK tissue.

References

[1] Melles GR, Eggink FA, Lander F, et al. A surgical technique for posterior lamellar keratoplasty. Cornea. 1998; 17(6):618–626

[2] Melles GR, Ong TS, Ververs B, van der Wees J. Descemet membrane endothelial keratoplasty (DMEK). Cornea. 2006; 25(8):987–990

[3] Agarwal A, Dua HS, Narang P, et al. Pre-Descemet's endothelial keratoplasty (PDEK). Br J Ophthalmol. 2014; 98(9):1181–1185

[4] Dua HS, Faraj LA, Said DG, Gray T, Lowe J. Human corneal anatomy redefined: a novel pre-Descemet's layer (Dua's layer). Ophthalmology. 2013; 120 (9):1778–1785

[5] Agarwal A, Agarwal A, Narang P, Kumar DA, Jacob S. Pre-Descemet Endothelial Keratoplasty With Infant Donor Corneas: A Prospective Analysis. Cornea. 2015; 34(8):859–865

[6] Agarwal A, Narang P, Kumar DA, Agarwal A. Trocar anterior chamber maintainer: Improvised infusion technique. J Cataract Refract Surg. 2016; 42 (2):185–18–9

[7] Price FW, Jr, Price MO. Descemet's stripping with endothelial keratoplasty in 200 eyes: Early challenges and techniques to enhance donor adherence. J Cataract Refract Surg. 2006; 32(3):411–418

[8] Huang T, Wang Y, Hu A, Luo Y, Chen J. Use of paediatric donor tissue in Descemet stripping endothelial keratoplasty. Br J Ophthalmol. 2009; 93(12):1625–1628

[9] Kim P, Yeung SN, Lichtinger A, Amiran MD, Rootman DS. Descemet stripping automated endothelial keratoplasty using infant donor tissue. Cornea. 2012; 31(1):52–54

[10] Sun YX, Hao YS, Hong J. Descemet membrane stripping endothelial keratoplasty with neonate donors in two cases. Br J Ophthalmol. 2009; 93 (12):1692–1693

10 Trocar Anterior Chamber Maintainer: An Improvised New Concept for Infusion and Endothelial Keratoplasty

Priya Narang and Amar Agarwal

10.1 Concept

The merits of a closed chamber infusion system that helps to maintain the tonicity of the globe throughout intraocular surgery cannot be overstated. Maintenance of a deep anterior chamber (AC) is a prerequisite for safe, smooth performance of intraocular surgery because it prevents inadvertent and harmful touch to the corneal endothelium and also to various other structures. For the same reason sodium hyaluronate was introduced and it served as a major breakthrough for all anterior segment intraocular surgeries.[1,2,3] Although the use of viscoelastic also plays an important role, its use for maintenance of an AC in corneal surgeries is not a prudent idea, more so with endothelial keratoplasty (EK) procedures.

Blumenthal devised a simple and practical method for maintaining the AC with a device that he called the anterior chamber maintainer (ACM), which was made from a 21-gauge scalp vein

(**butterfly**) set. Since the introduction of an ACM there have been various modifications to the ACM to suit the surgical condition of the eye. The ACM[4,5,6] and trocar cannula are the most common methods employed for infusion by anterior segment and posterior segment surgeons, respectively. Introduction of the trocar cannula was a monumental advance in ophthalmology because it allowed, for the first time, controlled access to the posterior segment of the eye. It is also an integral part of modern pars plana vitrectomy for maintaining infusion in the eye.[7,8,9,10,11] A 23-gauge (0.6 mm), 25-gauge (0.5 mm), or 27-gauge (0.4 mm) trocar system can be introduced transconjunctivally through the tenon's layer to expose the sclera. Instead, trocars are placed through the conjunctiva and sclera to afford access to the vitreous and also to maintain infusion in the eye. We designed a trocar AC maintainer (TACM) to help surgeons achieve better infusion (▶ Fig. 10.1). The TACM can be used by anterior segment surgeons for air/fluid infusion into the eye.[12]

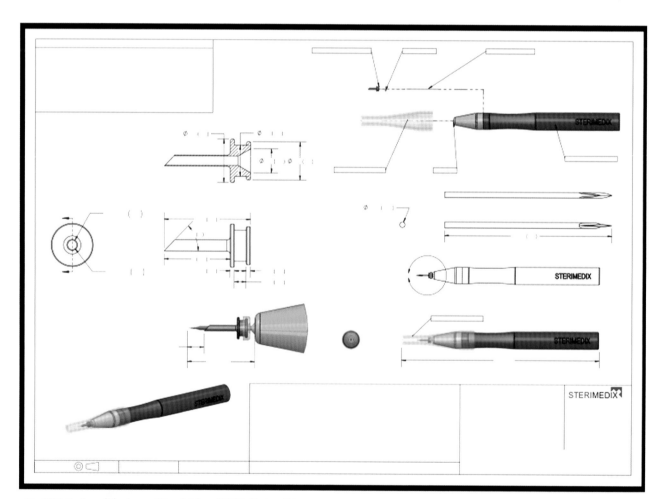

Fig. 10.1 Design of the trocar AC maintainer (TACM; Sterimedix).

10.2 Trocar Anterior Compartment Maintainer (TACM) Device

Taking into consideration the advantages of a trocar system, we employed a method of introducing the trocar cannula for AC maintenance that could be used by anterior segment surgeons with equal ease and élan. Initially we used normal trocars that were designed for posterior segment surgeries (▶ Fig. 10.2). Although we attained good infusion of air and fluid through it, we still felt the need for a trocar with a shorter blade so that any damage to the AC intraocular structures could be avoided (▶ Fig. 10.3).

10.3 Procedure of Positioning TACM in AC

Before cannula insertion, the conjunctiva is displaced with a cotton tip to keep the conjunctival puncture away from the sclera–limbal wound. The cannula (on a trocar) is inserted into the limbus approximately 1 mm away, usually at a 45-degree angle (depending on the gauge) and parallel to the limbus. The trocar is then turned directly toward the center of the globe so that it enters the AC in front of the iris tissue. It is advanced until the hub of the cannula is flush with the sclera. The trocar is then removed, leaving the cannula in place. This maneuver allows a longer scleral wound and carries a lower risk of wound leakage. The infusion line is attached to the stent of the cannula,

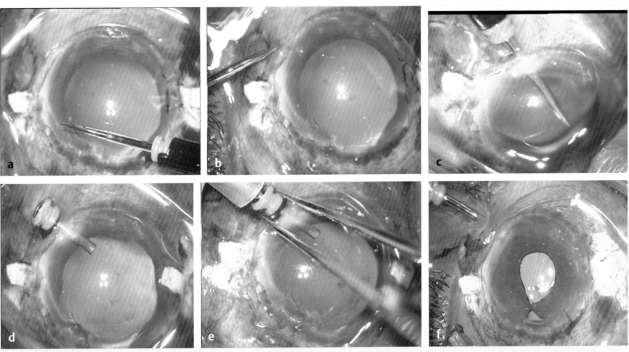

Fig. 10.2 A 23-gauge retinal trocar was used as the first trocar anterior chamber maintainer (TACM). **(a)** The 23-gauge trocar cannula system. **(b)** A trocar needle being inserted obliquely in the sclera about 1 mm away from the limbus. **(c)** The direction of the trocar needle is turned perpendicular toward the globe. The trocar is inserted in the eye so that it enters the eye in front of the iris. **(d)** The trocar is removed and the cannula is fixed in place. **(e)** The infusion line is attached to the cannula and the TACM is in place. **(f)** The cannula is removed and no active leakage is observed. The anterior chamber is well maintained.

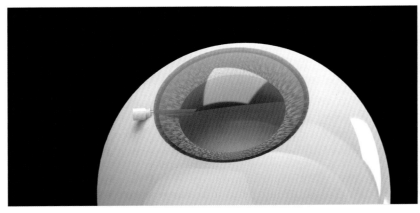

Fig. 10.3 Animation showing the trocar anterior chamber (AC) maintainer in place. Notice it passes through the sclera (about 0.5 to 1 mm from the limbus) and enters the AC above the iris.

and the infusion is turned on. At the end of the surgical procedure, the surgeon just withdraws the TACM, and, because the wound is self-sealing, no leakage is observed (▶ Fig. 10.4).

10.4 Advantages

The advantage of using a TACM is that it allows an easy, atraumatic transconjunctival entry into the anterior segment with better endurance and ability to create self-sealing ports, which are most desirable and are the hallmark of any intraocular surgery. Controlled access to the intraocular segment structures without running risk of hypotony is the prime concern of all surgeons. Valved trocars can offer better control of intraocular pressure and eye outflow during the surgery, although we have not yet exploited this option in our patients.

The TACM can also be employed for maintaining continuous air/fluid infusion in the eye in cases of corneal endothelial keratoplasty (▶ Fig. 10.5 and ▶ Fig. 10.6). This can prevent repeated shallowing and reforming of the AC and minimize the risk of iris damage, miosis, and lens damage in phakic eye procedures. Some surgeons even prefer using vitrectomy air exchange pumps for the same reason.[13] The various other advantages of the TACM are induction of less astigmatism because a corneal side port incision is prevented as is overcrowding of the AC and cornea in complicated cases, which provides more working space to the surgeon. Combined anterior segment and posterior segment surgeries can also be performed with the TACM in place.

10.5 Discussion

The maintenance of a deep AC is a prerequisite for a safe anterior segment surgery. The TACM helps prevent AC collapse, apart from serving as an important tool during intraocular lens (IOL) insertion, post-IOL insertion maneuvers, vitrectomy, or secondary IOL implantation, obviating the need for use of an ophthalmic viscosurgical device (OVD). Fluid is the natural milieu of the anterior segment, and its use during surgery does not disturb any of the anatomical relationships in the eye.[6] The surgical wound created for introduction of the ACM is a paracentesis wound with a side port incision in the peripheral cornea. The ACM must be exactly the right size, and the knife must be withdrawn along the tract of entry because any sidewise movement during entry or withdrawal will produce an incision that is too large and the ACM wound will leak. Suturing an incision is often required to prevent postoperative hypotony, and also to minimize the continuous leak and the induced postoperative astigmatism.[14] All these shortcomings are outweighed by the use of the TACM.

The TACM is placed in position during pre-Descemet endothelial keratoplasty (PDEK) surgery, and an air pump is connected to the TACM. This allows continuous air infusion into the eye during the process of recipient bed preparation that necessitates the performance of descematorhexis and peeling the diseased Descemet membrane (DM) from the recipient eye. After the insertion of the donor lenticule and partial unscrolling, the air pump is switched on again. Infusion of air at this

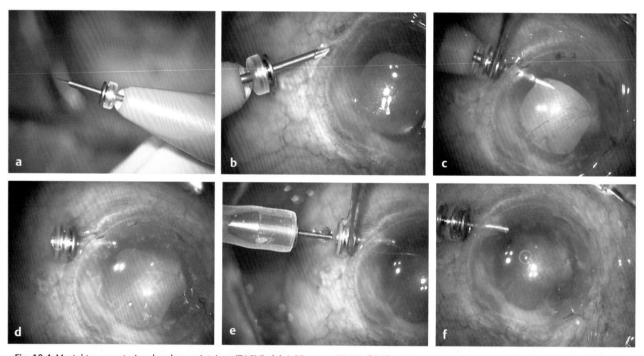

Fig. 10.4 Mastel trocar anterior chamber maintainer (TACM). **(a)** A 25-gauge TACM. **(b)** The TACM is passed 1 mm behind the limbus parallel to the limbus into a half-thickness of the sclera. **(c)** The TACM is rotated 90 degrees so that it passes into the anterior chamber above the iris. This creates a valvular effect in the sclera so that there is no leakage. **(d)** The trocar is removed and only the cannula is left. **(e)** The tubing connects to the cannula. **(f)** The TACM is in place. This can now pass fluid or air into the anterior chamber, depending on what the surgeon wants. In a glued intraocular lens or any surgery fluid can be passed, and in endothelial keratoplasty air can be passed via an air pump.

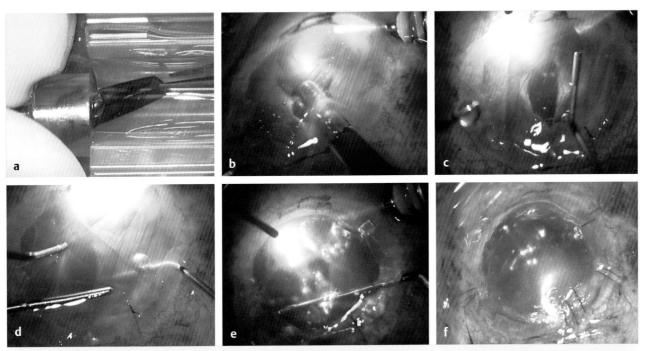

Fig. 10.5 The trocar anterior chamber maintainer (TACM) in pre-Descemet endothelial keratoplasty (PDEK) surgery. **(a)** A PDEK graft in the cartridge of an injector. **(b)** The PDEK graft is injected in the anterior chamber. Note the TACM is fixed. **(c)** The PDEK graft is unrolled. At this time no air is passed through the TACM. **(d)** The graft is unrolled and air will be injected under the graft. **(e)** The air pump is switched on so that air passes continuously through the TACM into the eye. **(f)** The TACM is removed, and the graft is attached fully.

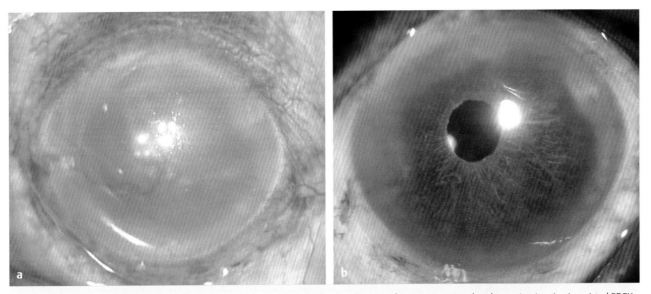

Fig. 10.6 Pre-Descemet endothelial keratoplasty (PDEK), pre- and postoperative after use of a trocar anterior chamber maintainer in air-assisted PDEK surgery. **(a)** Preoperative image. **(b)** Postoperative image at 1 month, with vision being 20/20.

stage helps the adherence of the donor lenticule to the recipient bed. When the graft is being unrolled, care should be taken to ensure that the tip of the TACM cannula does not collide with the donor lenticule, which can damage the endothelial cells and affect the visual outcome of the surgery.

With use of the TACM, an oblique incision parallel to the limbus displaces the circumferentially oriented scleral fibers laterally, rather than cutting them. Creation of a biplanar incision seals the wound perfectly. To conclude, the TACM helps to maintain the integrity and depth of the AC with great precision without compromising the amount of working space on the anterior corneal surface for the surgeon. It effectively allows the surgeon to switch over between air and fluid infusion as and when required.

References

[1] Pape LG, Balazs EA. The use of sodium hyaluronate (Healon) in human anterior segment surgery. Ophthalmology. 1980; 87(7):699–705

[2] Pape LG. Intracapsular and extracapsular technique of lens implantation with Healon R. J Am Intraocul Implant Soc. 1980; 6(4):342–343

[3] Miller D, Stegmann R. Use of sodium hyaluronate in human IOL implantation. Ann Ophthalmol. 1981; 13(7):811–815

[4] Thrasher B. Maintaining an anterior chamber with the Cavitron unit. J Am Intraocul Implant Soc. 1978; 4(4):220–221

[5] Lewicky AO, Lopez OI, Petkus RW, Stillerman ML. The Chamber Maintainer System (CMS). Ophthalmic Surg. 1982; 13(11):921–927

[6] Blumenthal M, Moisseiev J. Anterior chamber maintainer for extracapsular cataract extraction and intraocular lens implantation. J Cataract Refract Surg. 1987; 13(2):204–206

[7] Chen JC. Sutureless pars plana vitrectomy through self-sealing sclerotomies. Arch Ophthalmol. 1996; 114(10):1273–1275

[8] Kwok AK, Tham CC, Lam DS, Li M, Chen JC. Modified sutureless sclerotomies in pars plana vitrectomy. Am J Ophthalmol. 1999; 127(6):731–733

[9] de Juan E, Jr, Hickingbotham D. Refinements in microinstrumentation for vitreous surgery. Am J Ophthalmol. 1990; 109(2):218–220

[10] Fujii GY, De Juan E, Jr, Humayun MS, et al. A new 25-gauge instrument system for transconjunctival sutureless vitrectomy surgery. Ophthalmology. 2002; 109(10):1807–1812, discussion 1813

[11] Eckardt C. Transconjunctival sutureless 23-gauge vitrectomy. Retina. 2005; 25(2):208–211

[12] Agarwal A, Narang P, Kumar DA, Agarwal A. Trocar anterior chamber maintainer: Improvised infusion technique. J Cataract Refract Surg. 2016; 42(2):185:–1–89

[13] Leyland M. Anterior chamber maintenance during descemet stripping [letter]. Cornea. 2007; 26(10):1292–1293, author reply 1293

[14] Ashkenazi I, Avni I, Blumenthal M. Maintaining nearly physiologic intraocular pressure levels prior to tying the sutures during cataract surgery reduces surgically-induced astigmatism. Ophthalmic Surg. 1991; 22(5):284–286

11 Surgically Mastering Pre-Descemet Endothelial Keratoplasty in 15 Steps

Priya Narang and Amar Agarwal

The hallmark of any surgery is marked by its reproducibility in terms of surgical procedure and visual outcomes. Technical ease, availability of tissue donor, and the required hospital and surgical setup go a long way in the acceptance of any new surgical procedure. Among all the subtypes of endothelial keratoplasty (EK), Descemet membrane endothelial keratoplasty (DMEK) and pre-Descemet endothelial keratoplasty (PDEK) are met with the technical challenge of handling thin donor tissue and subsequently loading and unscrolling it in the eye, which can be even more unpredictable and challenging at times. Donor tissue characteristics[1,2] often affect and influence the tendency of some tissues to resist unscrolling and to behave in an inconsistent manner.

PDEK[3,4] combines a simplified technique of stripping the endothelium and Descemet membrane (DM) with the pre-Descemet layer (PDL) from the donor cornea, which is assisted by air dissection and creation of a type 1 bubble (bb).[5] PDEK allows closed chamber manipulation of the donor graft. It also successfully mitigates ocular surface complications and structural problems (including induced astigmatism and perpetually weak wounds), like other EK procedure subtypes, and also immunologic graft reactions and secondary glaucoma from prolonged topical corticosteroid use, unlike a penetrating keratoplasty (PK).

11.1 Donor Graft Preparation

This constitutes one of the most essential steps and the initial step of the surgery. The donor corneoscleral rim is obtained from the whole globe and is placed with the endothelial side up.

1. Bubble creation: A 30-gauge needle attached to an air-filled 5 mL syringe is introduced from the periphery of the corneoscleral rim of the graft up to the center. The needle is entered at a considerable depth below the DM so as to create a plane between the PDL and the residual stroma. The needle is introduced in a bevel-up position under direct supervision, and air is injected. A type 1 bubble is formed that characteristically spreads from the center to the periphery, is dome shaped, and is approximately 8 mm in diameter.

2. Staining and harvesting the graft: Staining the graft is essential for enhancing the visualization of the graft and to identify the correct orientation. The edge of the bb is entered with a side port blade, and trypan blue is injected inside to stain the graft. The graft is then cut with the corneoscleral scissors all around the periphery of the bb and is placed in the storage media (▶ Fig. 11.1).

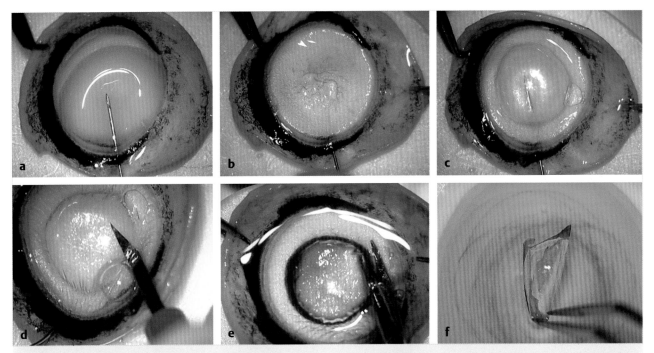

Fig. 11.1 Donor graft preparation. **(a)** A 5 mL air-filled syringe attached to a 30-gauge needle is introduced from the corneoscleral edge with the endothelial side up. **(b)** Air is being injected slowly and small bubbles start to form. **(c)** Air is injected and a type 1 bubble (bb) is formed. **(d)** The peripheral edge of the bb is ruptured with a side port blade. **(e)** Trypan blue is injected to stain the bubble. The edge of the bb is cut with the corneoscleral scissors. **(f)** The graft is placed in the storage media.

11.2 Recipient Bed Preparation and Graft Insertion

This procedure can be described in 15 steps that need to be followed sequentially in the following order:

- **Step 1:** Fix the infusion cannula. A trocar anterior chamber maintainer[6] (T-ACM) (▶ Fig. 11.2) or even a routine anterior chamber maintainer (ACM) can also be fixed if the surgeon is not well versed with the use of a T-ACM. Fixing up an infusion setup allows the surgeon to easily switch between an air or fluid infusion as and when required during the surgical procedure.
- **Step 2:** Switch on the air pump. Connect the T-ACM to an air pump (▶ Fig. 11.3). This facilitates continuous air infusion into the eye and helps to perform the procedure with an anterior chamber (AC) that is always well formed.
- **Step 3:** Frame the side port incisions. Two side port incisions are made at superotemporal and superonasal positions

(▶ Fig. 11.4). This is done so as to allow these sites to be used in the future for further intraocular manipulation.

- **Step 4:** Perform descemetorhexis. Descemetorhexis is performed with a reverse Sinskey hook (▶ Fig. 11.5). This step is essentially the same as in a DMEK procedure. Two Sinskey hooks are introduced from both the side port incisions, and the diseased DM is peeled and scraped off the recipient bed.
- **Step 5:** Frame the corneal incision tunnel. A 2.8 mm clear corneal incision is made, and the peeled DM–endothelium complex is removed (▶ Fig. 11.6). This site is further used for the introduction of the graft into the eye.
- **Step 6:** Inferior iridectomy. Inferior iridectomy is performed with a vitrector (▶ Fig. 11.7). This helps to prevent any incidence of pupillary blockage. The vitrectomy machine is set at low vacuum and at the cutter rate of around 20 cuts per minute. The cutter is then placed at the proposed iridectomy site, and the iris tissue is engaged into the cutter probe initially with the aspiration mode at a low setting. A low cutting rate ensures proper aspiration of the iris tissue into the cutter

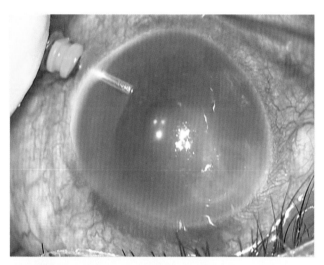

Fig. 11.2 The trocar anterior chamber maintainer is introduced into the eye.

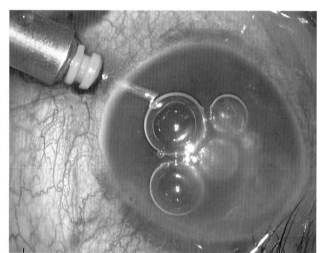

Fig. 11.3 The trocar anterior chamber maintainer is connected to the air pump.

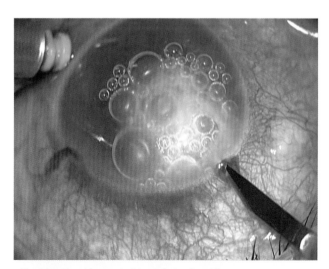

Fig. 11.4 The side port incision is being framed.

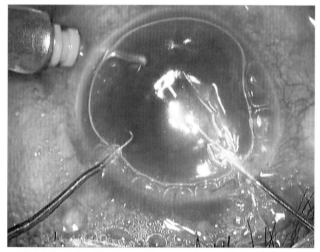

Fig. 11.5 Descemetorhexis is being performed with a reverse Sinskey hook.

followed by its cutting. The aspiration port is occluded by the iris stroma, and the iris is cut using the vitrectomy probe in a controlled manner under direct visualization, taking care not to disturb the angle structures. A customized iridectomy can thus be created in the desired quadrant, leaving the rest of the iris tissue undisturbed.

- **Step 7:** Loading the graft. Load the PDEK graft in the cartridge of the foldable intraocular lens (▶ Fig. 11.8; originally described by Francis Price). A few drops of balanced salt solution (BSS) can be added into the cartridge to keep the graft floating and to prevent it from adhering to the cartridge.
- **Step 8:** Switch off the air pump. This step (▶ Fig. 11.9) is performed before the graft is injected so that the force of the air does not displace the graft, and doing so also ensures that there is enough room for the graft to enter and be properly placed into the AC.
- **Step 9:** Graft injection. This is a critical step of the surgery, and the surgeon should avoid wound-assisted graft injection. The PDEK graft is injected in the AC (▶ Fig. 11.10) very slowly

and carefully. Maintaining an adequate depth of the AC is essential at this point in the surgery. If the AC is shallow then the assistant can inject a bit of fluid into the AC from the side port incision. Once the graft is injected and is seen floating in the AC, the cartridge and the injector are withdrawn from the AC.

- **Step 10:** Suture the clear corneal incision. The clear corneal incision is closed with a 10–0 nylon suture (▶ Fig. 11.11). This ensures there is no wound leakage and that the graft is placed in a well-formed AC.
- **Step 11:** Check the graft orientation. The correct orientation of the graft is checked (▶ Fig. 11.12); an endoilluminator can be used to facilitate this.[7] An obliquely directed endoilluminator light provides three-dimensional depth perception for the graft while allowing visualization of the entire graft. This allows proper comprehension of graft dynamics, morphology, and positioning, in turn leading to easier and faster surgery while potentially decreasing graft damage due to excessive manipulations.

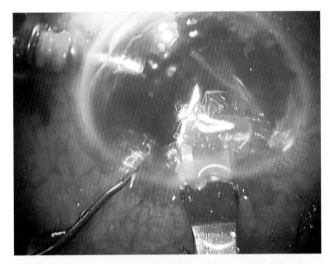

Fig. 11.6 The clear corneal incision is framed.

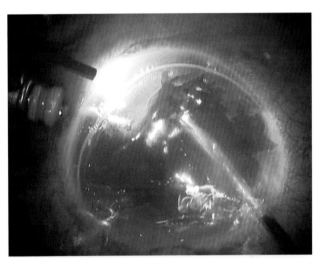

Fig. 11.7 Iridectomy is being performed with a vitrectomy probe.

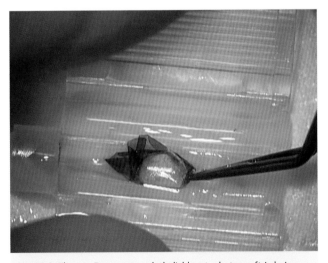

Fig. 11.8 The pre-Descemet endothelial keratoplasty graft is being loaded into the cartridge of the foldable intraocular lens.

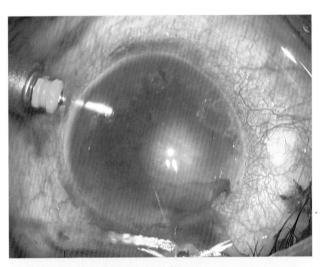

Fig. 11.9 The air pump is switched off.

- **Step 12:** Graft unrolling. After placing the graft in the correct orientation, the donor lenticule is centered and oriented with the rolls of the scroll facing upward using short bursts of BSS. After the graft unscrolls partially, a small air bubble is injected underneath the graft to sustain the correct membrane orientation. Unroll the graft and inject a bit of air beneath the graft (▶ Fig. 11.13).
- **Step 13:** Switch on the air pump. The air pump connected to the T-ACM or an ACM is switched on. This pushes the graft up and helps it to adhere to the corneal surface (▶ Fig. 11.14) of the recipient bed.
- **Step 14:** Unroll the peripheral curls of the graft. This is an extremely important step of the surgery that helps to eliminate and curb the incidence of postoperative rebubbling. The edges of the donor graft have a tendency to curl up and push the graft away from the recipient corneal bed. These peripheral edges, if not totally unrolled, can lead to small peripheral separations that usually do not seal down on their own and need to be treated. A reverse Sinskey hook is used to unroll

the peripheral edges of the donor graft. The entire process is done very gently, taking care to minimize the endothelial contact. The graft is then centered (▶ Fig. 11.15). Corneal massage is performed to adjust the centered position of the donor graft and to eliminate residual fluid at the donor graft–recipient interface. Residual interface fluid can also be drained through corneal venting incisions.

- **Step 15:** Suture all the wounds. All the corneal wounds are sutured to ensure tight closure of the globe to prevent any inadvertent air leakage from the AC. The infusion is stopped and the T-ACM is removed (▶ Fig. 11.16).

11.3 Discussion

The visual outcomes with the PDEK procedure have been reported to be very good, with good patient satisfaction. It is therefore reasonable for many surgeons to continue performing PDEK given the overall satisfactory results.

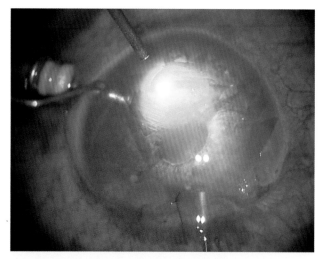

Fig. 11.10 The pre-Descemet endothelial keratoplasty graft is being injected into the anterior chamber.

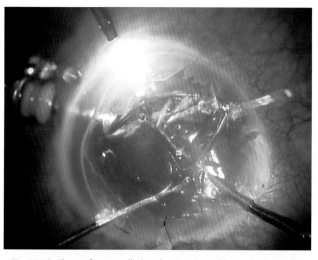

Fig. 11.11 The corneal incision is sutured to seal the anterior chamber.

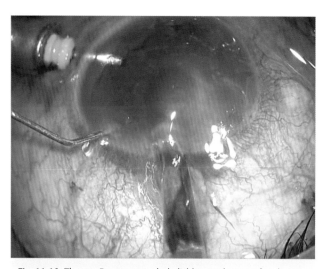

Fig. 11.12 The correct orientation of the graft is checked with an endoilluminator.

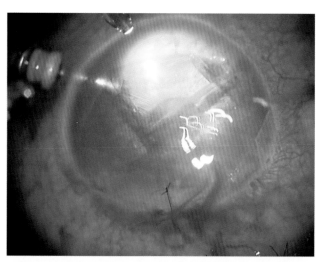

Fig. 11.13 The graft is unrolled and air is injected beneath the graft.

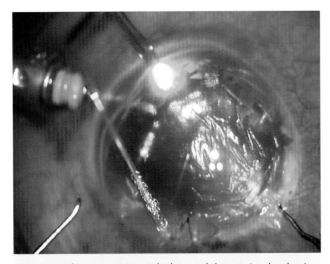

Fig. 11.14 The air pump is switched on, and the anterior chamber is filled with air to facilitate further adhesion of the graft to the endothelial surface.

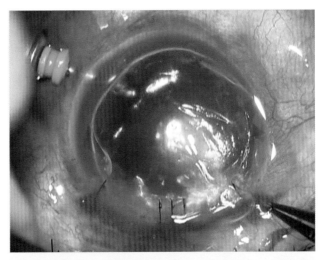

Fig. 11.15 The graft is centered.

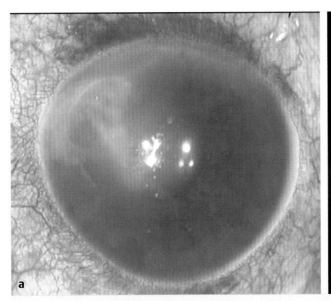

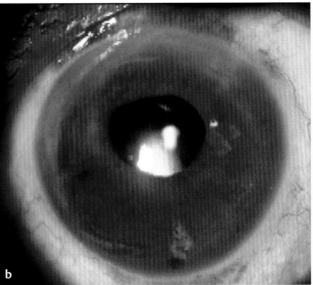

Fig. 11.16 Follow-up images. (a) Preoperative image. (b) At 3 months the postoperative image shows clearance of the corneal haze.

The early postoperative period is crucial following a PDEK procedure due to the issue of adequate adherence of the donor lenticule to the recipient bed. The tendency of donor lenticule to curl up and push itself away from the recipient cornea, if noted, suggests an impending partial detachment of the graft. This often requires air injection into the AC.

The depth of the AC should be properly gauged before the graft is injected, as an optimal depth is needed for the graft to unfold. In eyes with a deep AC, it is often difficult to unfold the graft, and these eyes also typically require an extra amount of air fill for graft adherence. Placing an infusion line connected to an air pump allows a continuous and adequate amount of air to be instilled into the AC.

Care should also be taken while positioning the graft because there is a chance of the graft colliding with the cannula of the ACM that is placed in the AC. The incidence is lessened with the use of the T-ACM because the T-ACM enters the AC from the sclera, does not encroach the anterior corneal surface, and is peripherally placed from the limbus. Pupilloplasty should always be performed in eyes with large iris defects because the graft may accidentally dislodge into the vitreous cavity. Pupil reconstruction also helps to maintain the depth of the AC throughout the surgery.

PDEK has extended itself as a lexicon among various EK subtypes that allows the use of adult and infant donor tissue.[3,4] The technique of PDEK scores higher than DMEK in this respect because older donor tissue is usually preferred for DMEK given that the thickness of DM increases with age,[8] which leads to less curling of the donor lenticule edges. The issue of tearing of the DM due to projection of the stromal collagen fibrils into the interfacial matrix of the DM[9] during peeling from the underlying stroma is also not encountered with PDEK.

As the experience with PDEK grows, surgical results improve due to continuous improvisation with and improvement on the surgical technique. This improvement will likely continue as more surgeons adopt the technique and add their valuable input.

References

[1] Price MO, Giebel AW, Fairchild KM, Price FW, Jr. Descemet's membrane endothelial keratoplasty: prospective multicenter study of visual and refractive outcomes and endothelial survival. Ophthalmology. 2009; 116(12):2361–2368

[2] Dirisamer M, Ham L, Dapena I, et al. Efficacy of descemet membrane endothelial keratoplasty: clinical outcome of 200 consecutive cases after a learning curve of 25 cases. Arch Ophthalmol. 2011; 129(11):1435–1443

[3] Agarwal A, Dua HS, Narang P, et al. Pre-Descemet's endothelial keratoplasty (PDEK). Br J Ophthalmol. 2014; 98(9):1181–1185

[4] Agarwal A, Agarwal A, Narang P, Kumar DA, Jacob S. Pre-Descemet Endothelial Keratoplasty With Infant Donor Corneas: A Prospective Analysis. Cornea. 2015; 34(8):859–865

[5] Dua HS, Faraj LA, Said DG, Gray T, Lowe J. Human corneal anatomy redefined: a novel pre-Descemet's layer (Dua's layer). Ophthalmology. 2013; 120 (9):1778–1785

[6] Agarwal A, Narang P, Kumar DA, Agarwal A. Trocar anterior chamber maintainer: Improvised infusion technique. J Cataract Refract Surg. 2016; 42 (2):185–189

[7] Jacob S, Agarwal A, Agarwal A, Narasimhan S, Kumar DA, Sivagnanam S. Endoilluminator-assisted transcorneal illumination for Descemet membrane endothelial keratoplasty: enhanced intraoperative visualization of the graft in corneal decompensation secondary to pseudophakic bullous keratopathy. J Cataract Refract Surg. 2014; 40(8):1332–1336

[8] Murphy C, Alvarado J, Juster R. Prenatal and postnatal growth of the human Descemet's membrane. Invest Ophthalmol Vis Sci. 1984; 25(12):1402–1415

[9] Schlötzer-Schrehardt U, Bachmann BO, Laaser K, Cursiefen C, Kruse FE. Characterization of the cleavage plane in DESCemet's membrane endothelial keratoplasty. Ophthalmology. 2011; 118(10):1950–1957

12 Air-Pump-Assisted Endothelial Keratoplasty

Brandon James Baartman and William J. Dupps, Jr.

12.1 Introduction

One of the great challenges faced by surgeons performing corneal endothelial transplantation is ensuring proper positioning and lasting adherence of the transplanted endothelial graft. Accomplishing donor adherence was noted as one of the largest early challenges in the successful development of the technique and remains a critical step of the procedure today.[1] The importance of attaining adequate intraoperative placement is underscored by the rate of endothelial graft dislocations, which have been reported as high as 25% in Descemet stripping automated endothelial keratoplasty (DSAEK) and higher still in Descemet membrane endothelial keratoplasty (DMEK) and other more selective forms of endothelial transplantation.[2]

A number of techniques have been employed to promote graft adhesion, most of which focus on enhancing the dehydration of the donor–recipient interface. Classically, this has been achieved by a combination of air tamponade for 10 to 15 minutes and massage of the corneal surface to facilitate removal of sequestered fluid. The air tamponade is generally achieved via manual injection of air from a syringe. Price and Price described the utility of occasional supplementation of air with an infusion cannula through the paracentesis.[1,3]

Manual air insufflation presents some limitations. Fluctuations in intraocular pressure (IOP) with manual insufflation occur during the course of the air tamponade, limiting the amount of pressure exerted on the donor graft and decreasing adherence. The anterior chamber can collapse or decompress during attempts at corneal massage, which limits the effectiveness of compressive maneuvers at best and can result in intraoperative graft decentration or dislocation and the need for graft repositioning, associated surgical delays, or occult retention of interface fluid that increases the risk of postoperative nonadherence.

12.2 Continuous Air Infusion for Graft Adherence

To counter these limitations, Meisler et al described a technique for continuous pumping of filtered air into the anterior chamber via a 30-gauge needle passed through a self-sealing corneal tract at the nasal limbus (▶ Fig. 12.1).[4] Citing the use of this principle to provide retinal tamponade and subretinal fluid evacuation in vitreoretinal surgery, it was suggested that a similar technique could be applied to the fluid in the donor–recipient interface. Following graft insertion and manual injection of an initial bubble through a paracentesis, air was continuously pumped into the anterior chamber with a vitreoretinal surgical system (Accurus, Alcon Surgical) to maintain IOP between 30 and 40 mm Hg for 10 to 15 minutes, with occasional spikes to 50 or 60 mm Hg as needed, ensuring constant pressure application to the donor–recipient interface. Once this "press" had taken place, air was then partially exchanged for a slow influx of balanced salt solution (BSS) facilitated by gentle manual release of the air through the paracentesis until the residual bubble diameter is achieved at the desired end point pressure. The

same-sized corneal entry site of the 30-gauge needle and its long path length into the cornea provided an airtight seal that facilitated chamber stability and limited pressure fluctuations upon needle removal. The use of a continuous and titratable infusion of air during the procedure demonstrated promising early results in the first 12 consecutive eyes, none of which experienced graft dislocation.

Recent developments in intraoperative optical coherence tomography (iOCT) have allowed for more objective analysis of the interface fluid dimensions and the impact of surgical interventions on interface fluid and dislocation rates. Xu and colleagues used iOCT to collect spatial and volumetric data of the donor–recipient interface at various points during the DSAEK procedure in 28 eyes, demonstrating a significant decrease in the height of interface fluid after pressure elevation with the continuous air pump technique.[5] Although the trend toward reduced interface fluid volume after pressure elevation alone was not statistically significant in this series, the combination of pressure elevation via the air pump technique and manual corneal sweep with a flat irrigation cannula did demonstrate a significant decrease in interface fluid volume. This study provided quantitative data to support the use of continuous air pump for dehydration of the donor–recipient interface and the success of the technique in reducing early graft dislocations.

iOCT has also been used to compare the air pump technique (also referred to as the active air infusion technique) to the manual corneal sweep alone.[6] While both techniques independently produced a significant decrease in interface fluid, the air pump technique demonstrated a significantly smaller maximum interface fluid area, mean fluid thickness, maximum fluid thickness, and final interface fluid pocket volume compared to the manual corneal sweep, resulting in a trend toward overall

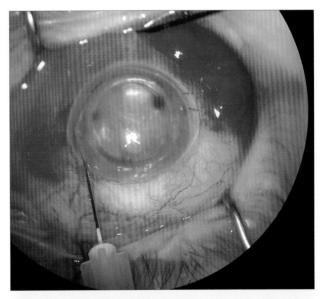

Fig. 12.1 Intraoperative view of a 30-gauge needle inserted through a self-sealing nasal tract for continuous, active air infusion and controlled air–fluid exchange.

less total interface fluid volume. Studies of continuous air infusion with iOCT imaging in the setting of DMEK are under way at our institution.

12.3 Current Technique Summary

The technique currently used by the senior author (WD) is an adaptation of the original technique description informed by observations from our experience in a large-scale prospective study of iOCT in DSAEK. After insertion of the graft, a bent 30-gauge needle on an air-filled syringe is used to (1) unfold the graft with a carefully deployed air bubble, (2) center the graft, and (3) secure its position with additional air injection as needed to fill the anterior chamber and deliver some initial compressive force.[7] For active infusion and air–fluid exchange, we have migrated to the VersaVIT Vitrectomy System (Synergetics) for several reasons, including the end of product support and disposable pack production for the Alcon Accurus, the much smaller footprint of the VersaVIT, and the lower cost of disposables for the VersaVIT. After airflow through the 30-gauge needle is confirmed in a cup of BSS (patency of the 30-gauge needle to airflow should not be assumed without testing), the tubing attaching the 30-gauge needle to the VersaVIT is laid on the main surgical drapes, run around the face, and redirected inferiorly toward the eye with the stopcock accessible for converting from air to fluid. The needle is then inserted into the angle through a long nasal corneal tunnel with a tangential orientation to the graft circumference and at least 1 mm away from the lenticule edge. The bevel of the needle is directed away from the graft during insertion, and air pressure is typically set to 20 mm Hg just prior to insertion. If the lenticule is dislocated prior to infusion needle insertion, the air pressure should be set to zero for insertion to avoid inadvertent air delivery into the interface, and/or manual reinjection of an air bubble to elevate the graft should be considered first. It is helpful to grasp the sclera adjacent to the site of entry of the needle and to insert the needle using a force directed away from the point of fixation. This puts the tissue on stretch and avoids compressing the cornea, which reduces the risk of inadvertent air escape or destabilizing corneal folds during needle insertion. Air infusion may not be visible initially if the pressure in the anterior chamber is below the infusion pressure. Careful visualization is needed to avoid advancing the needle through the iris, which can inadvertently deliver air to the posterior segment and lead to peripheral iris apposition and angle closure. If the peripheral corneal view is poor, the needle should be inserted with the pressure off and position confirmed prior to pressurization. With appropriate layout of the tubing and the friction of the long insertion tract, the needle can usually be retained in a hands-free fashion without tape.

Air pressure is then increased to 40 mm Hg. A visible reduction in lenticular folds is often appreciated, and we speculate that this smoothing effect on the posterior corneal surface could have some visual quality benefits. Within a minute, the pressure is then increased to 50 or 60 mm Hg, and slow, centripetal corneal strokes with a flat irrigating BSS cannula are performed for about 1 minute with irrigation to avoid inadvertent epithelial debridement. In the absence of hypotony, iOCT generally confirms an immediate apposition of the graft with this maneuver. With the pressure elevated, it is useful to irrigate the paracenteses and primary wound to inspect for air leakage, which may indicate the need for additional sutures. The ability to test the integrity of the wounds under pressurization is a distinct advantage of the technique that likely reduces the risk of postoperative hypotony due to wound leakage. Once apposition is confirmed, the pressure is lowered to 40 mm Hg, and any additional surgical maneuvers such as suture placement, suture burial, or subconjunctival injections can be performed with the advantage that chamber collapse is far less likely than without infusion. We no longer wait 5 to 10 minutes once apposition is confirmed, and immediately proceed to air–fluid exchange. The fluid pressure is set to 30 mm Hg on the vitrectomy unit, and then the stopcock is opened to fluid. Intermittent, gentle insertion of a 30-gauge BSS cannula into a paracentesis is performed until the air bubble diameter is at the desired level and the IOP has equilibrated to the predetermined pressure. The surgeon should wait several seconds after each burping maneuver before repeating since the surface tension of fluid in the tubing and needle is high and flow rates are low. Pressure can be increased above 30 mm Hg if flow is impeded, and the tip of the needle should be rotated or moved slightly to ensure that the tip is not occluded by apposition to the peripheral cornea. The needle is then very slowly withdrawn through the tract, again directing the bevel away from the graft, with the fluid pressure maintained to facilitate hydration of the tract.

12.4 Other Applications of the Air Pump in Endothelial Keratoplasty

The application of continuous air injection into the anterior chamber has found its way into additional steps of the Descemet stripping endothelial keratoplasty (DSEK)/DSAEK procedure, including the descemetorhexis. In the more traditional approach to the stripping of host Descemet membrane, an ophthalmic viscoelastic device (OVD) or air is used to maintain anterior chamber depth. However, many authors have noted difficulties with the use of OVD in DSAEK/DSEK, citing problems with visualization of the Descemet membrane during descemetorhexis and incomplete removal of the OVD leading to donor dislocation.[8,9] Therefore, some have applied the use of a continuous air infusion to maintain the anterior chamber depth through small incision during the descemetorhexis. Mehta and colleagues used an anterior chamber maintainer with an air-filled 60 mL syringe and three-way tap to produce a constant injection of air, which required a surgical assistant. Similar to the use of a continuous pump as in the air pump technique described earlier, Leyland also reported the use of an air exchange pump to maintain anterior chamber depth during descemetorhexis.[10] It is not known if the use of a continuous air pump during this stage of the procedure affects clinical outcome, but it is suggested that it may improve the ease of the procedure and consistency of the results.

References

[1] Price FW, Jr, Price MO. Descemet's stripping with endothelial keratoplasty in 200 eyes: Early challenges and techniques to enhance donor adherence. J Cataract Refract Surg. 2006; 32(3):411–418

[2] Suh LH, Yoo SH, Deobhakta A, et al. Complications of Descemet's stripping with automated endothelial keratoplasty: survey of 118 eyes at One Institute. Ophthalmology. 2008; 115(9):1517–1524

[3] Price MO, Price FW. Descemet's stripping endothelial keratoplasty. Curr Opin Ophthalmol. 2007; 18(4):290–294

[4] Meisler DM, Dupps WJ, Jr, Covert DJ, Koenig SB. Use of an air-fluid exchange system to promote graft adhesion during Descemet's stripping automated endothelial keratoplasty. J Cataract Refract Surg. 2007; 33(5):770–772

[5] Xu D, Dupps WJ, Jr, Srivastava SK, Ehlers JP. Automated volumetric analysis of interface fluid in descemet stripping automated endothelial keratoplasty using intraoperative optical coherence tomography. Invest Ophthalmol Vis Sci. 2014; 55(9):5610–5615

[6] Hallahan KM, Cost B, Goshe JM, Dupps WJ Jr, Srivastava SK, Ehlers JP. Intra-operative Interface Fluid Dynamics and Clinical Outcomes for Intraoperative OCT-Assisted DSAEK from the PIONEER Study. Am J Ophthalmol. 2016; doi: 10.1016/j.ajo.2016.09.028.

[7] Koenig SB, Dupps WJ, Jr, Covert DJ, Meisler DM. Simple technique to unfold the donor corneal lenticule during Descemet's stripping and automated endothelial keratoplasty. J Cataract Refract Surg. 2007; 33(2):189–190

[8] Mehta JS, Hantera MM, Tan DT. Modified air-assisted descemetorhexis for Descemet-stripping automated endothelial keratoplasty. J Cataract Refract Surg. 2008; 34(6):889–891

[9] Leyland M. Anterior chamber maintenance during descemet stripping. Cornea. 2007; 26(10):1292–1293, author reply 1293

[10] Leyland M. Syringe or pump for air-assisted DSAEK. J Cataract Refract Surg. 2009; 35(1):2–, author reply 2

13 Endoilluminator-Assisted Descemet Membrane Endothelial Keratoplasty and Endoilluminator-Assisted Pre-Descemet Endothelial Keratoplasty

Soosan Jacob and Amar Agarwal

Endothelial keratoplasty has evolved from Descemet layer endothelial keratoplasty (DLEK) to Descemet stripping automated endothelial keratoplasty (DSAEK) to Descemet membrane endothelial keratoplasty (DMEK) and Pre-Descemet endothelial keratoplasty (PDEK).[1] DSAEK is popular and has become universally accepted and practiced due partly to the ease of the surgery and the short learning curve. However, DMEK/PDEK is practiced in few centers, mainly because of the greater difficulty in performing the surgery. This difficulty is often compounded by the low visibility of the graft through a hazy cornea. Moreover, the graft is transparent, thin, and flimsy. Therefore, it is difficult to visualize the graft clearly in the anterior chamber after insertion. To overcome this, the graft can be stained with trypan blue. Despite this staining, good visualization often remains challenging through an edematous cornea. Also, the dye washes off in time, and, in the case of a longer surgical time, the inserted graft becomes too difficult to visualize. This chapter describes a technique, endoilluminator-assisted DMEK (E-DMEK) and endoilluminator-assisted PDEK (E-PDEK)[2,3] that enables easy identification of the orientation and visualization of the graft during all surgical steps. It uses oblique light from a vitreoretinal light pipe or an endoilluminator for better visualization.

13.1 Background

The endoilluminator has been used to provide an oblique source of illumination in anterior segment surgery since 1993. It has been used to visualize the anterior capsular flap during capsulorrhexis in hypermature cataracts, to perform cataract surgery in the presence of corneal opacity, for irrigation and aspiration during combined 23-gauge sutureless vitrectomy and cataract surgery, and as an endoilluminated infusion cannula for bimanual anterior chamber vitrectomy. Chandelier illumination has been used during DSAEK since 2011 via a chandelier illumination fiber inserted through the corneal side port to provide sclerotic scattering-like illumination from the sclerocorneal margin and endoillumination from the anterior chamber, resulting in excellent visibility for Descemet stripping and intraocular manipulation without obstruction from a hazy cornea. However, it has not been reported in patients undergoing DMEK/PDEK. The use of the endoilluminator for DMEK/PDEK is a logical extension of its previous uses. Because DMEK/PDEK is more challenging, the use of an endoilluminator is comparatively more valuable. E-DMEK/E-PDEK makes surgery simpler by allowing good visualization and better surgeon understanding of graft morphology and dynamics.

13.2 Surgical Technique

One of the key steps in DMEK/PDEK is determining the descemetic side of the graft. The descemetic side needs to face the overlying corneal stroma. This will allow the graft to be appropriately apposed to the stroma on injection of an air bubble. The key to being sure about the correct orientation of the graft is to look at the direction toward which the edges of the graft are curling. Because the Descemet membrane is an elastic structure, the graft edges always curl toward the stroma. Therefore, intraoperatively, the graft must be oriented with the curve facing upward. This is often difficult to confirm with the current techniques. Because the graft is transparent, it is difficult to ascertain the direction of the curvature of the edges, even in an eye with good visibility.

In DMEK the graft is prepared as usual with the submerged cornea using backgrounds away (SCUBA) technique described by Gimbel et al.[4,5] This allows easy preparation of the graft with less chance of damage and tearing. Another technique is to punch the donor to the desired size, followed by submerging the button in storage medium. The edge of the Descemet membrane is then gently grasped with a fine, nontoothed forceps and stripped from all sides, carefully avoiding any uncontrolled tears (▶ Fig. 13.1a, b). The graft is sized 0.5 mm smaller than the proposed recipient bed. The recipient bed is prepared by externally marking the surface of the cornea with a blunt trephine. The Descemet membrane is then scored with a reverse Sinskey hook and stripped. Once this is done, the DMEK graft is stained with trypan blue 0.1%. The graft is loaded into an injector using the technique described by Price et al. The spring coil is removed from the Viscoject injector (Medicel), and the silicone tip is replaced (▶ Fig. 13.1c, d). The graft is then placed into the 1.8 mm Viscoglide cartridge (Medicel) (▶ Fig. 13.1e, f). The cartridge is loaded onto the injector (▶ Fig. 13.1g). A microincision keratome is used to create a 2.2 mm temporal clear corneal incision, and a paracentesis is created 90 degrees away temporally. A small inferior peripheral iridectomy is created now (it may also have been created preoperatively using a neodymium:yttrium-aluminum-garnet (Nd:YAG) laser. Using the injector, the surgeon gently injects the graft into the anterior chamber, and the incisions are sutured (▶ Fig. 13.1h). At this point, the microscope light is turned off, and the endoilluminator or light probe (20, 23, or 25 gauge) is used as an oblique source of illumination to enhance visualization. It is held externally by the surgeon or by an assistant while the surgeon continues surgery bimanually. The tangential light provided by the endoilluminator is used to show details of the graft, folds in the grafts, and the position and orientation of the Descemet membrane in relation to the corneal stroma. The tip of the light probe is moved around the limbus while focusing it tangentially to allow good visualization and three-dimensional perception. The direction of graft edge curvature, and thereby graft orientation, is confirmed by tapping the host cornea gently and appreciating the reflexes created by the light bouncing off the edges of the graft and by seeing the movement induced in the graft (▸ Fig. 13.2 and ▸ Fig. 13.3). Using endoillumination, the graft is oriented the right way up and centered under the stripped recipient site, after which an air bubble is injected under the graft to float it up against the overlying stroma. At any time during the surgery, the surgeon can switch back and forth between the microscope light and the endoilluminator. Intraocular pressure and light perception are checked before closing the eye. The patient is asked to maintain a strict supine position for the first 24 hours.

13.3 Advantages of the Endoilluminator-Assisted Procedure

The tangential light provided by the endoilluminator details the graft, the folds in the graft, its position, and the orientation of the Descemet membrane. Moving the tip of the light probe around the limbus while keeping it tangentially focused allows good visualization and three-dimensional depth perception. Keeping only the operating microscope light on makes it difficult to determine whether the edges are curving upward or downward. It also decreases the unusually clear three-dimensional depth perception of the surgeon because of the transparent nature of the graft. Even in a nonedematous, clear cornea, it is often difficult to confirm the direction of the curvature of the

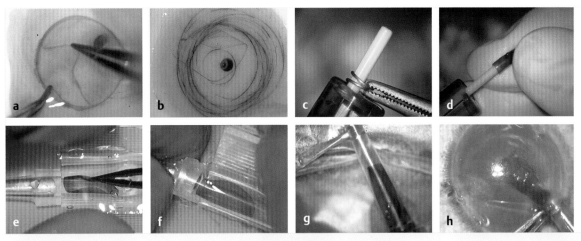

Fig. 13.1 (a) The Descemet membrane endothelial keratoplasty (DMEK) graft is prepared by keeping the corneoscleral button submerged in storage medium. The edge of the Descemet membrane is held and gently separated from the stroma. (b) The DMEK graft is seen with its edges curving toward the Descemet membrane. (c) The spring coil of a Viscoject injector (Medicel) is removed. (d) The soft silicone tip is replaced. (e) The DMEK graft is loaded into the Viscoglide cartridge (Medicel) with the correct orientation. (f) The cartridge is closed and loaded onto the injector. (g) The DMEK graft is injected forward to the tip of the cartridge. (h) The graft is injected into the anterior chamber.

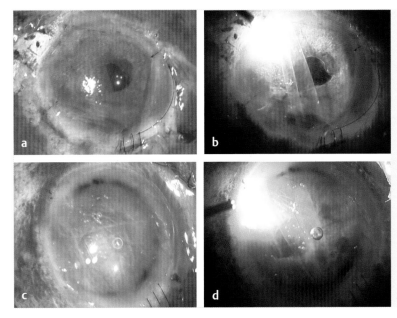

Fig. 13.2 (a) Media opacity prevents clear and adequate visualization of the Descemet membrane endothelial keratoplasty (DMEK) graft under the microscope light. (b) In the endoilluminator-assisted DMEK (E-DMEK) technique, using an obliquely directed endoilluminator and switching off the microscope light provides three-dimensional depth perception of the graft while allowing visualization of the entire graft and views from different angles. This allows better surgeon comprehension of graft dynamics, morphology, and positioning, in turn leading to easier and faster surgery while potentially decreasing graft damage due to prolonged surgery and excessive manipulations. (c) The graft viewed under microscope light, which decreases visualization. (d) The graft viewed with an endoilluminator is clearer.

scrolled edges with the operating microscope light alone, and the surgeon may have to use an instrument inserted under the scroll edge to confirm the direction of the roll (Moutsouri's sign).[6] With E-DMEK, the light reflexes that are created by the tangential endoilluminator light falling on the folds and edges of the graft allow confirmation of the direction of the curvature of the graft edges and thereby graft orientation while maintaining a no-touch technique, thus decreasing cell loss in the graft. E-DMEK also allows movements induced in the graft during various maneuvers to be easily seen by the surgeon. The handheld slit beam technique for DMEK surgery was described by Burkhart et al in 2013.[7] However, E-DMEK has the advantages of allowing views of the entire graft rather than only a slit view and not requiring scanning across the graft for a more complete view. The endoilluminator gives a clear view of the entire graft. The strong, focused light of the probe is able to pierce through the edematous cornea and allow easy visualization. The authors prefer holding the endoilluminator close to the corneal surface externally as opposed to inserting it into the anterior chamber, where it produces excessive sclerotic scattering of the light. When directed tangentially, it provides excellent visualization. Inserting the endoilluminator into the anterior chamber also tends to cause wound leakage and shallowing of the anterior chamber, and it occupies space within the anterior chamber, thus interfering with the free movement of the graft and hindering graft flotation.

E-DMEK allows better three-dimensional visualization and depth perception, thereby providing a better understanding of graft morphology, position, orientation, and dynamics. It is a valuable technique to enhance surgical ease, speed, and success for the DMEK surgeon. Potential graft damage caused by excessive handling and maneuvering within the eye is decreased (▸ Fig. 13.4).

PDEK also needs an endoilluminator for visualization, and the same principle is used as in E-DMEK (▸ Fig. 13.5 and ▸ Fig. 13.6)

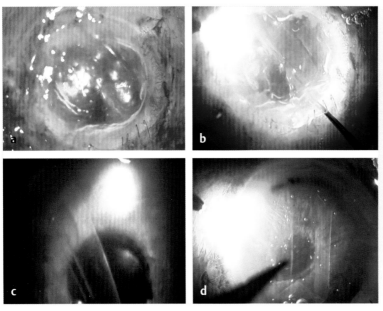

Fig. 13.3 **(a)** The graft is seen under the microscope light after apposition to the overlying stroma with an air bubble. **(b)** In the same eye, the folded edge at the inferior aspect is seen well only with endoilluminator-assisted Descemet membrane endothelial keratoplasty (E-DMEK). **(c)** Folds and edges in the graft bounce light and create reflections, which allows easier perception of orientation. **(d)** Graft details through an edematous cornea via E-DMEK.

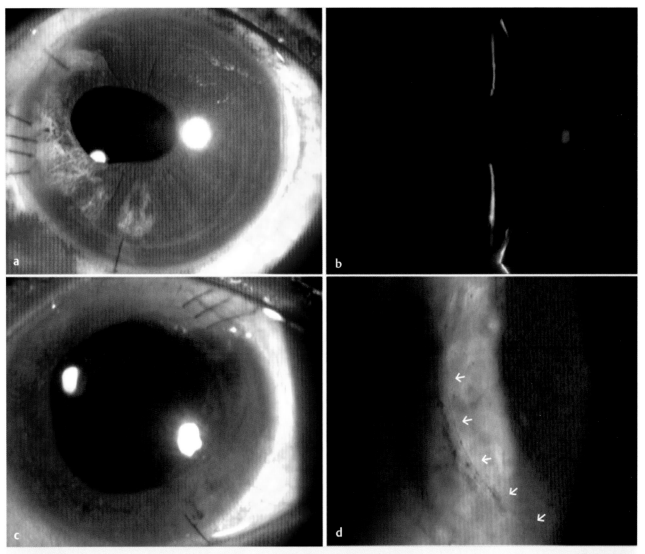

Fig. 13.4 (a) Appearance of the cornea at 1 month postoperative follow-up. (b) Slit view of the same patient shows a nonedematous cornea and attached graft. The inferior edge of the graft can be seen. (c) Appearance of a clear cornea in a different patient on postoperative day 10. (d) The attached graft margin is shown (arrowheads).

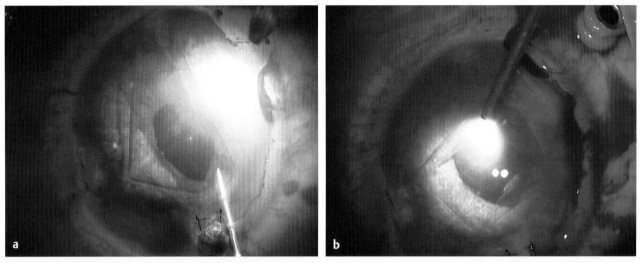

Fig. 13.5 Endoilluminator assisted pre-Descemet endothelial keratoplasty (E-PDEK). **(a)** Note that, when using an endoilluminator one can see the edges are rolled inward. This indicates the PDEK graft is upside down. **(b)** The edges of the PDEK graft are rolled upward, which is now the correct side.

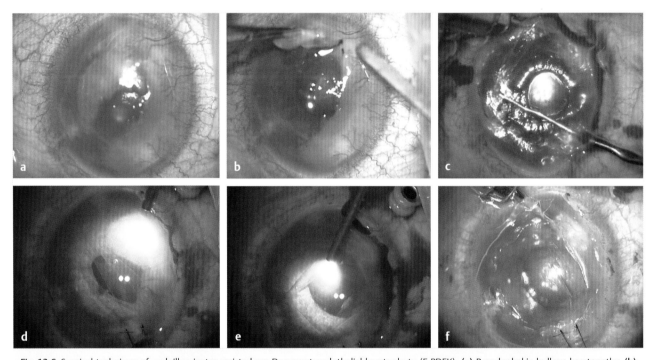

Fig. 13.6 Surgical technique of endoilluminator-assisted pre-Descemet endothelial keratoplasty (E-PDEK). **(a)** Pseudophakic bullous keratopathy. **(b)** Epithelium removed. **(c)** Descematorhexis. **(d)** PDEK graft inside the anterior chamber. E-PDEK checks graft is correctly oriented. **(e)** Graft opening up and seen clearly with E-PDEK. **(f)** PDEK graft attached.

References

[1] Dua HS, Faraj LA, Said DG, Gray T, Lowe J. Human corneal anatomy redefined: A novel pre-Descemet's layer (Dua's layer). Ophthalmology. 2013; 120 (9):1778–1785

[2] Agarwal A, Dua HS, Narang P, et al. Pre-Descemet's endothelial keratoplasty (PDEK). Br J Ophthalmol. 2014; 98(9):1181–1185

[3] Jacob S, Agarwal A, Kumar DA. Endoilluminator-assisted Descemet membrane endothelial keratoplasty and endoilluminator-assisted pre-Descemet endothelial keratoplasty. Clin Ophthalmol. 2015; 9:2123–2125

[4] SCUBA technique for DMEK donor preparation. https://www.youtube.com/watch?v=vpToO8PFsvI. Accessed on 23/11/16

[5] Brissette A1, Conlon R, Teichman JC, Yeung S, Ziai S, Baig K. Evaluation of a new technique for preparation of endothelial grafts for Descemet Membrane Endothelial Keratoplasty. Cornea. 2015 May;34(5):557-9.

[6] Dapena I, Moutsouris K, Droutsas K, Ham L, van Dijk K, Melles GRJ. Standardized 'no touch' technique for Descemet membrane endothelial keratoplasty (DMEK). http://2012.eeba.eu/files/presentation_IV.a_key_note_Dapena_Standardized_no_touch_technique_for_DMEK.pdf. Accessed on 23/11/16

[7] Burkhart, ZN, Feng, MT, Price, MO, Price, F.W. Handheld slit beam techniques to facilitate DMEK and DALK. Cornea 2013;32(5):722-724.

14 Descemet Membrane Endothelial Keratoplasty Modifications and Nonkeratoplasty Concepts: Hemi-DMEK and Descemet Membrane Endothelial Transfer

Salvatore Luceri, Lamis Baydoun, Isabel Dapena, and Gerrit R.J. Melles

The introduction of the Descemet membrane keratoplasty (DMEK) resulted in the improvement of postoperative clinical outcomes and a reduction of complication rates as compared to previous techniques, especially in eyes with Fuchs endothelial corneal dystrophy (FECD).[1] In addition, DMEK also provided new insight into corneal endothelial cell biology and physiology.[2] Clinical observations after standard (circular) DMEK suggested that corneal clearing may not only depend on complete coverage of the denuded stroma after removal of the diseased Descemet membrane and endothelium (descemetorhexis). In eyes with decentered grafts, corneal clearance was also observed in bare stromal area between the graft and the edge of the descemetorhexis.[3] Furthermore, corneal clearing may also not rely on complete donor-to-host apposition, as seen in eyes with a (partially) detached DMEK graft.[4,5] These observations led to further modifications of the standard DMEK technique, such as using half-moon-shaped grafts (hemi-DMEK), and nonkeratoplasty surgical approaches, such as performing a descemetorhexis only or a descemetorhexis with a free-floating graft secured in the main incision (Descemet membrane endothelial transfer [DMET]).

14.1 Hemi-Descemet Membrane Endothelial Keratoplasty (Hemi-DMEK)

A recent modification of DMEK, the so-called hemi-DMEK, was based on (1) the clinical observation that no complete coverage of the entire denuded recipient stroma by a graft is required in order to achieve corneal clearance, and (2) the idea to reduce endothelial tissue shortage.[3,6,7,8] With the introduction of DMEK, more efficient use of corneal donor tissue became feasible because it was now possible to generate two transplants from one donor cornea. The donor cornea could be split in such a way that the posterior part of the donor cornea could be used as a DMEK graft, and the remaining anterior part could be used as a transplant for deep anterior lamellar keratoplasty (DALK).[9,10,11,12] This approach, however, could not reduce endothelial tissue shortage because only one endothelial graft could be obtained from one donor cornea.

For penetrating keratoplasty (PK) and Descemet stripping (automated) endothelial keratoplasty (DSEK/DSAEK), where the graft is generally thicker at the periphery than in the center, a centrally trephined transplant is required for optical reasons. A DMEK graft, however, is evenly thin over its whole surface area because it consists only of Descemet membrane and endothelium. Therefore, for DMEK, the peripheral portions of the graft could also be used without resulting in optical impairment. Thus, in 2014 the Melles group introduced the concept of hemi-DMEK, in which a half-moon-shaped (semicircular) Descemet

membrane graft is prepared from one untrephined 11.5 to 12 mm (full) diameter donor Descemet membrane sheet (▶ Fig. 14.1). In contrast to standard DMEK graft preparation, where only the trephined central 8.5 to 9.5 mm circular DMEK graft is used and the outer Descemet membrane rim is discarded, in hemi-DMEK, two semicircular grafts for two recipients may be used from one *untrephined*, full-diameter Descemet membrane sheet, potentially doubling the number of endothelial grafts harvested from the same donor pool.[13] Since the total surface area of the half-moon-shaped graft is similar to the standard (circular) DMEK graft, the graft shape may be the main difference between both techniques. As a result, for the first time two endothelial transplants could be obtained from one donor corneal button.

A small case series of patients with FECD showed that visual outcomes at 6 and 12 months after hemi-DMEK are comparable to those after standard DMEK.[14,15,16]

Despite the shape mismatch between the circular descemetorhexis and the semicircular hemi-DMEK graft, corneal clearance occurred over the entire cornea by 3 to 6 months postoperatively (▶ Fig. 14.2), also over initially bare stromal areas (denuded of Descemet membrane).[14,15] Similar observations have been made after standard DMEK in eyes with a decentered graft or a partially detached DMEK graft, suggesting that, besides donor endothelium, host endothelial cells may also be actively involved in corneal clearance after endothelial keratoplasty.[3,5] It should be noted, however, that endothelial cell density after hemi-DMEK appears to be lower for the currently available study group as compared to endothelial cell density after standard DMEK. Longer follow-up data may show whether further endothelial cell density decline is comparable for hemi-DMEK and standard DMEK.

Longer follow-up data and data of larger study groups should show whether, besides visual outcomes, allograft rejection rates and graft survival in hemi-DMEK prove to be similar to standard DMEK. Hemi-DMEK could then become the next step in endothelial keratoplasty for the treatment of FECD, potentially doubling the pool of endothelial graft tissue.

14.2 Descemet Membrane Endothelial Transfer (DMET)

The observation that complete donor–to-host apposition may not (always) be required for corneal transparency and deturgescence after posterior lamellar keratoplasty in eyes with graft detachment after DSAEK[17] and DMEK[4,5] has questioned the concept of keratoplasty.[2]

In eyes with 50% graft detachment/apposition after DMEK, endothelial cells were also detected over the recipient bare stroma underlying the detachment, suggesting an active role of endothelial cells in migration and redistribution as a healing

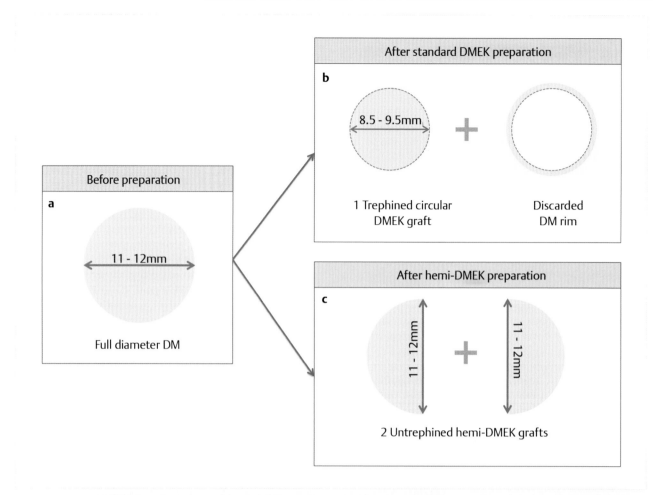

Fig. 14.1 Graft preparation from **(a)** a full diameter (11–12 mm) corneoscleral button to achieve **(b)** one single (trephined) standard Descemet membrane endothelial keratoplasty (DMEK) graft or **(c)** two (untrephined) semicircular hemi-DMEK grafts. The overall endothelial surface area of each untrephined hemi-DMEK graft is similar to that of a trephined circular standard DMEK graft. Assuming a transplant with a homogeneous curvature, the posterior corneal curvature can be calculated using the formula for calculating the surface area of a spherical cap,[29] which gives a posterior corneal surface area for a standard circular DMEK (9 mm) of 73 mm^2 and of 69 mm^2 for a hemi-DMEK graft (11.5 mm). (Figure has been published in Lam et al[15]; reproduced with permission of Graefes Arch Clin Exp Ophthalmol.)

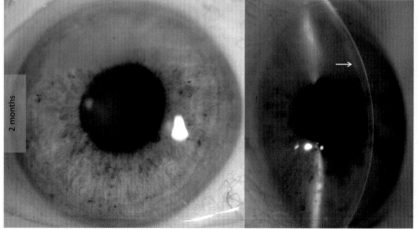

Fig. 14.2 Slit-lamp image at 2 months after hemi-DMEK. In this case, the graft has been positioned horizontally with its straight edge inferiorly, the latter initially being underlined by pigment deposition. Denuded stromal areas in the inferior cornea showed slower clearance than the central cornea, but it was complete by 2 months. Superior cornea, edematous in the area overlying an initial small peripheral graft detachment (white arrow), was the last to clear up. Best-corrected visual acuity was 20/22 (0.9) at 2 months postoperatively.

response after keratoplasty.[3] These observations suggested that it is possible to reestablish corneal clearance in the presence of at least some physical contact between the donor graft and host stroma.

These observations led to the concept of Descemet membrane endothelial transfer (DMET). This new nonkeratoplasty concept introduced by Melles and colleagues is based on injecting a Descemet roll into the anterior chamber and securing it in the main incision after performing a descemetorhexis to remove the diseased tissue (▶ Fig. 14.3).[5,18,19] This technique would be an immense simplification of standard DMEK because challenging surgical steps, such as graft unfolding and graft attachment, may be skipped and surgery duration would be significantly shortened. However, corneal clearance in DMET may take up to 6 months, and endothelial cell densities may be significantly lower at 6 months postoperatively.[5,19]

Key to DMET is a repopulation of the posterior stroma by endothelial cells, either from the graft or from the recipient Descemet rim or both. In a first series of 12 eyes comparing DMET clinical outcomes in eyes with FECD (primarily a

Descemet membrane disorder) and with bullous keratopathy (primarily an endothelial depletion), the surgery was effective only in the first group in terms of reendothelialization of the recipient bare posterior stroma and corneal clearance. No improvement was reported in eyes with bullous keratopathy, thus allegedly indicating a primary role of the recipient endothelium in achieving corneal clearance.[5]

If migration of the remaining peripheral host endothelial cells in eyes with FECD would potentially allow repopulation of the posterior stroma after a central descemetorhexis, that is, by eliminating the guttae, which presumably are the pathological and physical barrier for cells to migrate,[20] then, like DMET, a descemetorhexis alone could be another possible treatment approach. However, until now there are only anecdotal cases of corneal clearance after a descemetorhexis without graft implantation, so that there is no consistent proof for its efficacy.[21,22,23,24,25]

Although DMET and descemetorhexis alone have not been implemented as nonkeratoplasty treatment options in clinical practice, DMET may have questioned the description of FECD as

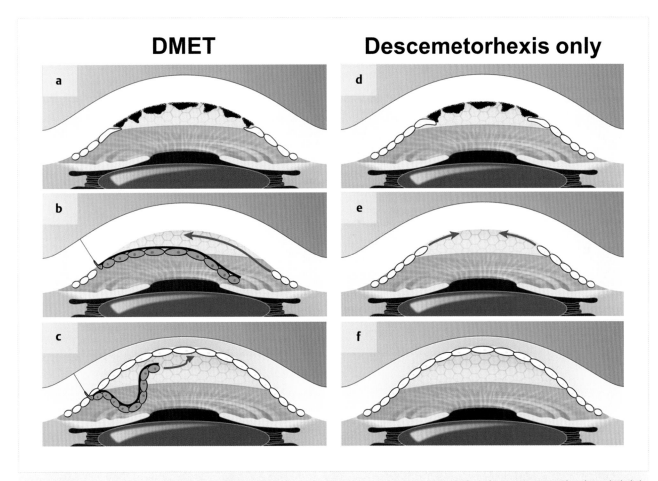

Fig. 14.3 Mechanisms behind Descemet membrane endothelial transfer (DMET) and a descemetorhexis-only in the management of Fuchs endothelial corneal dystrophy. Regarding DMET, the donor graft is thought to induce recipient endothelial migration. **(a)** Regarding descemetorhexis, clinical observations indicate that by removing the guttae that may act as barriers to the migration of peripheral stemlike cells, and **(b)** by inserting a free-floating donor tissue (green) attached to the incision, migration of the recipient endothelial cells should be induced. **(c)** Consequently, recipient endothelial cells may be more effective than donor ones in covering the bare stroma and restoring corneal transparency. **(d, e, f)** In early stages of Fuchs endothelial corneal dystrophy (FED) the guttae have not progressed to the far periphery; thus a sufficient amount of peripheral stemlike cells might be sufficient to induce recipient endothelial migration. Consequently, descemetorhexis would act as a simple removal of a physical barrier to the proliferation and migration of peripheral recipient endothelial cells. (Figure has been published in Bruinsma et al[2]; reproduced with permission of EYE.)

a dystrophy and allowed us to gain a deeper understanding of the processes involved in endothelial cell wound healing. This insight might also have led to further developments for the treatment of FECD and potential alternative approaches, such as cell injections or drug therapies.[26,27,28]

14.3 Conclusion

Clinical observations after DMEK have led to a better understanding of the corneal endothelium and opened the door to alternative treatment options. Modifications of the standard DMEK technique might simplify existing surgical techniques and also allow for a more efficient use of donor tissue.

References

[1] Rodríguez-Calvo-de-Mora M, Quilendrino R, Ham L, et al. Clinical outcome of 500 consecutive cases undergoing Descemet's membrane endothelial keratoplasty. Ophthalmology. 2015; 122(3):464–470

[2] Bruinsma M, Tong CM, Melles GRJ. What does the future hold for the treatment of Fuchs endothelial dystrophy; will 'keratoplasty' still be a valid procedure? Eye (Lond). 2013; 27(10):1115–1122

[3] Dirisamer M, Dapena I, Ham L, et al. Patterns of corneal endothelialization and corneal clearance after Descemet membrane endothelial keratoplasty for fuchs endothelial dystrophy. Am J Ophthalmol. 2011; 152(4):543–555.e1

[4] Balachandran C, Ham L, Verschoor CA, Ong TS, van der Wees J, Melles GR. Spontaneous corneal clearance despite graft detachment in Descemet membrane endothelial keratoplasty. Am J Ophthalmol. 2009; 148(2):227–234.e1

[5] Dirisamer M, Yeh RY, van Dijk K, Ham L, Dapena I, Melles GR. Recipient endothelium may relate to corneal clearance in Descemet membrane endothelial transfer. Am J Ophthalmol. 2012; 154(2):290–296.e1

[6] Tourtas T, Heindl LM, Kopsachilis N, Bachmann BO, Kruse FE, Cursiefen C. Use of accidentally torn Descemet membrane to successfully complete descemet membrane endothelial keratoplasty. Cornea. 2013; 32(11):1418–1422

[7] Gaum L, Reynolds I, Jones MN, Clarkson AJ, Gillan HL, Kaye SB. Tissue and corneal donation and transplantation in the UK. Br J Anaesth. 2012; 108 Suppl 1: i43–i47

[8] Vajpayee RB, Sharma N, Jhanji V, Titiyal JS, Tandon R. One donor cornea for 3 recipients: a new concept for corneal transplantation surgery. Arch Ophthalmol. 2007; 125(4):552–554

[9] Lie JT, Groeneveld-van Beek EA, Ham L, van der Wees J, Melles GR. More efficient use of donor corneal tissue with Descemet membrane endothelial keratoplasty (DMEK): two lamellar keratoplasty procedures with one donor cornea. Br J Ophthalmol. 2010; 94(9):1265–1266

[10] Heindl LM, Riss S, Laaser K, Bachmann BO, Kruse FE, Cursiefen C. Split cornea transplantation for 2 recipients - review of the first 100 consecutive patients. Am J Ophthalmol. 2011; 152(4):523–532.e2

[11] Heindl LM, Riss S, Bachmann BO, Laaser K, Kruse FE, Cursiefen C. Split cornea transplantation for 2 recipients: a new strategy to reduce corneal tissue cost and shortage. Ophthalmology. 2011; 118(2):294–301

[12] Groeneveld-van Beek EA, Lie JT, van der Wees J, Bruinsma M, Melles GR. Standardized 'no-touch' donor tissue preparation for DALK and DMEK: harvesting undamaged anterior and posterior transplants from the same donor cornea. Acta Ophthalmol (Copenh). 2013; 91(2):145–150

[13] Lie JT, Lam FC, Groeneveld-van Beek EA, van der Wees J, Melles GRJ. Graft preparation for hemi-Descemet membrane endothelial keratoplasty (hemi-DMEK). Br J Ophthalmol. 2016; 100(3):420–424

[14] Lam FC, Baydoun L, Dirisamer M, Lie J, Dapena I, Melles GR. Hemi-Descemet membrane endothelial keratoplasty transplantation: a potential method for increasing the pool of endothelial graft tissue. JAMA Ophthalmol. 2014; 132 (12):1469–1473

[15] Lam FC, Baydoun L, Satué M, Dirisamer M, Ham L, Melles GR. One year outcome of hemi-Descemet membrane endothelial keratoplasty. Graefes Arch Clin Exp Ophthalmol. 2015; 253(11):1955–1958

[16] Gerber-Hollbach N, Parker J, Baydoun L, et al. Preliminary outcome of hemi-Descemet membrane endothelial keratoplasty for Fuchs endothelial dystrophy. Br J Ophthalmol. 2016; pii. DOI: doi:10.1136/bjophthalmol-2015–307783

[17] Zafirakis P, Kymionis GD, Grentzelos MA, Livir-Rallatos G. Corneal graft detachment without corneal edema after descemet stripping automated endothelial keratoplasty. Cornea. 2010; 29(4):456–458

[18] Dirisamer M, Ham L, Dapena I, van Dijk K, Melles GRJ. Descemet membrane endothelial transfer: "free-floating" donor Descemet implantation as a potential alternative to "keratoplasty". Cornea. 2012; 31(2):194–197

[19] Lam FC, Bruinsma M, Melles GRJ. Descemet membrane endothelial transfer. Curr Opin Ophthalmol. 2014; 25(4):353–357

[20] Moshirfar M, Kim G. The role of host endothelial cell proliferation in descemet membrane endothelial transfer. Cornea. 2013; 32(2):218–219

[21] Ham L, Dapena I, Moutsouris K, Melles GR. Persistent corneal edema after descemetorhexis without corneal graft implantation in a case of fuchs endothelial dystrophy. Cornea. 2011; 30(2):248–249

[22] Shah RD, Randleman JB, Grossniklaus HE. Spontaneous corneal clearing after Descemet's stripping without endothelial replacement. Ophthalmology. 2012; 119(2):256–260

[23] Bleyen I, Saelens IE, van Dooren BT, van Rij G. Spontaneous corneal clearing after Descemet's stripping. Ophthalmology. 2013; 120(1):215

[24] Arbelaez JG, Price MO, Price FW, Jr. Long-term follow-up and complications of stripping descemet membrane without placement of graft in eyes with Fuchs endothelial dystrophy. Cornea. 2014; 33(12):1295–1299

[25] Fernández E, Lam FC, Bruinsma M, Baydoun L, Dapena I, Melles GRJ. Fuchs endothelial corneal dystrophy: current treatment recommendations and experimental surgical options. Expert Rev Ophthalmol. 2015; 10:301–312

[26] Patel SV, Bachman LA, Hann CR, Bahler CK, Fautsch MP. Human corneal endothelial cell transplantation in a human ex vivo model. Invest Ophthalmol Vis Sci. 2009; 50(5):2123–2131

[27] Okumura N, Koizumi N, Ueno M, et al. ROCK inhibitor converts corneal endothelial cells into a phenotype capable of regenerating in vivo endothelial tissue. Am J Pathol. 2012; 181(1):268–277

[28] Koizumi N, Okumura N, Ueno M, Kinoshita S. New therapeutic modality for corneal endothelial disease using Rho-associated kinase inhibitor eye drops. Cornea. 2014; 33 Suppl 11:S25–S31

[29] Quilendrino R, Höhn H, Tse WH, et al. Do we overestimate the endothelial cell "loss" after descemet membrane endothelial keratoplasty? Curr Eye Res. 2013; 38(2):260–265

15 Endothelial Keratoplasty Including Pre-Descemet Endothelial Keratoplasty with Glued Intraocular Lens

Ashvin Agarwal, Priya Narang, and Amar Agarwal

15.1 Introduction

Glued intraocular lens (IOL) was introduced in 2007 as a technique for sutureless scleral fixation of the IOL via trans-scleral haptic tuck in patients with absent or deficient capsular support.[1,2,3,4,5,6,7,8,9,10,11,12,13] This may be done as a primary procedure during cataract extraction in case of posterior capsular rupture (PCR) and deficient capsule or as a secondary procedure in an aphakic patient. It may also be used for closed chamber translocation of a malpositioned or subluxated three-piece IOL. However, many of these patients who need primary or secondary glued IOL implantation have already undergone complicated cataract surgery with an inability to implant an IOL in the bag during the cataract extraction. Therefore the chances of endothelial damage and the consequent need for a keratoplasty are also higher in these patients. Depending on the severity of endothelial damage and corneal scarring the patient may require either a penetrating keratoplasty (PK) or an endothelial keratoplasty (EK).

15.2 Glued IOL with Penetrating Keratoplasty

Glued IOL may be combined with PK when there is associated stromal scarring. The PK can be done with the help of a femtosecond laser. The advantages of glued IOL with PK as compared to other forms of secondary IOL fixation are the relatively short open-sky time as well as the sturdy fixation of the IOL.

15.3 Glued IOL with Endothelial Keratoplasty

In patients with predominantly endothelial damage, EK may be performed instead of PK. The advantages over PK include a closed chamber technique with faster visual recovery, better vision quality, less induction of irregular astigmatism, decreased chances of rejection, and fewer surface and suture-related problems. There is also likely to be less postoperative refractive surprise with EK as compared to PK. Glued IOL can be combined with Descemet stripping automated endothelial keratoplasty (DSAEK), Descemet membrane endothelial keratoplasty (DMEK), or pre-Descemet endothelial keratoplasty (PDEK). It may also be done as a staged procedure, with the glued IOL performed first and EK in a second sitting.

15.4 Principles of Combining Glued IOL with Endothelial Keratoplasty

In aphakic eyes, a loss of bicamerality of the eye leads to posterior migration of the air bubble used for attaching the EK graft. This increases the risk for a consequent postoperative partial or total graft detachment, forward bowing of the iris, iris–graft touch, graft dislocation into the vitreous, and so on, all of which can necessitate secondary procedures, such as refloating, rebubbling, vitrectomy, anterior chamber (AC) formation, and so on, in turn increasing graft endothelial cell loss. An effective compartmentalization of the eye can be obtained through the glued IOL technique. The glued IOL offers advantages of posterior chamber IOL placement, ease of centration, scleral fixation, as well as stable and sturdy fixation without pseudophakodonesis. It is therefore our preferred technique when combining with EK unlike AC IOL placement, which has disadvantages of decreased AC space, iris-fixated IOLs (which require intact iris all around), as well as sutured scleral-fixated IOL (which has disadvantages of greater pseudophakodonesis and greater difficulty in centration) (▶ Fig. 15.1, ▶ Fig. 15.2, ▶ Fig. 15.3).

The procedure is started as a conventional glued IOL. An AC maintainer or a trocar AC maintainer is inserted. Conjunctival flaps and lamellar scleral flaps are made 180 degrees apart. Sclerotomies (20/22 gauge) are made under the scleral flap ~ 1 mm from the limbus. This is followed by a limited 23-gauge vitrectomy through the sclerotomies followed by glued IOL implantation. The haptics are tucked in the Scharioth pockets, and the flaps may be glued down. As the posterior capsule is unlikely to be intact, there is still a chance of posterior migration of air that is injected into the AC for graft support. Migration of air behind the IOL leads to insufficient support for the graft with consequent graft detachment. It is therefore imperative to have a good iris–IOL diaphragm separating the anterior chamber from the vitreous cavity. Therefore, when combining a glued IOL with EK, the sclerotomy should be made slightly closer to the limbus than usual in order to decrease the potential gap between the iris and the IOL. At the same time, an iridoplasty should be done to obtain a round pupil that overlaps the IOL optic all around. Once this is done the adequacy of air fill is checked by turning off the infusion and checking for the air fill. If inadequate, the pupil may need to become smaller or the IOL may need to come closer to the iris. A well formed iris–IOL diaphragm prevents air from going back into the vitreous cavity and allows good postoperative support for the graft. Once the air fill is found to be adequate, air is attached to the AC maintainer (ACM) through an air pump, and host descemetorhexis is

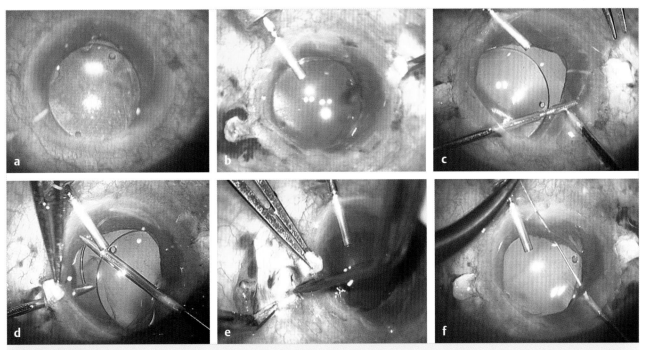

Fig. 15.1 Pre-Descemet endothelial keratoplasty (PDEK) with glued intraocular lens (IOL) (Part 1). **(a)** Pseudophakic bullous keratopathy. Note the corneal haze and a single-piece, nonfoldable posterior chamber IOL in the anterior chamber (AC). **(b)** AC maintainer fixed. One can also fix a trocar AC maintainer or a trocar cannula in the pars plana. Two sclera flaps created 180 degrees apart and a 20/22-gauge sclerotomy created with a needle 1 mm from the limbus. **(c)** After vitrectomy, the haptics are grasped with glued IOL forceps and externalized using the handshake technique. **(d)** One should be careful when externalizing the haptics because this is a single-piece, nonfoldable IOL. If the haptic breaks the IOL can be explanted and replaced with a three-piece IOL. **(e)** Scharioth pocket created with a 26-gauge needle and haptics tucked within them. **(f)** Pupilloplasty done.

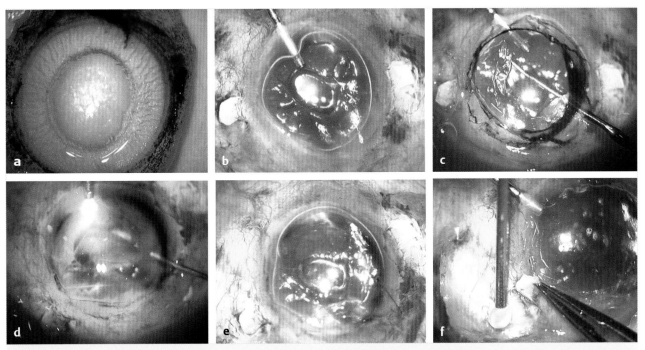

Fig. 15.2 Pre-Descemet endothelial keratoplasty (PDEK) with glued intraocular lens (IOL) (Part 2). **(a)** Type 1 big bubble is created. The PDEK can be performed in one sitting with the glued IOL. It is better to do in two steps so that the glued IOL heals well and a month later PDEK is performed. Another advantage is that donor corneas are not readily available and one can do the glued IOL and wait for a good donor cornea to do the PDEK. **(b)** Air pump–assisted PDEK. The air pump is connected to the trocar anterior compartment (AC) maintainer or AC maintainer so that air is continuously flowing inside the AC. If one is doing PDEK with glued IOL in one sitting it is better to have a trocar cannula in the pars plana with fluid being passed inside and an AC maintainer or a trocar AC maintainer in the AC passing air. This way there will not be any hypotony and one can control the amount of fluid being passed inside the eye. **(c)** Descemetorhexis. **(d)** The PDEK graft is injected inside the AC and unrolled with the help of endoilluminator-assisted PDEK. **(e)** The graft is attached. **(f)** Glue is applied.

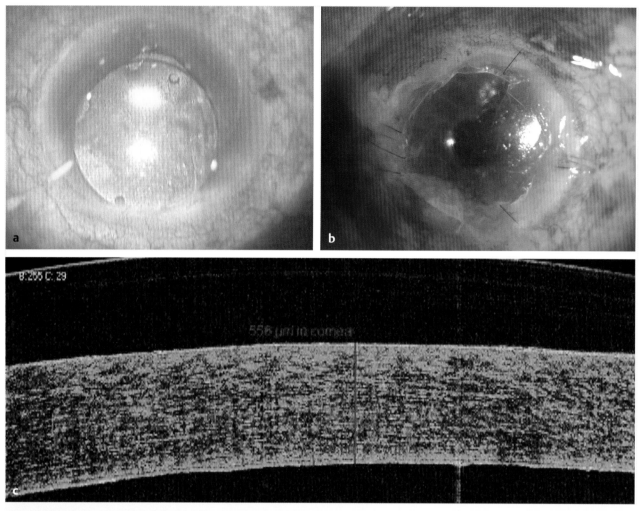

Fig. 15.3 Pre Descemet's Endothelial Keratoplasty (PDEK) with glued IOL (Part 3) **(a)** Pre op **(b)** One day post op **(c)** Anterior segment OCT shows an attached graft.

performed. The EK graft is then injected into the AC, unfolded, and floated up using air. In cases with subluxated or dislocated three-piece IOL needing EK, a closed chamber translocation of the subluxated IOL into a glued IOL may be done using the handshake technique. This is followed by iridoplasty, if required, and EK.

Cases with a malpositioned single-piece IOL requiring explantation or an AC IOL need an enlargement of the wound followed by explantation of the IOL. This is followed by the technique already described. Construction of a scleral tunnel for IOL explantation or a 3 mm L-shaped scleral tunnel incision gives very good wound closure and excellent AC stability.

A potential complication that may occur on combining a glued IOL with EK is the risk for hypotonous and subsequent graft detachment in the postoperative period. Hypotony can lead to detachment of the EK graft from the eyelids pushing on the cornea with normal lid movements. This risk can be decreased by making sure that the globe is adequately pressurized at the end of surgery. As noted, this is done by achieving an adequately tight air bubble in the AC. If the globe still feels hypotonic, air is injected through the pars plicata into the vitreous cavity with a 30-gauge needle under direct visualization of the needle tip in the vitreous cavity. At the conclusion of

surgery, it should also be ensured that the sclerotomies are well sealed by the scleral flaps using fibrin glue. All corneal incisions should be leakproof and may also be sealed using fibrin glue to avoid any postoperative leakage of aqueous or escape of air, which could increase the risk of detachment. Patients undergoing the procedure therefore need to be watched more closely after surgery to look for any evidence of partial or total graft detachments and taken for rebubbling if required.

A properly positioned IOL and a good iridoplasty decrease the chances of the graft slipping into the vitreous cavity during surgery. However, this possibility should be kept in mind, and care should be taken to avoid any inappropriate fluidics, which may cause a graft drop.

15.5 Glued IOL with Descemet Stripping Endothelial Keratoplasty

Descemet stripping endothelial keratoplasty (DSEK) can be combined effectively with glued IOL. The glued IOL is put in place and followed by iridoplasty, host descemetorhexis, insertion, and flotation of the DSEK graft. DSEK has disadvantages of causing more induced hyperopia as compared to DMEK and

PDEK but may be preferred in cases with an incomplete iris–IOL diaphragm, large-sector iridectomies, or traumatic/congenital aniridia. The standard DSAEK graft or the ultrathin DSEK graft may be used. The DSEK graft may be inserted using the taco technique with forceps, Busin glide, Tan EndoGlide (Angiotech), or suture pull-through technique.

DSEK is a partial-thickness corneal graft operation in which the inner endothelial layer is replaced.

Two partial-scleral-thickness flaps approximately 2.5 by 2.5 mm are made 180 degrees opposite to each other. An ACM is introduced in the inferior quadrant. A circular mark is placed on the patient's corneal surface, and it serves as a guide for removal of the recipient Descemet membrane. The anterior chamber is entered through a peripheral stab incision, and the Descemet membrane is scored and detached as a single disc. It is important not to damage the inner surface of the patient's cornea during this step of the Descemet membrane removal because the inner corneal stroma will form half of the donor–recipient interface. A sclerotomy wound is created with a 20-gauge needle ~ 1 mm away from the limbus beneath the scleral flaps, and the entire glued IOL surgery is performed until the haptics are tucked into the scleral pockets. An inferior peripheral iridectomy is performed to prevent postoperative air bubble–associated pupillary block glaucoma attack. The ACM helps to maintain the AC throughout the surgery. The use of viscoelastic is deterred because it is important not to leave residual viscoelastic in the AC; it is thought to potentially hamper good adhesion between the donor corneal disc and the recipient corneal stroma.

Next, the donor cornea is mounted within an artificial AC and pressurized. Manual dissection is used to remove the anterior corneal stroma. The dissected donor corneal tissue is then placed with the epithelial side down, and trephination is carried out from the endothelial side using a disposable trephine. The diameter of the trephine matches the diameter of the circular mark placed on the corneal epithelium of the recipient cornea made at the beginning of the procedure. The donor disc is about 150 µm thick.

A small amount of viscoelastic is placed on the endothelial surface of the donor corneal disc. The donor corneal disc is then introduced into the AC with a taco-fold technique using a forceps, or it is inserted using a surgical glide or an inserter in its unfolded or partially folded state. Once within the AC, the donor disc is attached to the recipient's inner corneal stroma using a large air bubble. The donor–recipient interface is formed between donor and recipient corneal stroma. The donor disc is then centered to the recipient cornea using the pre-placed epithelial circular mark. A wait of ~ 10 minutes facilitates initial donor recipient corneal disc adherence. Postoperatively, the patient is asked to lie flat in the recovery room for about an hour and also to lie flat for the most part during the first postoperative day.

15.6 Glued IOL with Descemet Membrane Endothelial Keratoplasty

Gerritt Melles described DMEK, which refers to transplantation of the Descemet membrane with endothelium.[14,15] It has advantages over DSAEK with respect to visual quality,

absence of hyperopization, and lower rates of graft rejection. The DMEK graft may be harvested directly by the operating surgeon or may be ordered from the eye bank. The submerged cornea using backgrounds away (SCUBA) technique, as described by Art Giebel, is used to harvest the DMEK graft.[16] It is more easily harvested from older donor corneas due to weaker attachments in older corneas between the Descemet membrane and overlying stroma. Corneas younger than 40 are therefore generally not suitable for DMEK. The DMEK graft is more fragile than the DSAEK and PDEK grafts and is more likely to tear during graft preparation and manipulation if handled inappropriately. Extreme care in handling should therefore be exercised.

Glued IOL implantation and air fill check are followed by host descemetorhexis and DMEK graft implantation. Perception of light and IOP are checked, and the patient maintains a supine position for 24 hours (▶ Fig. 15.4).

In patients with compromised endothelium (▶ Fig. 15.4a) it has a tremendous potential for faster recovery. The recipient corneal dissection in DMEK is similar to the above two procedures, resulting in the exposure of the patient's uncut inner corneal stroma. An inferior peripheral iridectomy is performed as in DSEK and DSAEK procedures. The donor Descemet membrane is scored, partially detached under fluid, and trephined from the endothelial side. A Sinskey hook is used to lift up the edge of the cut Descemet membrane. Once an adequate edge is lifted, a nontoothed forceps is used to gently grab the Descemet membrane at its very edge and the graft (▶ Fig. 15.7b) is separated from the underlying stroma in a capsulorhexis-like circumferential manner. The Descemet membrane with the healthy donor corneal endothelium is removed as a single donor disc without any donor corneal stroma. Hence there is no need for an artificial AC or a microkeratome in the donor tissue preparation. This donor Descemet membrane/endothelial complex is stained with a vital dye, such as trypan blue, for visualization.

An ACM is introduced, and all the steps of glued IOL surgery are followed consecutively, beginning from 180-degree-opposite scleral marking to the externalization and tucking of haptics (▶ Fig. 15.4c, d).

The graft is then carefully loaded into a Visian ICL injector (Staar Surgical) (▶ Fig. 15.4e) with the cartridge tip held occluded with a finger. It is then injected gently into the AC by plunging the soft-tipped injector, taking care not to fold the graft. Wound-assisted implantation is avoided, and the ACM flow is titrated carefully to prevent backflow and extrusion of the graft through the incision. The default shape of the donor disc is a coiled circular tube. This donor disc is then uncoiled using fluidics, and the surgeon must avoid for the most part any direct instrument contact to the donor endothelium. Proper orientation is essential prior to attaching the donor Descemet membrane to the exposed recipient bare corneal stroma. The graft orientation is then checked, and it is unfolded gently using a small air bubble as described by Melles. Once unfolded, an adequately tight air bubble is injected under the graft to float it up against the stroma (▶ Fig. 15.4f). Fibrin glue is finally used to seal the lamellar scleral flaps, conjunctiva, and clear corneal incisions.

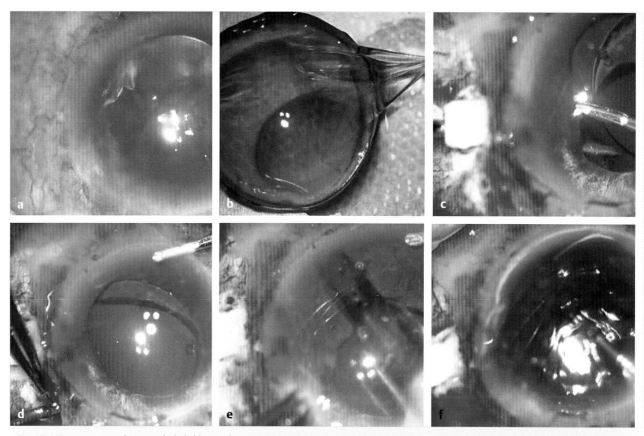

Fig. 15.4 Descemet membrane endothelial keratoplasty (DMEK) with glued intraocular lens (IOL). (a) Preoperative pseudophakic bullous keratopathy. Posterior chamber (PC) IOL implanted in the anterior chamber (AC). (b) DMEK graft being prepared. (c) PC IOL implanted in AC leading to corneal decompensation. The same PC IOL is being relocated into the PC using a closed-globe glued IOL technique. The haptic is grabbed from over the iris using a glued IOL forceps and with the handshake technique is transferred between the two hands until the tip of the haptic is held. (d) The haptic is exteriorized through the sclerotomy made under the scleral flap. The same procedure is followed for the second haptic, which is exteriorized through a sclerotomy under a second scleral flap created 180 degrees away from the first. Each haptic is then tucked into a scleral tunnel created at the edge of the scleral flap. (e) The DMEK graft is loaded in a Visian ICL injector and is injected into the AC. (f) The DMEK graft is unrolled and an air bubble is used to appose it against the overlying stroma.

15.7 It Takes Two to Tango—Pre-Descemet Endothelial Keratoplasty with Glued IOL

Amar Agarwal and Harminder Dua described PDEK, in which the newly described pre-Descemet layer, the Descemet membrane, and the endothelium are transplanted after host Descemet membrane stripping. The combination of PDEK with glued IOL (▶ Fig. 15.5, ▶ Fig. 15.6, ▶ Fig. 15.7) serves the purpose of simultaneously handling corneal endothelial dysfunction and secondary IOL fixation.[6]

15.8 Technique

A trephine of suitable diameter is used to mark the anterior corneal surface for Descemet stripping. The desired diameter of the graft should be about 0.5 mm smaller than the recipient eye. The PDEK graft is then prepared. A 30-gauge needle attached to an air-filled 5 mL syringe is introduced in a bevel-up position into the donor corneoscleral rim, placed endothelial side up. Air is then injected to form a type 1 bubble of the

desired diameter. The type 1 bubble consists of the pre-Descemet layer, the Descemet membrane, and the endothelium and is seen as a dome-shaped elevation that is ~ 7 to 8 mm in diameter. It typically enlarges from the center to the periphery and has a distinct edge all around. Trypan blue is then used to stain the graft with a 26-gauge needle introduced into the edge of the bubble. A Vannas scissor is used to cut the graft all around the edges of the bubble, and the graft is harvested and placed in a bowl containing the storage medium. If a type 2 bubble consisting of only Descemet membrane and endothelium is formed, surgery may be continued as a DMEK. The type 2 bubble is larger and enlarges from the periphery to the center. It lacks a clearly defined edge and is more likely than a type 1 bubble to burst; therefore care should be taken while expanding it.

The recipient eye is prepared as described previously by stripping the Descemet membrane. When combining with a glued IOL, the IOL implantation is completed, followed by iridoplasty and PDEK graft implantation. The graft is loaded into an IOL injector as described by Francis Price and injected into the AC. Graft orientation is confirmed followed by the graft unfolding and floating up using an air bubble.[11]

The PDEK graft has advantages over the DMEK graft in being more robust, stronger, and less likely to tear. It also allows the

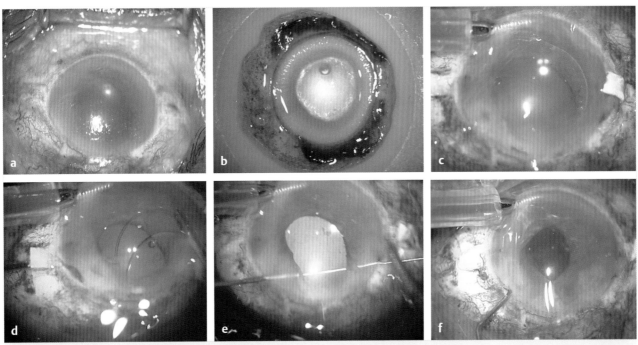

Fig. 15.5 It takes two to tango—pre-Descemet endothelial keratoplasty (PDEK) with glued intraocular lens (IOL) (Part 1). **(a)** Preoperative photograph of the cornea of a patient with pseudophakic bullous keratopathy. Posterior chamber (PC) IOL in anterior chamber (AC). **(b)** A type 1 big bubble (bb) is formed between the pre-Descemet layer (Dua layer) and stroma. Note the bb does not reach the periphery of the cornea because there are firm adhesions between the pre-Descemet layer and stroma in the periphery. If a bubble is created that extends to the corneoscleral limbus it is a type 2 (pre-Descemet) bb. This means the air has formed between the Descemet membrane and the pre-Descemet layer. **(c)** AC maintainer is fixed and scleral flaps created. **(d)** Glued IOL surgery is performed and haptics are externalized. **(e)** Pupilloplasty. **(f)** Pupilloplasty completed with glued IOL in place. Eye is now ready for PDEK surgery.

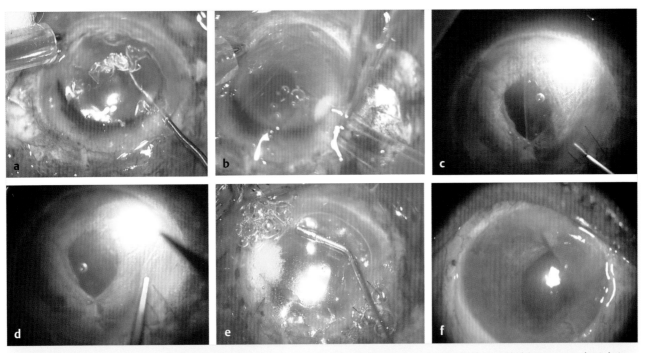

Fig. 15.6 It takes two to tango—pre-Descemet endothelial keratoplasty (PDEK) with glued intraocular lens (IOL) (Part 2). **(a)** Descemetorhexis being performed. **(b)** The PDEK graft is injected into the anterior chamber with the help of the injector. **(c)** Graft is subsequently unrolled with air and fluidics. An endoilluminator is used to help in ascertaining orientation and checking the unrolling of the graft (E-PDEK). **(d)** The graft is unrolled after checking correct orientation. **(e)** Air is injected under the graft to appose it to the cornea. PDEK graft is attached to the cornea with a complete air fill of the anterior chamber. Then glue is applied to the scleral flaps. **(f)** Postoperative at 1 week.

use of young donor grafts of any age, thereby allowing the transfer of a greater quantity of endothelial cells. This, in turn, allows the use of better-quality donor grafts as compared to DMEK grafts.

An AC IOL, if present, should be explanted followed by the performance of vitrectomy with glued IOL. Pupilloplasty should be performed if necessary, followed by the PDEK procedure. (▶ Fig. 15.8, ▶ Fig. 15.9, ▶ Fig. 15.10).

15.9 Advantages

The glued IOL can be done in much less open-sky time as compared to other secondary IOL fixation techniques. Once the haptics have been exteriorized, the optic acts as a tamponade and is helpful in preventing expulsive hemorrhage. It can also be done with any available three-piece IOL without the need for a special IOL with eyelets on the haptic. The glued IOL may be done even in hypotonous eyes, and centration can be adjusted once the graft is sutured and the globe is formed. Lack of

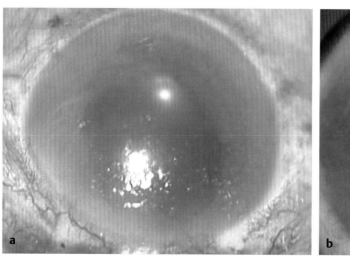
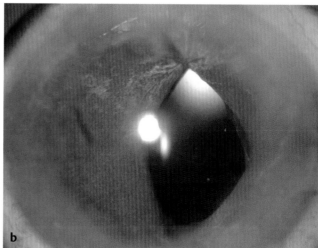

Fig. 15.7 It takes two to tango—pre-Descemet endothelial keratoplasty (PDEK) with glued intraocular lens (IOL) (Part 3). (a) Preoperative case of pseudophakic bullous keratopathy with a posterior chamber IOL placed in the anterior chamber. (b) Postoperative at 1 year, 20/30 vision.

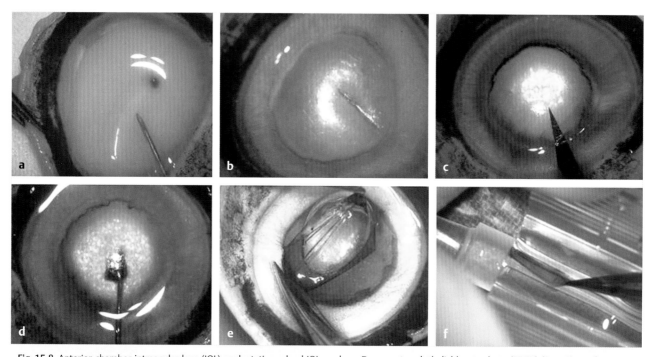

Fig. 15.8 Anterior chamber intraocular lens (IOL) explantation, glued IOL, and pre-Descemet endothelial keratoplasty (PDEK) (Part 1)—graft preparation of PDEK. (a) A 30-gauge needle injects air inside the stroma of the donor cornea with needle bevel facing upward. Donor cornea seen with endothelium facing upward. (b) Type 1 big bubble created. Note that the bubble does not go to the periphery. If the bubble went to the periphery it would be a type 2 big bubble, meaning we would then create a Descemet membrane endothelial keratoplasty (DMEK) graft. (c) Knife entry into the big bubble. (d) Trypan blue stain injected into the big bubble. (e) Vannas scissor dissects the PDEK graft. (f) PDEK graft loaded on the IOL cartridge.

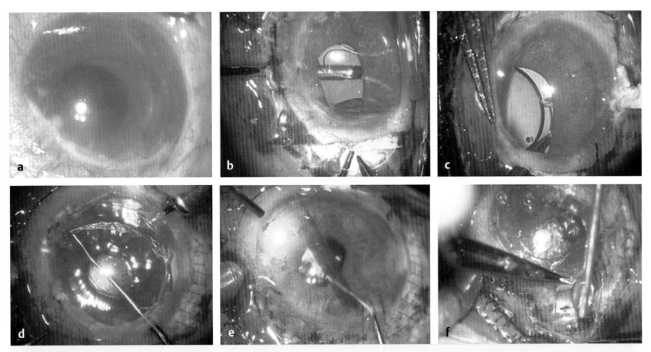

Fig. 15.9 Anterior chamber (AC) intraocular lens (IOL) explantation, glued IOL, and pre-Descemet endothelial keratoplasty (PDEK) (Part 2)—glued IOL. (a) Pseudophakic bullous keratopathy with an AC IOL. (b) AC IOL explanted after vitrectomy. (c) Glued IOL. (d) Descemetorhexis. (e) PDEK graft injected. (f) Graft attached and glue applied in the scleral flaps.

pseudophacodonesis is another advantage in glued IOL as compared to other secondary IOL fixation techniques.

While doing scleral fixation with sutures, the surgeon must readjust the knots to maintain the central position of the IOL. In our procedure, simply manipulating the amount of externalization can cause proper centration of the IOL. The final tucking of the haptic provides further stabilization. A sutured scleral-fixated IOL hangs in the posterior chamber, with the sutures passing through the haptic eyes, similar to a hammock, causing dynamic torsional and anteroposterior oscillation. This pseudophacodonesis may result in progressive endothelial loss. However, in this technique, haptics are used for fixation on the scleral side and the stable optic–haptic junction prevents torsional and anteroposterior instability. Therefore, there is much less pseudophacodonesis (▶ Fig. 15.8). The haptics are covered in the scleral flap and tucked well inside the scleral pocket. There is an additional well-apposed layer of conjunctiva over the sclera. This further reduces the chances of haptic extrusion. Better dynamic stability of the glued IOL prevents pseudophacodonesis and may reduce endothelial cell loss or repositioning surgery. Combined, these two surgical modalities may improve results.

15.10 IPhone-Assisted High-Speed Photography for Glued IOL Understanding

High-speed photography is the art of photographing a rapidly occurring event by using a fast shutter speed to capture moments not appreciated with the naked eye. Scientists have used high-speed photography to study physical movement, measuring phenomena such as surface tension and gravitational effects. It is also employed for tracking the accuracy of missiles and rockets and to record the sequence of events at the core of nuclear explosions. Sports photographers use high-speed photography to record fast-moving sporting events and to analyze the speed and movements of athletes.

Human eyes are accustomed to viewing videos at 24 to 25 frames per second (fps), and it is believed that 30 fps is the final limit of a human eye to appreciate the sequence of movements. High-speed cameras with much faster shutter speeds are usually employed for recording videos to assess the fine details of any special event. IPhone 5S and the newer models thereafter have an inbuilt native feature of recording videos at 120 fps (iPhone 5S) and 240 fps (iPhone 6). Attaching an iPhone to the slit lamp or to a microscope with the help of an adapter can help in recording videos at higher fps on the "SLO-MO" mode of the video recorder. These videos capture 120 frames in 1 second, which provides a detailed analysis of the sequence of events that a normal human eye fails to appreciate. Clinically, the surgeon opens the "Camera" and goes to "SLO-MO" mode written just adjacent to "video" recording. The video at SLO-MO mode is recorded in the manner of a normal video recording by pressing the appropriate button. When this video is recorded at high fps and is later played, then it runs at an eye-friendly rate of 25 to 30 fps. Thus the surgeon can appreciate every minute detail that a normal eye fails to appreciate.

The presence of subtle movements of intraocular structures, such as the iris, lens, and capsular bag–IOL complex has crucial clinical implications. Preoperative detection of these subtle intraocular movements often goes unnoticed, and the surgeon confronts the surgical challenge intraoperatively. In our practice, we have used and exploited this scenario to detect subtle

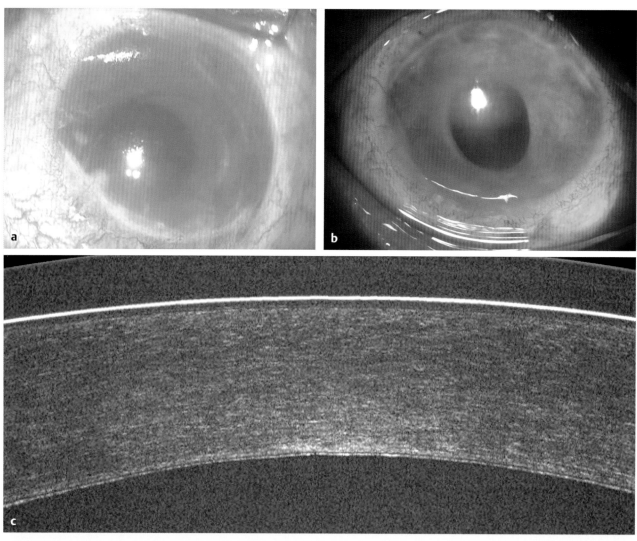

Fig. 15.10 Anterior chamber (AC) intraocular lens (IOL) explantation, glued IOL, and pre-Descemet endothelial keratoplasty (PDEK) (Part 3). **(a)** Preoperative. **(b)** One month postoperative. Note the cornea is cleared. **(c)** Anterior segment optical coherence tomography shows graft attached.

intraocular movements, such as iridodonesis, phacodonesis, and pseudophacodonesis. The presence of iridodonesis in an otherwise normal-looking eye should raise the suspicion of compromised zonules or lens instability, and the surgeon can be apprised of the impending intraoperative complication. We recommend that all cases of traumatic cataract or those associated with pseudoexfoliation or connective tissue disorders be evaluated with a high fps recording to detect subtle intraocular movements because this allows the surgeon to be ready with contingency plans if required. Detection of pseudophacodonesis is another important aspect of SLO-MO recording because it goes a long way in explaining the process of vitreous disturbance in the eye following a secondary IOL implantation that can eventually lead to cystoid macular edema. Higher fps recording allows pre-detection and warns the surgeon of the possible challenges inherent in such cases. Apprehending and anticipating a clinical entity and its subsequent repercussions allow the case to be handled in a better way and allow a thorough preparation for and consideration of adjunctive surgical devices

before surgery, while curbing the intraoperative surprise and making the surgery more predictable.

Surgeons who have an older iPhone can use third-party applications (e.g., SLO-PRO is an app that can be downloaded, and videos at high fps can be recorded with its help). Various apps are also available for android phone users. The use of smartphones obviates the need to purchase a high-speed camera and is comparatively cost-effective. Glued IOL fixation demonstrates iridodonesis, but no pseudophacodonesis is seen due to intrascleral haptic tuck. An AC IOL or a sutured IOL demonstrates pseudophacodonesis.

15.11 Conclusion

Thus we see that glued IOL can be combined with DSAEK, DMEK, and PDEK in a safe and effective manner. An iridoplasty should be performed when required. In complete aniridia, it may be required to be combined with an aniridia IOL or with an artificial iris.

References

[1] Agarwal A, Kumar DA, Jacob S, Baid C, Agarwal A, Srinivasan S. Fibrin glue-assisted sutureless posterior chamber intraocular lens implantation in eyes with deficient posterior capsules. J Cataract Refract Surg. 2008; 34(9):1433–1438

[2] Prakash G, Jacob S, Ashok Kumar D, Narsimhan S, Agarwal A, Agarwal A. Femtosecond-assisted keratoplasty with fibrin glue-assisted sutureless posterior chamber lens implantation: new triple procedure. J Cataract Refract Surg. 2009; 35(6):973–979

[3] Prakash G, Agarwal A, Jacob S, Kumar DA, Chaudhary P, Agarwal A. Femtosecond-assisted descemet stripping automated endothelial keratoplasty with fibrin glue-assisted sutureless posterior chamber lens implantation. Cornea. 2010; 29(11):1315–1319

[4] Jacob S, Agarwal A, Kumar DA, Agarwal A, Agarwal A, Satish K. Modified technique for combining DMEK with glued intrascleral haptic fixation of a posterior chamber IOL as a single-stage procedure. J Refract Surg. 2014; 30 (7):492–496

[5] McKee Y, Price FW, Jr, Feng MT, Price MO. Implementation of the posterior chamber intraocular lens intrascleral haptic fixation technique (glued intraocular lens) in a United States practice: Outcomes and insights. J Cataract Refract Surg. 2014; 40(12):2099–2105

[6] Agarwal A, Dua HS, Narang P, et al. Pre-Descemet's endothelial keratoplasty (PDEK). Br J Ophthalmol. 2014; 98(9):1181–1185

[7] Osher RH, Snyder ME, Cionni RJ. Modification of the Siepser slip-knot technique. J Cataract Refract Surg. 2005; 31(6):1098–1100

[8] Dua HS, Faraj LA, Said DG, Gray T, Lowe J. Human corneal anatomy redefined: a novel pre-Descemet's layer (Dua's layer). Ophthalmology. 2013; 120 (9):1778–1785

[9] Agarwal A, Jacob S, Kumar DA, Agarwal A, Narasimhan S, Agarwal A. Handshake technique for glued intrascleral haptic fixation of a posterior chamber intraocular lens. J Cataract Refract Surg. 2013; 39(3):317–322

[10] Gabor SGB, Pavlidis MM. Sutureless intrascleral posterior chamber intraocular lens fixation. J Cataract Refract Surg. 2007; 33(11):1851–1854

[11] Price FW, Jr, Price MO. Descemet's stripping with endothelial keratoplasty in 200 eyes: Early challenges and techniques to enhance donor adherence. J Cataract Refract Surg. 2006; 32(3):411–418

[12] Jacob S, Agarwal A, Agarwal A, Narasimhan S, Kumar DA, Sivagnanam S. Endoilluminator-assisted transcorneal illumination for Descemet membrane endothelial keratoplasty: enhanced intraoperative visualization of the graft in corneal decompensation secondary to pseudophakic bullous keratopathy. J Cataract Refract Surg. 2014; 40(8):1332–1336

[13] Schoenberg ED, Price FW, Jr. Modification of Siepser sliding suture technique for iris repair and endothelial keratoplasty. J Cataract Refract Surg. 2014; 40 (5):705–708

[14] Melles GR, Eggink FA, Lander F, et al. A surgical technique for posterior lamellar keratoplasty. Cornea. 1998;17:618-626.

[15] Melles GR, Ong TS, Ververs B, van der Wees J. Descemet membrane endothelial keratoplasty (DMEK). Cornea. 2006;25:987-990.

[16] Giebel AW, Grandin JC, Price FW. SCUBA technique for DMEK donor preparation [video]. YouTube. http://www.youtube. com/watch?v=vpToO8PFsvI.

16 Endothelial Keratoplasty in Glaucoma

Francis W. Price, Jr., and Marianne O. Price

16.1 Background

Endothelial keratoplasty (EK) has become the most frequently performed type of corneal transplant in the United States, with the most prevalent EK technique being Descemet stripping endothelial keratoplasty (DSEK).[1] EK is now used for over 90% of cases of endothelial failure, so it is not surprising that EK surgeries are being done in eyes with preexisting glaucoma. Moreover, we know that the long-term use of topical corticosteroids to prevent keratoplasty rejection often leads to the development of glaucoma. We have found that approximately one-third of patients without a preexisting history of glaucoma will develop increased intraocular pressure (IOP) during the first year after DSEK with a prednisolone acetate 1% dosing regimen of four times a day for 4 months, then tapering to three times a day for 1 month, twice a day for 1 month, and once a day through 1 year.[2] The percentage of eyes developing increased IOP can be higher with higher steroid dosing or lower if the dosing is decreased. Either way, glaucoma and keratoplasty are inextricably intertwined.

When examining 5-year DSEK survival rates, we as well as others have found that the most significant risk factor for graft failure is previous glaucoma filtration surgery, with tubes being associated with a higher rate of graft failure than trabeculectomies.[3,4,5] These findings have important implications when setting appropriate patient expectations for surgery. Patients who have a tube should be cautioned that the graft will likely need to be replaced within 5 years. Compared with penetrating keratoplasty (PK), an EK graft is much easier and less traumatic to replace. EK also provides quicker visual recovery than a full-thickness graft, which requires multiple sutures, each of which causes some scarring to the recipient cornea.

Why do grafts fail sooner in eyes with prior glaucoma filtration surgery? Whenever performing keratoplasty on an eye

with a tube, we trim the tube at the time of transplant surgery, or we reposition the tube a month ahead of time so that no tubes touch the cornea. So the increased risk of graft failure in these eyes is not attributable to the tube contacting the cornea. We have sampled anterior chamber fluid from eyes with tubes and trabeculectomies and found that eyes with tubes (both valved and nonvalved) have on average a 10-fold higher protein concentration in the aqueous humor, and eyes with a trabeculectomy have a 5-fold higher protein concentration than eyes undergoing routine cataract surgery in the absence of prior glaucoma surgery (▶ Fig. 16.1).[6] We believe that glaucoma filtration surgery produces an unhealthy aqueous environment for the corneal endothelium.

Early graft failure after tubes and trabeculectomies is an important demographic issue. In reviewing our PK cases performed between 1982 and 1996, we found that eyes with a history of prior glaucoma surgery accounted for only 3% of the pseudophakic corneal edema cases, whereas in our DSEK series performed between 2003 and 2005, eyes with prior glaucoma surgery accounted for 33% of the pseudophakic corneal edema cases.[3,7] Thus pseudophakic corneal edema is increasingly associated with prior glaucoma surgery. If the grafts in these eyes only last about 5 years on average, then we will see a large number of regrafts being performed for these problems. This will be aggravated by a switch that is occurring in the United States to make tubes the primary surgical procedure for glaucoma instead of trabeculectomies.

To put all this into prospective, our analysis of DSEK graft survival showed that the 5-year survival rate was 95% in eyes without a preexisting history of glaucoma and 90% in eyes with medically managed glaucoma, which was not a significant difference. However, the 5-year survival rate dropped to 59% in eyes with a prior trabeculectomy and was only 25% in those with a prior aqueous shunt (▶ Fig. 16.2).[3] When we analyzed

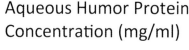

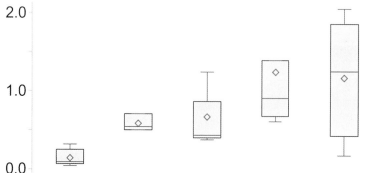

Fig. 16.1 The protein concentration of the aqueous humor is significantly elevated in eyes that have undergone glaucoma filtration surgery, such as Express or standard trabeculectomy, or implantation of an Ahmed or Baerveldt aqueous shunt, as compared with eyes without prior surgery (controls). In the box plots, the diamond shows the mean value, the horizontal line shows the median, the bottom and top of the boxes represent the 25th and 75th percentiles, respectively, and the vertical lines extend to the minimum and maximum sampled values.

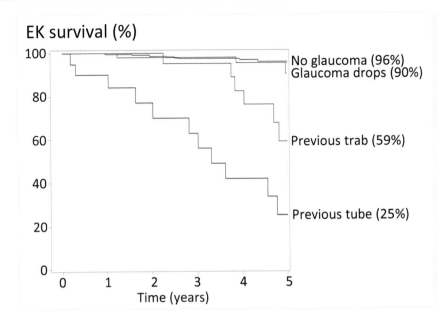

Fig. 16.2 Kaplan–Meier survival curves for Descemet stripping endothelial keratoplasty (DSEK) performed in eyes without any previous diagnosis of glaucoma, eyes with glaucoma managed with eyedrops, eyes with a previous trabeculectomy, and eyes with a previous aqueous shunt. EK, endothelial keratoplasty; trab, trabeculectomy.

graft survival in eyes with a previous failed PK that was treated with DSEK, we were surprised to find that the number of previous failed PKs and corneal neovascularization were not risk factors for graft failure—the only significant risk factor was a prior tube.[8] The 4-year survival rate of EK under a failed PK was 96% in eyes without a glaucoma filter but only 22% in eyes with a filter.[8] Filters are going to lead to many regrafts. They will also cause a lot of secondary corneal decompensation in virgin corneas. Tubes may become the most common cause for grafting corneas.

16.2 Surgical Considerations

16.2.1 Medically Managed Glaucoma Eyes

The procedure a surgeon offers a patient depends on the skill set and experience of the surgeon. For those with a skill set to offer Descemet membrane endothelial keratoplasty (DMEK), DMEK is the procedure of choice for uncomplicated eyes with medically managed glaucoma. (Pre-Descemet endothelial keratoplasty [PDEK] for all practical purposes is similar to DMEK.) With DMEK, only the healthy donor endothelium and Descemet membrane are transplanted. We have shown that, with similar corticosteroid dosing regimens, DMEK has a far lower rate of immunologic rejection episodes compared with PK or DSEK.[9] This is very important for glaucoma patients because it allows one to significantly decrease the strength of postoperative topical corticosteroids without increasing the risk of immunologic graft rejection episodes.[10,11] Furthermore, we evaluated the risk of immunologic graft rejection if corticosteroids are discontinued 1 year after DMEK—the risk of a rejection episode during the subsequent 12 months was 6%, and the risk of graft failure was 0.4% when steroids were discontinued versus 0% if a weak topical steroid continued to be used once a day.[12] Overall, the risk of immunologic graft rejection after stopping steroids is much less for DMEK than for PK.[9]

It is important to note that medically managed glaucoma significantly increases the risk of PK failure, whereas it does not significantly affect the risk of EK failure.[3,13] With PK the corneal nerves are severed so patients suffer from an anesthetic cornea. The toxic preservatives in glaucoma eyedrops are associated with increased risk of ocular surface disease and graft failure from ocular surface disease in PK eyes.[7] In contrast, EK eyes have a normal ocular surface and retain corneal sensation so chronic use of glaucoma eye drops does not significantly increase the risk of EK failure.[3]

16.2.2 Eyes with Trabeculectomies

Trabeculectomies offer a challenge in that any intraocular surgery runs the risk of causing the filter to fail from the bleb scarring down. EK surgery uses an air bubble rather than sutures to hold the graft in place. In our opinion, the longer the air bubble is in the eye, the higher the chance of filter failure. The air often can either block the filter or go up into the bleb. We recommend that if a bleb scars down, it should be needled and treated immediately to try and restore function. Eyes with low IOP (< 8 mm Hg) with a very large and thin bleb can pose a problem in that the low pressure makes it hard to get a firm air bubble to hold the graft in place. Lid squeezing or forced blinking can indent the cornea and dislodge the graft. Reinjections of air are often needed after EK in eyes with low IOP and filters.

16.2.3 Eyes with Tubes

Tubes present mechanical issues with both grafts and corneas in general. Because the implanting surgeon often judges the tube length after the eye is opened and partially deflated, there is a tendency to make tubes too long. Tube lengths should be determined before opening the eye and planned so that the tube sticks only about 1.5 to 2 mm into the anterior chamber. The tube should be orientated away from the cornea, otherwise any eye compression with blinking or rubbing can push the tube against the cornea.

Long tubes should be trimmed at the time of EK surgery. If the tube is against the cornea, then a month prior to EK surgery the tube should be repositioned away from the cornea

(▶ Fig. 16.3). Our preferred method of either placing a tube or repositioning a tube is the technique described by Alvarado et al.[14] No graft is required, and the tube is placed deep in the scleral tissue, exiting in the posterior chamber just behind the iris. This results in no tube elevation near the limbus, so it decreases the chance of erosions or irritation from the tube.[14] We prefer to reposition tubes a month ahead of EK surgery because the old track from which the tube was removed can often leak in the immediate postoperative period, causing hypotony. Wound leaks and hypotony are common causes of EK graft detachment. Placing a tube through the pars plana will definitely remove it from being near the cornea, but it requires a pars plana vitrectomy, and it does not really help long-term graft survival because the protein content in the unicameral eye is still elevated in the anterior chamber.[6,15]

Care should be taken not to allow the endothelium of the graft to come into contact with the tube because it will obviously damage the endothelial cells. This is more challenging with DMEK, and insertion techniques in which the endothelium faces inward instead of outward can be helpful for preventing endothelium–tube contact.[16]

16.3 Controlling Intraocular Pressure

16.3.1 Choosing the Right Glaucoma Drops

Different glaucoma eye drops have different effects on the cornea and anterior chamber. We typically like to start with a beta-blocker if someone does not have a contraindication, and then brimonidine, because neither of those drugs has a significant deleterious effect on the cornea, although they are not as potent as the prostaglandin analogues. Prostaglandin analogues are our third choice, because they can cause increased inflammation in and around the eye. Finally our last choice is a carbonic anhydrase inhibitor, because it can have a negative effect on the corneal endothelial pumping mechanism, especially in compromised corneas.[17]

16.3.2 When Drops Are Not Enough

Often we get into a balancing act between trying to taper corticosteroids to control IOP while still preventing graft rejection or intraocular inflammation. (This balancing act is easier with DMEK because it has less risk of rejection than DSEK or PK.) When we reach the point where we cannot medically control IOP and cannot further cut corticosteroids, we need to resort to surgery. Tubes and trabeculectomies are always options, but as already noted, each can cause a long-term compromise of the corneal endothelium as well as short-term complications from flat chambers or surgical misadventures. In the past, cyclodestructive procedures had substantial risk of hypotony, pain, bleeding, and inflammation. The new pulsed-laser cyclophotoactivated treatments with the MP3 laser (Iridex Corp.) do not appear to significantly cause any of those four problems while controlling the IOP. However, this treatment is relatively new, and longer follow-up is needed to see how it does long term. Selective laser trabeculoplasty (SLT) of the angle can also be tried, but often with EK surgery, especially DSEK, it can be hard to see well enough into the angle to perform adequate treatments.

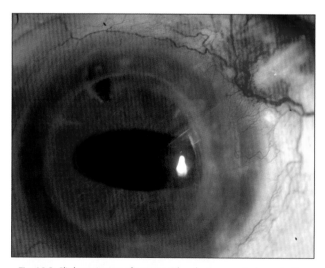

Fig. 16.3 Slit lamp image of an eye with a decompensated penetrating keratoplasty (PK) and an eroded and exposed tube that needs to be repositioned. Our treatment was two staged surgeries. First we repositioned the tube into the posterior chamber entering the anterior chamber through a peripheral iridectomy. One month later we performed Descemet membrane endothelial keratoplasty under the failed PK.

References

[1] Park CY, Lee JK, Gore PK, Lim CY, Chuck RS. Keratoplasty in the United States: a 10-year review from 2005 through 2014. Ophthalmology. 2015; 122 (12):2432–2442

[2] Vajaranant TS, Price MO, Price FW, Gao W, Wilensky JT, Edward DP. Visual acuity and intraocular pressure after Descemet's stripping endothelial keratoplasty in eyes with and without preexisting glaucoma. Ophthalmology. 2009; 116(9):1644–1650

[3] Anshu A, Price MO, Price FW. Descemet's stripping endothelial keratoplasty: long-term graft survival and risk factors for failure in eyes with preexisting glaucoma. Ophthalmology. 2012; 119(10):1982–1987

[4] Aldave AJ, Chen JL, Zaman AS, Deng SX, Yu F. Outcomes after DSEK in 101 eyes with previous trabeculectomy and tube shunt implantation. Cornea. 2014; 33 (3):223–229

[5] Nahum Y, Mimouni M, Busin M. Risk factors predicting the need for graft exchange after Descemet stripping automated endothelial keratoplasty. Cornea. 2015; 34(8):876–879

[6] Rosenfeld C, Price MO, Lai X, Witzmann FA, Price FW, Jr. Distinctive and pervasive alterations in aqueous humor protein composition following different types of glaucoma surgery. Mol Vis. 2015; 21:911–918

[7] Price MO, Thompson RW, Jr, Price FW, Jr. Risk factors for various causes of failure in initial corneal grafts. Arch Ophthalmol. 2003; 121(8):1087–1092

[8] Anshu A, Price MO, Price FW, Jr. Descemet's stripping endothelial keratoplasty under failed penetrating keratoplasty: visual rehabilitation and graft survival rate. Ophthalmology. 2011; 118(11):2155–2160

[9] Anshu A, Price MO, Price FW, Jr. Risk of corneal transplant rejection significantly reduced with Descemet's membrane endothelial keratoplasty. Ophthalmology. 2012; 119(3):536–540

[10] Price MO, Price FW, Jr, Kruse FE, Bachmann BO, Tourtas T. Randomized comparison of topical prednisolone acetate 1% versus fluorometholone 0.1% in the first year after descemet membrane endothelial keratoplasty. Cornea. 2014; 33(9):880–886

[11] Price MO, Feng MT, Scanameo A, Price FW, Jr. Loteprednol etabonate 0.5% gel vs. prednisolone acetate 1% solution after Descemet membrane endothelial keratoplasty. Prospective randomized trial. Cornea. 2015; 34(8):853–858

[12] Price MO, Scanameo A, Feng MT, Price FW, Jr. Descemet membrane endothelial keratoplasty: risk of immunologic rejection episodes after discontinuing topical corticosteroids. Ophthalmology. 2016; 123(6):1232–1236

[13] Sugar A, Tanner JP, Dontchev M, et al. Cornea Donor Study Investigator Group. Recipient risk factors for graft failure in the cornea donor study. Ophthalmology. 2009; 116(6):1023–1028

[14] Alvarado JA, Hollander DA, Juster RP, Lee LC. Ahmed valve implantation with adjunctive mitomycin C and 5-fluorouracil: long-term outcomes. Am J Ophthalmol. 2008; 146(2):276–284

[15] Anshu A, Price MO, Richardson MR, et al. Alterations in the aqueous humor proteome in patients with a glaucoma shunt device. Mol Vis. 2011; 17:1891–1900

[16] Busin M, Leon P, Scorcia V, Ponzin D. Contact lens-assisted pull-through technique for delivery of tri-folded (endothelium in) DMEK grafts minimizes surgical time and cell loss. Ophthalmology. 2016; 123(3):476–483

[17] Konowal A, Morrison JC, Brown SVL, et al. Irreversible corneal decompensation in patients treated with topical dorzolamide. Am J Ophthalmol. 1999; 127(4):403–406

17 Pre-Descemet Endothelial Keratoplasty in Failed Grafts

Athiya Agarwal, Dhivya Ashok Kumar, and Amar Agarwal

17.1 Background

Graft failure in any circumstances can take place due to intrinsic defects in the donor graft or preexisting pathology in the recipient. Inherent graft issues, such as low endothelial count, surgical trauma, and donor endothelial disease, can lead to early graft failure.[1,2,3,4] Graft rejection is one of the common etiologies of secondary graft failure, especially in full-thickness or penetrating keratoplasty (PK).[1,2] Lamellar keratoplasties have also shown fewer incidences; but still rejection has been noticed after deep lamellar keratoplasty or endothelial keratoplasty.[5] Corneal stroma is often the culprit recognized as the cause of rejection because of its antigenic nature. A failed penetrating graft can be replaced by another penetrating full-thickness graft or by an endothelial graft.[6,7,8,9,10,11] Subsequent PK has a higher failure rate and exposes the patient to an additional period of a prolonged visual recovery, the creation of an unstable wound, and further ocular surface disruption. On the other hand, secondary endothelial keratoplasty (EK) has the advantage of less surgical manipulation, no suture-related inflammation or astigmatism, and early visual recovery.[12,13,14,15,16] In this section we will be discussing our experience of pre-Descemet endothelial keratoplasty (PDEK) in previous failed grafts.

17.2 Graft Failure

Graft failure can be primary or secondary in origin. Primary graft failure is defined as failure of the graft to clear after surgery due to endothelial dysfunction and presenting with persistent, nonresolving corneal edema.[2] Primary graft failure presents as a failure to show improvement in visual acuity after the initial surgery. Endothelial trauma, elderly donor, and donor tissue diseases have been hypothesized for the cause of primary failure. Secondary failure refers to failure of graft after an initial period of clearance or normal function. High-risk keratoplasties, repeat PKs, postoperative conditions associated with glaucoma, retinal surgery, suture problems, persistent epithelial defect, infectious keratitis, and graft rejection can be significant causes of failure.[1,2] Persistent ocular surface problem and recurrence of host disease can also cause secondary graft failure in some cases. Even though the incidence of endothelial rejection is lower, graft rejection has been reported with EK. Penetrating keratoplasty is associated with stromal rejection, which demands measures to reduce the incidence be taken in patients post-PK. However, prolonged steroid use places the patient at risk of ocular hypertension and sometimes steroid-induced glaucoma and secondary cataracts, which in turn threaten best corrected vision.

17.3 Resurgery in Graft Failure

In challenging cases the ophthalmologist must decide whether to proceed with another surgery in the event of a failed graft. A failed PK can be corrected by repeat PK or primary endothelial keratoplasty. The advantages of endothelial keratoplasty in the case of a failed PK is the (1) closed-globe procedure, (2) lowered risk of graft rejection, (3) fewer surgical maneuvers, and (4) absence of complications inherent to PK (e.g., suture infection, glaucoma, astigmatism). However, performing endothelial keratoplasty requires suitable training skills, immense ground knowledge, and confidence.

17.4 Pre-Descemet Endothelial Keratoplasty in Failed Graft

17.4.1 Donor Selection

It is always better to use young donor grafts with an endothelial cell count > 2800 cells/mm²) and hexagonality > 40% in failed graft procedures. Exclude eyes with low cell count, elderly donors, and prolonged storage time.

17.4.2 Donor Graft Preparation

Donor graft preparation is the same as that for any PDEK procedure and has been explained previously.[17,18] A 30-gauge needle attached to a 5 mL syringe is inserted from the limbus into the midperipheral stroma (▶ Fig. 17.1). Air is slowly injected into the donor stroma until a type 1 big bubble[1] is formed. Viscoelastics can also be used for big bubble formation in eyes with difficulty in pneumatic dissection. The bubble wall is penetrated at the extreme periphery, and trypan blue is injected to stain the graft, which is then cut with a pair of corneoscleral scissors and covered with the tissue culture medium.

17.4.3 Recipient Bed Preparation

Under peribulbar anesthesia, initially a trocar anterior chamber maintainer (TACM) is placed at the limbus. The Descemet membrane (DM) is scored all around, with the diameter being smaller than that of the PK graft (▶ Fig. 17.2). The graft–host junction should not be disturbed with undue force or manipulation. The DM is then stripped off and gently removed via the main port. The donor PDEK lenticule is inserted into the anterior chamber (AC) with a customized injector. It is attached to the recipient bed by careful unrolling with an air bubble and attached to the overlying recipient stroma. The margins are swept in cases of a tight roll on the endothelial side under air with a reverse Sinskey hook. Intrachamber positive pressure is maintained thereafter for a short time by an air pump connected to the TACM. The main wound is closed with 10–0 monofilament nylon interrupted sutures, and the previous graft–host interface is rechecked for any leaks. The patient is laid supine for 30 minutes in the operating room and then shifted.

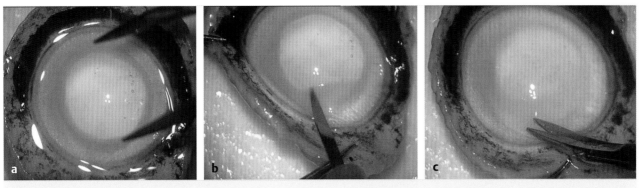

Fig. 17.1 **(a)** A type 1 big bubble formed in donor cornea using viscoelastics. **(b)** Bubble pierced with knife at the margin. **(c)** Graft is gently cut with curved Vannas scissors.

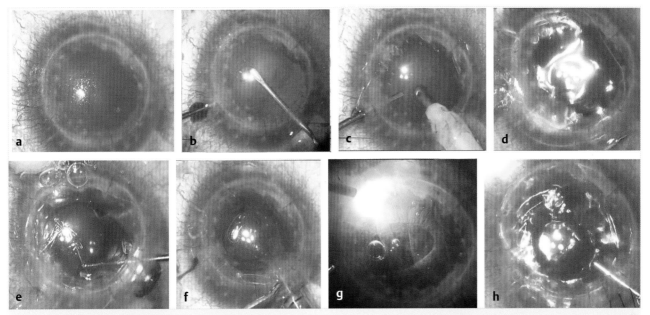

Fig. 17.2 **(a)** Preoperative image of failed penetrating keratoplasty in an eye with coexisting cataract **(b)** Capsulorhexis and **(c)** phacoemulsification performed to remove the lens. **(d)** Air injected to fill the anterior chamber by the end of intraocular lens implantation. **(e)** Anterior chamber maintainer is inserted and Descemet membrane is scored all around the recipient bed and stripped. **(f)** Graft loaded in a customized injector is injected into the anterior chamber. **(g)** Endoilluminator is used to visualize the graft in corneal edema and graft is positioned. **(h)** Air is injected beneath the lenticule to appose it with the overlying host stroma.

17.5 Results and Outcomes

In our experience of PDEK on failed grafts, 13 eyes have been operated. It included the previous primary PK (n = 7, 53.8%), Descemet stripping automated endothelial keratoplasty (DSAEK) (n = 2, 15.4%), and Descemet membrane endothelial keratoplasty (DMEK) (n = 4, 30.7%). Seven of 13 eyes (53.8%) presented as secondary graft failure (graft rejection being common post-PK), and the remaining 6 eyes (46.1%) had no clear graft following surgery. All the 6 eyes with no significant improvement in best corrected visual acuity (BCVA) after primary surgery had elderly donors (> 50 years). There was significant improvement (▶ Fig. 17.3) in BCVA (p = 0.003). The mean preoperative and postoperative BCVA in Snellen's decimal equivalent was 0.02 ± 0.1 and 0.23 ± 0.2, respectively. The preoperative central corneal thickness was 758.3 ± 75.8 μm, and postoperatively it was 594.2 ± 52.6 μm. There was a significant fall in central corneal thickness in the immediate postoperative period in all the eyes (p = 0.001) (▶ Fig. 17.4). There was graft detachment in one eye, and air injection was performed (▶ Fig. 17.5). Intraoperative difficulty in graft unfolding and wound dehiscence of previous PK graft was noted in one eye each. A postoperative grade 4 AC reaction was seen in one patient and was treated with medical management by steroids. Graft size larger than the previous PK graft was noted in one eye, which was noted as a postoperative folded graft in anterior segment optical coherence tomography (OCT) (▶ Fig. 17.6). There was no improvement in vision in 2 of 13 eyes (15.4%). Primary graft failure was seen in 2 eyes post-PK (n = 2) and post-DMEK (n = 1). Two eyes required repeat PK, one eye required repeat PDEK, and one eye required keratoprosthesis. Recurrence of primary corneal disease (dystrophy) was seen in 1 eye. Out of 13 eyes, there were 3 eyes with a donor age < 20 years. On analyzing the lens status and other procedures status, of 13

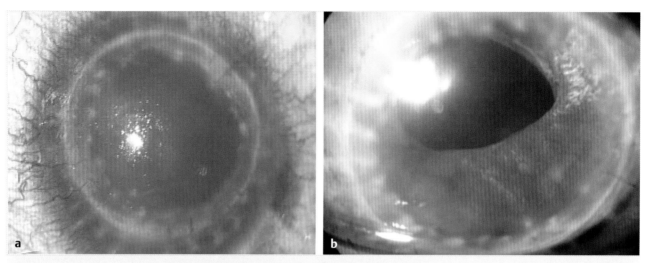

Fig. 17.3 (a) In an eye with macular dystrophy, postoperative corneal clarity (b) **postoperative PDEK** shows good graft adhesion in failed primary penetrating keratoplasty.

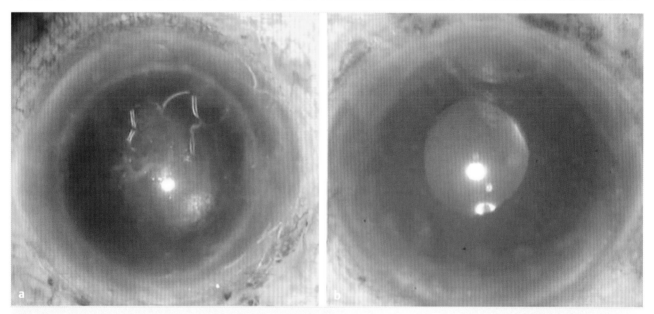

Fig. 17.4 (a) A post-Descemet stripping endothelial keratoplasty failed graft and (b) postoperative pre-Descemet endothelial keratoplasty in the same eye.

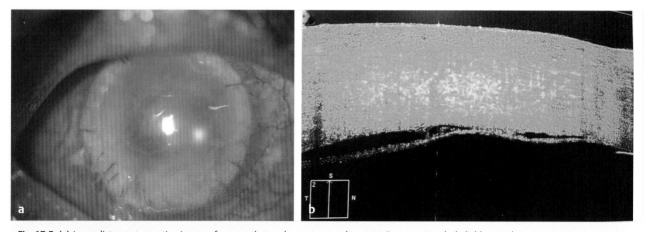

Fig. 17.5 (a) Immediate postoperative image of an eye that underwent secondary post-Descemet endothelial keratoplasty in primary penetrating keratoplasty. (b) Graft detachment seen in optical coherence tomography.

eyes, 1 eye had combined cataract surgery, 2 eyes had a glued intraocular lens (IOL) prior to the secondary PDEK (3 months earlier), 1 eye had a previous glaucoma valve implant (▶ Fig. 17.7), and 9 eyes had a posterior chamber IOL in situ.

17.6 Precautions in Failed Grafts

In an eye with previous DSAEK, the DM stripping can release the adhesion of the old DSAEK graft; hence care is taken not to apply excess pressure. Loose adhesion and early postoperative secondary PDEK can also predispose this. DSAEK might possibly modify the stromal proteins and thereby impair the adhesion of the PDEK graft as well. Good intraoperative air pressure and proper postoperative positioning will aid in strong adherence. When the size of the PDEK graft is smaller than the DSAEK graft, the postoperative migration and endothelial cell morphological changes will usually compensate for corneal recovery. The PDEK graft showed a significant difference in graft thickness (▶ Fig. 17.8) and good postoperative adhesion as compared to the DSAEK graft (▶ Fig. 17.9).

In eyes with PK, the graft–host junction is usually not interrupted intraoperatively. The PDEK graft is preferably smaller than the PK graft because there can be rolled edges or folds in

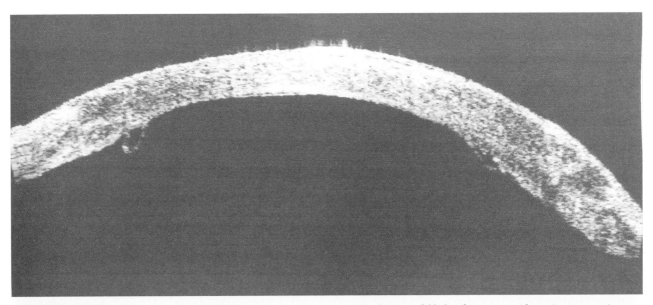

Fig. 17.6 Immediate postoperative anterior segment optical coherence tomography showing a folded graft in an eye with previous penetrating keratoplasty.

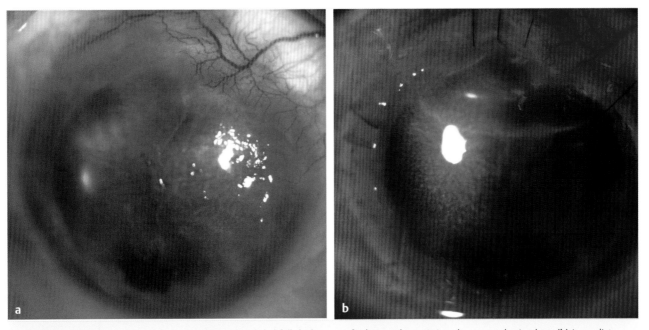

Fig. 17.7 (a) Preoperative image of an eye with primary failed full-thickness graft along with coexisting glaucoma valve implant. (b) Immediate postoperative image after secondary pre-Descemet endothelial keratoplasty.

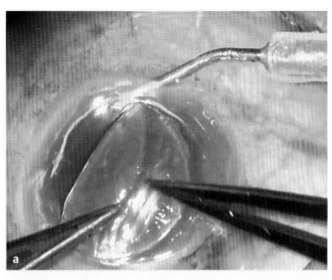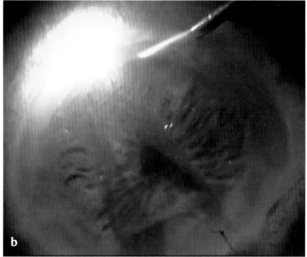

Fig. 17.8 Intraoperative image showing the difference in thickness of (a) Descemet stripping automated endothelial keratoplasty and (b) pre-Descemet endothelial keratoplasty graft.

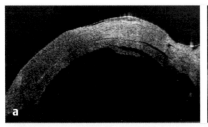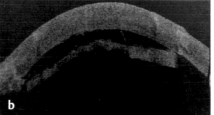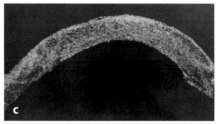

Fig. 17.9 (a,b) Immediate postoperative anterior segment optical coherence tomography of primary Descemet stripping automated endothelial keratoplasty (DSAEK). (c) Comparison with secondary pre-Descemet endothelial keratoplasty (PDEK) graft in the same eye. Note: See the poor early DSAEK graft adhesion and bulky graft as compared to good graft apposition of the thin PDEK graft.

large grafts that may not fit into the curvature of the original stroma. If the primary PK graft gives way intraoperatively, the wound has to be sutured to maintain wound stability (▶ Fig. 17.5). Other postoperative complications (e.g., graft detachment, dislocation, and reverse flap) can also happen when one is operating on failed grafts. Donor grafts that are smaller than the host PK and the presence of prior glaucoma drainage devices are risk factors for higher rates of graft dislocation. Nonvisualization during surgery has been one of the challenges faced by surgeons in operating on failed grafts; however, the advantage of PDEK with an endoilluminator helps in visualization of the graft, even in cases with corneal edema (▶ Fig. 17.2).[19]

Timing of the secondary surgery has always been the diagnostic dilemma in failed grafts. For DMEKs, if the graft does not become attached or clear after a minimum of 3 months postsurgery, one can proceed with a secondary PDEK. In long-standing corneal edema, stromal fibrosis and anterior surface irregularities might occur that limit the visual outcome of repeat surgery.[12,13] This is similar for secondary PDEK as well. Loss of endothelial cells, presence of fibrocellular tissue on the stromal surface, retained DM on the stromal surface, and epithelial ingrowth can be some of the reasons for primary endothelial graft failure. Nonadhesion of the graft is one of the main challenges after DMEK, which can happen due to adhesion difficulties between the DM and stroma (of the failed graft). This issue has been optimized by the use of a PDEK graft that contains an additional layer (pre-Descemet layer) along with the DM, which aids in adhesion. Though ultrathin-DSAEK shares the improved visual outcome and lower immunologic rejection rate of DMEK over DSAEK while minimizing all types of postoperative complications, PDEK does not require the advanced instrumentation required for DSAEK.[15]

17.7 Conclusion

Operating in an eye to reverse the stromal changes in a failed graft is far different from operating on a virgin cornea (▶ Fig. 17.10). Surgical skills and patient selection along with choosing the type of surgery to best suit the particular eye with fewer complications is vital. PDEK has the advantage of a thinner graft (unlike DSAEK) and less endothelial loss due to less intraoperative tissue trauma (unlike DMEK); therefore is a promising surgery in cases of failed previous keratoplasty.

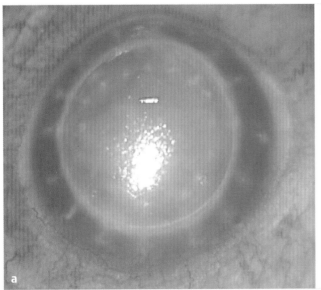 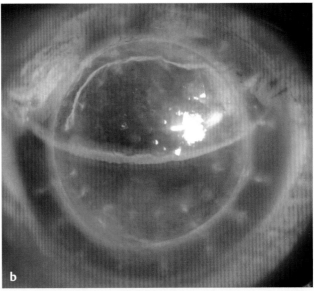

Fig. 17.10 Pre-Descemet endothelial keratoplasty (PDEK) with a young donor in a failed penetrating keratoplasty case. **(a)** Preoperative image. Note the white cornea. **(b)** Three days post-PDEK. The donor was a young person. This eye came from Miracle in Sight and in collaboration with Duke University.

References

[1] Hjortdal J, Pedersen IB, Bak-Nielsen S, Ivarsen A. Graft rejection and graft failure after penetrating keratoplasty or posterior lamellar keratoplasty for fuchs endothelial dystrophy. Cornea. 2013; 32(5):e60–e63

[2] Yu AL, Kaiser M, Schaumberger M, Messmer E, Kook D, Welge-Lussen U. Perioperative and postoperative risk factors for corneal graft failure. Clin Ophthalmol. 2014; 8:1641–1647

[3] Ang M, Htoon HM, Cajucom-Uy HY, Tan D, Mehta JS. Donor and surgical risk factors for primary graft failure following Descemet's stripping automated endothelial keratoplasty in Asian eyes. Clin Ophthalmol. 2011; 5:1503–1508

[4] Ćirković A, Schlötzer-Schrehardt U, Weller JM, Kruse FE, Tourtas T. Clinical and ultrastructural characteristics of graft failure in DMEK: 1-year results after repeat DMEK. Cornea. 2015; 34(1):11–17

[5] Ezon I, Shih CY, Rosen LM, Suthar T, Udell IJ. Immunologic graft rejection in descemet's stripping endothelial keratoplasty and penetrating keratoplasty for endothelial disease. Ophthalmology. 2013; 120(7):1360–1365

[6] Nahum Y, Mimouni M, Busin M. Risk Factors Predicting the Need for Graft Exchange After Descemet Stripping Automated Endothelial Keratoplasty. Cornea. 2015; 34(8):876–879

[7] Patel NP, Kim T, Rapuano CJ, Cohen EJ, Laibson PR. Indications for and outcomes of repeat penetrating keratoplasty, 1989–1995. Ophthalmology. 2000; 107(4):719–724

[8] Ang M, Ho H, Wong C, Htoon HM, Mehta JS, Tan D. Endothelial keratoplasty after failed penetrating keratoplasty: an alternative to repeat penetrating keratoplasty. Am J Ophthalmol. 2014; 158(6):1221–1227.e1

[9] Rapuano CJ, Cohen EJ, Brady SE, Arentsen JJ, Laibson PR. Indications for and outcomes of repeat penetrating keratoplasty. Am J Ophthalmol. 1990; 109(6):689–695

[10] Al-Mezaine H, Wagoner MD, King Khaled Eye Specialist Hospital Cornea Transplant Study Group. Repeat penetrating keratoplasty: indications, graft survival, and visual outcome. Br J Ophthalmol. 2006; 90(3):324–327

[11] Ghosheh FR, Cremona FA, Rapuano CJ, et al. Trends in penetrating keratoplasty in the United States 1980–2005. Int Ophthalmol. 2008; 28(3):147–153

[12] Weller JM, Tourtas T, Kruse FE, Schlötzer-Schrehardt U, Fuchsluger T, Bachmann BO. Descemet membrane endothelial keratoplasty as treatment for graft failure after descemet stripping automated endothelial keratoplasty. Am J Ophthalmol. 2015; 159(6):1050–1057.e2

[13] Kymionis GD, Kankariya VP, Diakonis VF, Karavitaki AE, Siganos CS, Pallikaris IG. Descemet stripping automated endothelial keratoplasty in a child after failed penetrating keratoplasty. J AAPOS. 2012; 16(1):95–96

[14] Yoeruek E, Bartz-Schmidt KU. Secondary descemet membrane endothelial keratoplasty after failed primary descemet membrane endothelial keratoplasty: clinical results. Cornea. 2013; 32(11):1414–1417

[15] Busin M, Albé E. Does thickness matter: ultrathin Descemet stripping automated endothelial keratoplasty. Curr Opin Ophthalmol. 2014; 25(4):312–318

[16] Clements JL, Bouchard CS, Lee WB, et al. Retrospective review of graft dislocation rate associated with descemet stripping automated endothelial keratoplasty after primary failed penetrating keratoplasty. Cornea. 2011; 30(4):414–418

[17] Agarwal A, Dua HS, Narang P, et al. Pre-Descemet's endothelial keratoplasty (PDEK). Br J Ophthalmol. 2014; 98(9):1181–1185

[18] Kumar DA, Dua HS, Agarwal A, Jacob S. Postoperative spectral-domain optical coherence tomography evaluation of pre-Descemet endothelial keratoplasty grafts. J Cataract Refract Surg. 2015; 41(7):1535–1536

[19] Jacob S, Agarwal A, Kumar DA. Endoilluminator-assisted Descemet membrane endothelial keratoplasty and endoilluminator-assisted pre-Descemet endothelial keratoplasty. Clin Ophthalmol. 2015; 9:2123–2125

18 Pre-Descemet Endothelial Keratoplasty in Scarred Cornea

Priya Narang and Amar Agarwal

18.1 Introduction

The cornea is a transparent structure that allows passage of light into the eye and forms the first refractive media that the ray of light embarks upon before hitting the lens and retina. Any disruption in the normal architecture of the corneal lamellae leads to scarring of the corneal stroma, which can be a response to surgery, trauma, or viral or bacterial keratitis. Trauma to the clear cornea often leads to opacity and scarring, which vary in intensity depending on the type and duration of the episode of injury. The cells responsible for scar deposition are fibroblastic cells derived from stromal keratocytes.[1] Following trauma the proximal keratocytes undergo apoptosis, and keratocytes that are distal to the wound become active fibroblasts.[1,2] Healed corneal scars are often long-lasting and disrupt vision for millions of patients worldwide.

Currently, surgical replacement of the stroma is the only successful approach for restoration of vision in scarred corneas. The treatment of corneal scars depends on the depth of the scar and fibrosis. Superficial keratectomy is performed for scar tissue that lies close to the epithelium and is quite superficial. The corneal epithelial surface cells are first removed, and then scar tissue is peeled off the front of the cornea. The epithelial cells then heal over the wound, usually in about a week's time. Phototherapeutic keratectomy is often employed when the corneal scar tissue extends into the upper parts of the corneal stroma or is very irregular in nature. Anterior lamellar keratoplasty is performed for corneal scars that involve the stroma and have a healthy endothelium. Involvement of the endothelium with the stromal scar necessitates an endothelial keratoplasty (EK) procedure along with the removal of scarred corneal tissue. The surgical procedure to be performed in such a scenario depends on the extent of corneal involvement, and it may range from penetrating keratoplasty (PK) to Descemet stripping endothelial keratoplasty (DSEK), Descemet membrane endothelial keratoplasty (DMEK), Descemet stripping automated endothelial keratoplasty (DSAEK), or Descemet membrane automated endothelial keratoplasty (DMAEK). Pre-Descemet endothelial keratoplasty (PDEK)[3,4] is a new variant of EK procedures that, unlike other EK procedures, facilitates the use of infant, young, and adult donor tissue.

PK as a procedure is faced with several difficulties, including the shortage of donor tissue, postsurgical complications associated with the use of drugs to prevent immune rejection, and a significant increase in the occurrence of glaucoma. On the other hand, EK procedures focus on the transplant of corneal endothelium, yielding better visual results but still facing the need for donor tissue. Because PDEK allows the use of infant and young donor tissue[4] it increases the donor tissue pool, which is seen as advantageous.

18.2 Our Surgical Experience

The use of infant donor tissue for scarred cornea cases has helped a great deal in the clearance of corneal scar due to bullous keratopathy. The infant donor tissue is virtually rich in endothelial cell density count that probably translates into faster and better visual recovery (▶ Fig. 18.1, ▶ Fig. 18.2, ▶ Fig. 18.3, ▶ Fig. 18.4).

Adequate visualization of the intraocular structures is essential in complex cases of scarred cornea. An endoilluminator facilitates surgery because the scarred cornea, when illuminated by obliquely falling light, allows better visualization and comprehension of graft orientation and positioning.[5]

Correction of any other associated intraocular condition, such as lens removal and intraocular lens (IOL) placement, should be performed before a PDEK procedure to enhance the chances of graft survival and mitigate the issue of constant irritation, which could be of concern at a later stage. In cases associated with IOL decentration, subluxation, or the need for a secondary IOL fixation, glued IOL fixation is performed in all cases, followed by pupilloplasty, which helps to narrow the pupil.[6] This facilitates adequate formation of the anterior chamber and also prevents air diversion in the vitreous cavity.

18.3 Discussion

Aphakic and pseudophakic bullous keratopathy is one of the major indications for corneal grafting in many developing countries,[7,8,9] and many patients in developing countries (e.g., India) do not seek surgical treatment until their bullous lesions are severe and the disease is advanced.

The advantages of performing a PDEK in complex cases of bullous keratopathy is that PDEK requires a smaller incision rather than an "open-sky" condition, and the integrity of the corneal surface in PDEK eyes is preserved without corneal incisions or sutures, eliminating the epithelium-related complications (e.g., epithelial defect and ulcer) and the suture-related complications (e.g., loose suture, infection, and neovascularization) of conventional PK.

However, in cases of bullous keratopathy with severe subepithelial opacity and/or obvious stromal scar, we always scrape off the epithelium to enhance the intraoperative visualization of intraocular structures. This may often function as superficial keratectomy. The corneal surface can be reepithelialized in 3 to 4 days.

Although PDEK has unique advantages, it is a more technically challenging procedure in the treatment of complex bullous keratopathy because combined procedures (e.g., anterior vitrectomy, IOL removal, etc.) are necessary in eyes with intraocular comorbidities. Because PDEK is more difficult to perform than PK, the combined procedures will definitely challenge the surgeon's skills.

Another problem challenging PDEK surgeons is the assessment of postoperative functional vision before PDEK surgery. Because complicated intraocular comorbidities accompany bullous keratopathy, a clear cornea does not guarantee good postoperative vision. It is difficult for surgeons to choose the perfect time for IOL implantation.

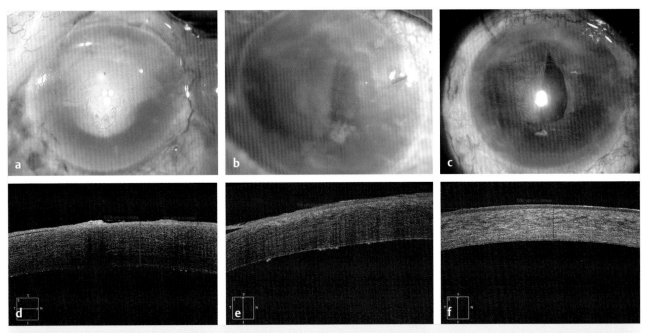

Fig. 18.1 Serial clinical slit lamp photography and anterior segment optical coherence tomography images of a scarred cornea with pseudophakic bullous keratopathy. (a,d) Preoperative image before glued intraocular lens (IOL) fixation showing corneal edema with subepithelial haze. (b,e) Images after glued IOL fixation and before endothelial keratoplasty showing persistent corneal edema and subepithelial haze with bullae. (c,f) After Pre-Descemet endothelial keratoplasty showing resolved corneal edema and resolved haze. The vision is 20/20.

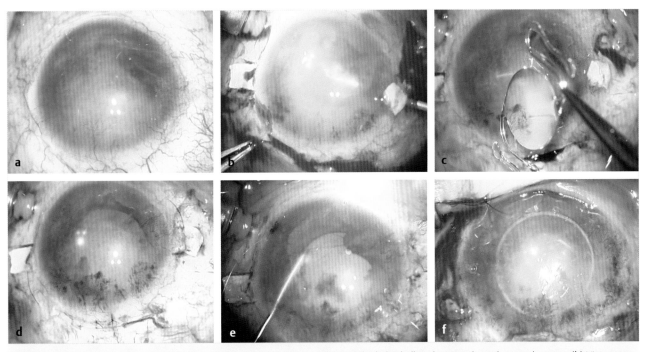

Fig. 18.2 Scarred cornea with pseudophakic bullous keratopathy (part 1). (a) Pseudophakic bullous keratopathy with scarred cornea, (b) Vitrectomy being performed. Note the scleral flaps for glued intraocular lens (IOL) fixation. Also note the trocar infusion cannula for fluid infusion. (c) Anterior chamber IOL explanted. Visualization is aided using an endoilluminator. (d) Glued IOL. Note the three-piece IOL haptics externalized. (e) Pupilloplasty. (f) Fibrin glue is applied and the scleral flaps are sealed.

In our series, secondary IOL implantation with a glued IOL technique was performed along with pupilloplasty to narrow the iris diaphragm. This indirectly helps to maintain the integrity of the anterior chamber and an ensure adequate air filling in the postoperative period. PDEK is often performed as a second-stage procedure in cases with other comorbidities. Combining PDEK with other intraocular surgeries is a feasible and effective procedure for complex bullous keratopathy with severe vision loss.

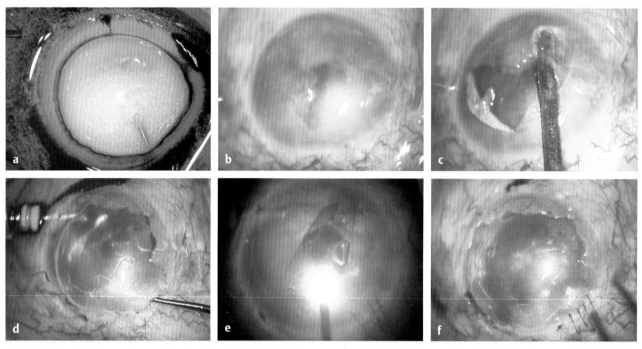

Fig. 18.3 Scarred cornea with pseudophakic bullous keratopathy (part 2). **(a)** A type 2 big bubble forms so a Descemet membrane endothelial keratoplasty graft (young donor) is prepared. **(b)** Scarred cornea after 1 month of glued intraocular lens fixation. **(c)** The epithelium is removed. **(d)** A trocar anterior chamber maintainer is fixed. Descemetorhexis is being performed. **(e)** The graft is inserted inside the anterior chamber. **(f)** The graft is attached.

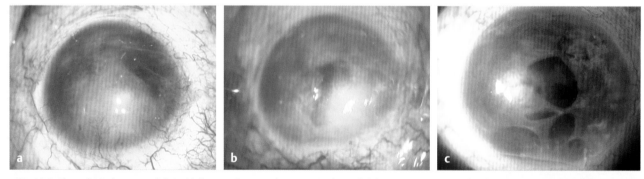

Fig. 18.4 Chronological pattern of clinical follow-up of a scarred cornea case (part 3). **(a)** Preoperative image that demonstrates severe corneal edema and scar with corneal vascularization. **(b)** Image of the same patient after glued intraocular lens fixation and vitrectomy. **(c)** Postoperative image after Descemet membrane endothelial keratoplasty with young donor graft. Resolution of corneal edema with minimal haze is seen at 6 months follow-up.

References

[1] Funderburgh JL, Mann MM, Funderburgh ML. Keratocyte phenotype mediates proteoglycan structure: a role for fibroblasts in corneal fibrosis. J Biol Chem. 2003; 278(46):45629–45637

[2] Wilson SE. Analysis of the keratocyte apoptosis, keratocyte proliferation, and myofibroblast transformation responses after photorefractive keratectomy and laser in situ keratomileusis. Trans Am Ophthalmol Soc. 2002; 100:411–433

[3] Agarwal A, Dua HS, Narang P, et al. Pre-Descemet's endothelial keratoplasty (PDEK). Br J Ophthalmol. 2014; 98(9):1181–1185

[4] Agarwal A, Agarwal A, Narang P, Kumar DA, Jacob S. Pre-Descemet Endothelial Keratoplasty With Infant Donor Corneas: A Prospective Analysis. Cornea. 2015; 34(8):859–865

[5] Jacob S, Agarwal A, Agarwal A, Narasimhan S, Kumar DA, Sivagnanam S. Endoilluminator-assisted transcorneal illumination for Descemet membrane endothelial keratoplasty: enhanced intraoperative visualization of the graft in corneal decompensation secondary to pseudophakic bullous keratopathy. J Cataract Refract Surg. 2014; 40(8):1332–1336

[6] Narang P, Agarwal A, Dua HS, Kumar DA, Jacob S, Agarwal A. Glued intra-scleral fixation of intraocular lens with pupilloplasty and pre-Descemet endothelial keratoplasty: a triple procedure. Cornea. 2015; 34(12):1627–1631

[7] Maeno A, Naor J, Lee HM, Hunter WS, Rootman DS. Three decades of corneal transplantation: indications and patient characteristics. Cornea. 2000; 19 (1):7–11

[8] Xie LX, Wang FH, Shi WY. Analysis of causes for penetrating keratoplasty at Shandong Eye Institute from 1997 to 2002 in Chinese]. Zhonghua Yan Ke Za Zhi. 2006; 42(8):704–708

[9] Chu W. The past twenty-five years in eye banking. Cornea. 2000; 19 (5):754–765

Part IV

Surgical Outcomes, Complications, and Future Trends

19 Optical Coherence Tomography in Endothelial Keratoplasty

Yuri McKee, Evan D. Schoenberg, and Francis W. Price, Jr.

19.1 Introduction

First described by Huang et al[1] in 1991, the application of optical coherence tomography (OCT) in the measurement and imaging of ophthalmic systems has revolutionized the approach to many aspects of eye disease. As a noncontact imaging modality OCT confers a distinct advantage over ultrasound and confocal biomicroscopy. The rapid, noninvasive, and high-resolution qualities of modern OCT make for an excellent adjunct to the diagnostic modalities available to the modern corneal surgeon. This chapter uses a case-based approach to demonstrate the utility of OCT in the management of endothelial keratoplasty (EK).

The initial iteration of anterior segment OCT (AS-OCT) was labeled time-domain OCT (TD-OCT). Carl Zeiss Meditec introduced the Visante TD-OCT as a tool for precise anterior segment imaging in 2005. The Visante uses a 1310 nm wavelength that can penetrate the cornea and some limbal structures to give a limbus-to-limbus view of the anterior segment with spatial resolution as fine as 15 μm. The Visante can demonstrate two-dimensional corneal shape, corneal opacities, corneal pachymetry, anterior chamber depth, iris–corneal angle anatomy, iris anatomy, and structures adjacent to the anterior lens capsule, such as a phakic intraocular lens (IOL). Newer Fourier-domain OCT (FD-OCT) devices (e.g., Avanti, OptoVue; Cirrus, Carl Zeiss Meditec) use an 830 μm wavelength that is popular for retinal imaging. Although resolution improves to as good as 5 μm, the scan length is more limited. Special attachment lenses are required to image the anterior segment with most models of FD-OCT. Although current technology does not allow FD-OCT to span the entire corneal diameter, the improved resolution of corneal and angle structures is quite useful.

EK has been rapidly growing in popularity worldwide in the past several years for the treatment of cornea endothelial dysfunction. First described by Melles et al,[2] EK confers significant advantages over penetrating keratoplasty (PK), such as stronger postoperative integrity of the globe, less induced astigmatism, faster visual recovery, and significantly reduced episodes of immune graft rejection.[3] With the advances in EK technique have come challenges in securing the posterior corneal graft to the host cornea. Preoperative, intraoperative, and postoperative imaging of the anterior segment with OCT has proven critical in many cases. Currently, the two most popular iterations of EK are Descemet stripping automated endothelial keratoplasty (DSAEK) and Descemet membrane endothelial keratoplasty (DMEK). In our practice DMEK is the preferred EK technique due to vastly lower rejection rates, smaller incision size, rapid visual recovery, and better visual potential. DMEK is technically more difficult than DSAEK and thus is not suitable in eyes with a discontinuous iris–lens diaphragm, aphakia, aniridia, or extensive posterior corneal irregularity that may preclude DMEK graft adhesion. Unless a surgeon is highly experienced in DMEK technique DSAEK may also be preferable in eyes with a history of filtering glaucoma surgery, penetrating keratoplasty, vitrectomy, and significant corneal edema that limits the view of the anterior chamber.

19.2 Preoperative OCT Imaging in EK

In the presence of significant corneal edema AS-OCT may provide critical information regarding the anatomy of the anterior segment and the suitability for EK surgery in a particular eye. Significant peripheral anterior synechiae, a shallow anterior chamber, large iris defects, and posterior corneal irregularities may all increase the complexity of EK surgery. In eyes where slit lamp examination is limited by media opacities an AS-OCT can demonstrate these potential problems preoperatively and assist in proper surgical planning. When treating endothelial failure of a previous PK graft, AS-OCT provides valuable information regarding the potential for posterior apposition of the graft to the host, which can guide surgical planning and help predict postoperative difficulties with adherence. Some authors have suggested a role for AS-OCT to determine DSAEK graft diameter.[4] We prefer DMEK in most cases but will choose DSAEK if there is a very significant graft–host mismatch as evidenced on AS-OCT.

19.3 Intraoperative OCT Imaging in EK

The use of OCT during ophthalmic surgery has been previously reported by using a handheld OCT device or an OCT device attached to a C-arm in the operative suite. Use of OCT in this manner required a pause in surgery and repositioning of the surgical microscope to allow for OCT imaging.[5,6] Another approach to intraoperative OCT was described by Geerling et al, coupling a TD-OCT unit with a dielectric mirror to a surgical microscope. This produced two-dimensional images with a number of limitations, including difficulty orienting the image and poor light penetration, but it served as a proof of concept.[7] Recently OCT has been incorporated into a commercially available surgical microscope in the Haag-Streit intraoperative OCT (iOCT) system. This device allows for real-time images of the anterior or posterior segment during surgical maneuvers as the OCT scanning beam is incorporated into the microscope and projected though the main objective lens. A small LCD screen near the surgeon allows for easy viewing of the OCT image with minimal head movement during surgery. Intraoperative OCT confers advantages in many different aspects of ophthalmic surgery. Specific advantages during EK include visualization of interface fluid during DSAEK, determination of proper graft orientation in DMEK, and visualization of posterior corneal deformities that may preclude proper graft positioning or adherence in either iteration of EK.[8]

19.4 Postoperative OCT Imaging in EK

The most popular use for OCT in EK is postoperative evaluation of the graft. Corneal edema may preclude a detailed slit lamp view of graft position or adhesion. OCT is commonly used to evaluate the cause of graft detachment,[9] confirm proper graft orientation,[10] and guide postoperative decision making in cases of graft malfunction. OCT can also accurately follow graft and host thickness during the immediate postoperative period[11,12] or later during episodes of graft rejection or graft failure. Other potential complications, including epithelial ingrowth,[13] interface opacification,[14] and retained Descemet membrane,[15] may also be elucidated with AS-OCT.

A recent study by Dr. Gerrit Melles' group (Yeh et al.) evaluated the predictive value of AS-OCT in DMEK graft attachment, comparing graft attachment on AS-OCT at 1 hour, 1 week, and 1 month postoperatively to attachment at 6 months. This study, in which no air reinjection was performed at any time point, concluded that DMEK graft attachment at 1 week had excellent predictive value for continued attachment through 6 months. Grafts that were attached at 1 hour but significantly detached at 1 week were likely to spontaneously reattach, whereas grafts detached at both time points were less likely to undergo spontaneous reattachment.[16] This provides insight into the evolution of graft adherence and may guide decision making in certain circumstances. It is worth noting that, in our practice, we reinject air for any significant detachment rather than awaiting spontaneous clearance. In our analysis of 673 eyes with at least 6 months' follow-up, this achieves visual improvement sooner and is not associated with decreased endothelial cell counts nor increased incidence of any complications.[17]

19.5 Case Studies of OCT in EK

19.5.1 Case 1: Uncomplicated Normal DSEK

In this case a normal postoperative DSEK is demonstrated (▶ Fig. 19.1). The central cornea is clear, and there is a thin, well-centered graft without folds or detachment. The graft edge is clearly seen at the slit lamp and on OCT. Graft and host thickness can easily be measured individually on OCT. Ultrasonic pachymetry will only yield the total thickness of the graft–host complex. The Visante TD-OCT demonstrates the entire width of the graft and easily penetrates deep into the anterior chamber with the longer 1310 nm wavelength. Some detail is lost in the lower resolution with the longer wavelength. Graft and host thickness can be easily measured at any point using the "Flap Tool" function (not shown) that was originally designed to measure LASIK flap thickness.

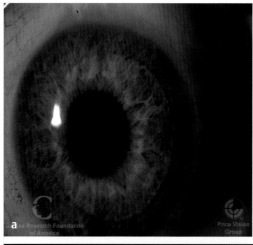

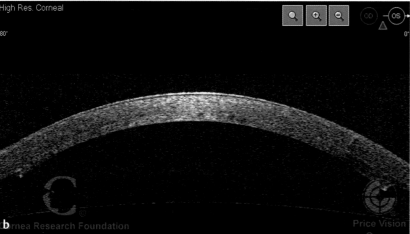

Fig. 19.1 **(a)** Color photo of a normal Descemet stripping automated endothelial keratoplasty (DSAEK) after complete healing. **(b)** Time-domain optical coherence tomography of a normal DSAEK.

19.5.2 Case 2: Uncomplicated DMEK

Here a postoperative day 1 DMEK (▶ Fig. 19.2) is still supported by an air bubble and is fully attached as demonstrated by the Avanti FD-OCT (Optovue). Notice the maximum scan diameter is 8 mm instead of 12 mm, as in a Visante scan, accompanied by a corresponding decrease in scan depth. The FD-OCT imparts higher resolution due to the shorter 830 nm wavelength of the scanning source. The DMEK graft adheres in such a seamless manner that it is nearly impossible to notice a difference between a graft and a virgin cornea.

This Visante TD-OCT demonstrates the normal appearance of a postoperative DMEK graft with good graft adhesion, centration, and function. This patient has no air left in the anterior

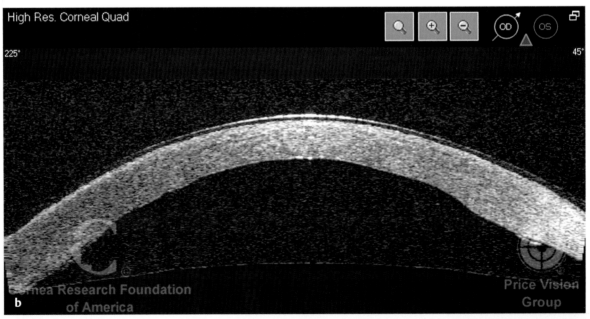

Fig. 19.2 (a) A normal postoperative day 1 Descemet membrane endothelial keratoplasty (DMEK) as seen on Fourier-domain optical coherence tomography (OCT). The air bubble is not visible on this image of the OCT, but the edge of a bubble can be seen in certain frames. Do not confuse the edge of an air bubble with an inverted graft or a graft detachment. **(b)** A normal DMEK on time-domain OCT at postoperative day 5.

chamber, and a contact lens is still in place, consistent with a postop day 5 OCT. The faint edge lift noted superiorly is inconsequential and may be observed in the course of normally scheduled postoperative visits. The surface hyperreflectivity in the AS-OCT is due to the bandage contact lens (BCL) placed at the conclusion of surgery because the patient underwent simultaneous superficial keratectomy.

19.5.3 Case 3: Small DMEK Detachment Requiring Observation Only

Two days status post–uncomplicated DMEK, this patient was found to have a localized inferior detachment of the graft (▶ Fig. 19.3). Small detachments such as this one are common and typically inferiorly where the air bubble spends less time even with good reported compliance to supine positioning. The detachment was fully resolved by postoperative day 5. TD-OCT provides visualization of even subtle detachments and may be used to objectively follow their extent. Note the gentle curve of the detached portion of the DMEK graft toward the stroma, confirming that the graft is in the proper orientation.

19.5.4 Case 4: DMEK Detachment Requiring Air

In this example, 3 days after DMEK, a large undulating DMEK graft detachment is demonstrated under an area of corneal edema (▶ Fig. 19.4a). This patient demonstrated an immediate benefit from an additional air injection and supine positioning. Careful inspection of the detached graft edge reveals a slight upward curl toward the corneal stroma. This finding confirms that the graft is in the correct orientation with endothelium facing the iris. In general, our criteria for air reinjection for DMEK are as follows:

1. Absence of adequate anterior chamber air bubble to completely cover a detachment (typically < 30–40% air bubble)
2. Graft detachment > 2 clock hours or an expanding detachment
3. Significant edema over a graft detachment
4. Graft detachments that threaten the visual axis

Small, nonprogressive, peripheral detachments without overlying stromal edema that do not threaten the visual axis may be safely observed.

In another example a DMEK was done in a patient (▶ Fig. 19.4b) who had a history of pars plans vitrectomy and a well-functioning trabeculectomy. The inability to shallow the anterior chamber during surgery in a patient without a vitreous body greatly increases the complexity and operating time of DMEK. In addition, a well-functioning trabeculectomy can quickly cause dissipation of even a full air fill. This can leave very little air contact time for the graft and increase the chance of a need for repeat air injection. The use of 16% sulfur hexafluride (SF6), a nonexpensive concentration of an inert gas, helps to increase the graft contact time of the inert gas, but caution must be used in the setting of a trabeculectomy. The inert gas absorbs much more slowly and can occlude the sclerostomy or fill the bleb with gas, resulting in a dangerous elevation of intraocular pressure. Inferior graft detachments are the most common as patients often have trouble abiding by a strict supine positioning regimen. When upright, the bubble will continue to support the superior graft, but the inferior graft will be supported only when the patient is supine. Occasionally supine positioning with a chin-up posture is required to ensure that the inferior aspect of the graft is fully supported by the air bubble. Face-down positioning should be avoided because this can lead to air migrating posterior to the iris.

19.5.5 Case 5: Postoperative Bullae after DSAEK

Bullae and stromal edema can make evaluation of graft position difficult, especially with a thin-cut DSAEK or DMEK. If the involved area is covered by the graft, this may indicate graft dysfunction or failure. On the other hand, if the involved area is outside the graft, observation and temporizing measures, such as hypertonic saline drops, should be advised because endothelial cells may migrate from the graft over time. AS-OCT can demonstrate the graft position even through a hazy cornea while also visualizing the bullae themselves (▶ Fig. 19.5). In this case inferior corneal edema after a DSAEK proved to be related to a superior displacement of the graft but no graft detachment.

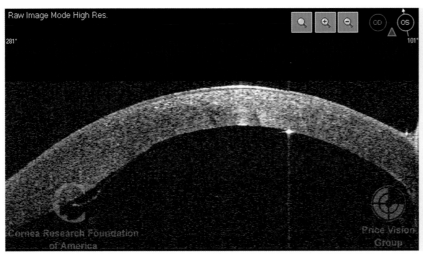

Fig. 19.3 A small peripheral Descemet membrane endothelial keratoplasty graft detachment demonstrated by time-domain optical coherence tomography. This can be observed at normally scheduled visits.

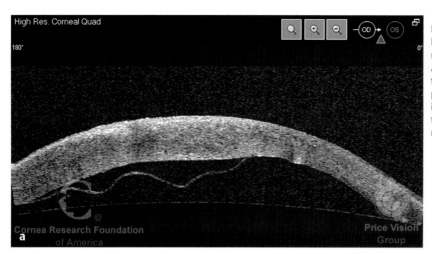

Fig. 19.4 **(a)** A large temporal Descemet membrane endothelial keratoplasty (DMEK) detachment that resolved with a repeat air injection. **(b)** A DMEK graft with a large inferior detachment that required SF6 to resolve the detachment. The patient was carefully monitored following the injection of SF6 due to the presence of a trabeculectomy, which can be occluded by inert non-expansile gases.

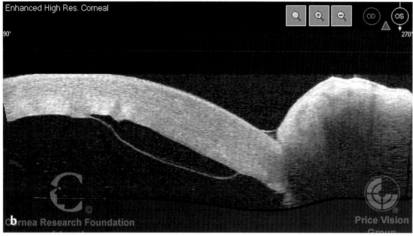

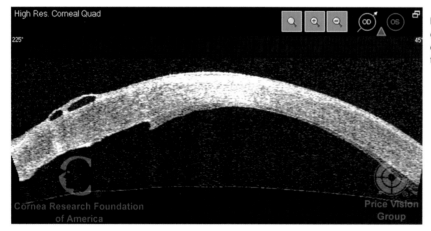

Fig. 19.5 Corneal edema and epithelial bullae due to superior displacement of the graft as demonstrated by time-domain optical coherence tomography.

Observation and conservative measurements eventually resulted in resolution of the edema.

19.5.6 Case 6: Persistent DSAEK Detachment

This patient underwent a combined phacoemulsification, IOL insertion, and DSAEK procedure for cataract and Fuchs endothelial dystrophy. The central corneal edema quickly cleared, but a persistent area of temporal corneal edema over the surgical wound persisted. Most DSAEK detachments will spontaneously clear without additional air injection over a few days to a few weeks at most. Although the patient achieved excellent vision she did report a slight visual distortion temporally as well as a foreign body sensation associated with the edema. When the edema failed to clear an AS-OCT was done with a Cirrus FD-OCT (Carl Zeiss Meditec). While the scan size is much less with FD-OCT, the resolution is much greater, allowing for the visualization of details that may be missed on TD-OCT. This detachment was shown to be the result of a curl of host Descemet membrane and likely a small amount of posterior stroma that was repelling the edge of the DSAEK graft

(▶ Fig. 19.6a). Corneal edema over the graft detachment precluded visualization of the true nature of this problem. The OCT images proved that a repeat air injection would not resolve this detachment. The patient was taken back to the operating room where the offending tissue scroll was removed with microforceps, and then an air bubble was placed to promote graft edge adhesion (▶ Fig. 19.6b). Postoperatively the patient reported rapid resolution of her discomfort and visual disturbance.

19.5.7 Cases 7 and 8: DMEK under PK

Placing a DMEK graft under a failed PK confers many advantages over replacing the entire graft, including a lower rejection rate, small incision, and quick recovery. Thus rescuing a PK from endothelial failure becomes a much lower risk surgery with a better long-term rejection profile. As a trade-off placing a DMEK under a PK requires significant experience with the surgical technique and closer postoperative follow-up due to the higher risk of graft edge detachment. The use of SF6 gas to increase the contact time of the anterior chamber gas bubble may be useful in cases of DMEK under PK, especially when a

significant posterior contour discrepancy exists in the graft–host interface. Preoperative evaluation of the graft–host interface can assist with surgical planning. A significant posterior discontinuity may be reason to use a graft with a diameter equal to or less than the original PK graft. However, we have observed that using EK grafts < 8 mm may lead to a higher rate of failure, presumably due to fewer overall endothelial cells in smaller grafts. Consequently, DMEK grafts may need to bridge the graft–host interface, leading to challenges in promoting graft edge adhesion. In questionable cases the surgeon may opt for a DSAEK graft instead of a DMEK graft under a PK because the surgical technique is less demanding, and obtaining stable graft adhesion may be less difficult. The following cases demonstrate some challenges in placing a DMEK under PK and how the AS-OCT can be useful in management of these cases.

19.5.8 Case 7

The first patient was referred for a slowly failing PK that was placed more then 20 years previously. The falling endothelial

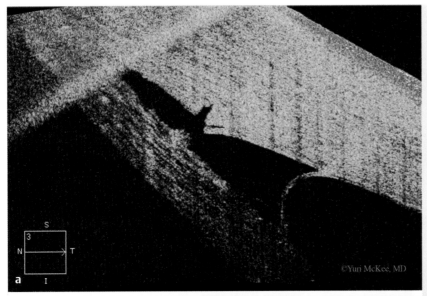
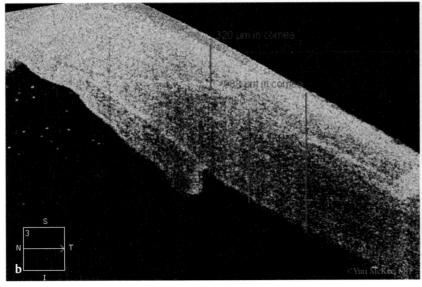

Fig. 19.6 **(a)** A peripheral Descemet stripping automated endothelial keratoplasty (DSAEK) graft detachment near the main surgical wound due to a curl of posterior stroma and Descemet membrane (DM). **(b)** After surgical removal of the residual DM tissue and an additional air injection the temporal graft detachment rapidly cleared along with the host stromal edema. Optical coherence tomography also demonstrates our preferred wound construction for a DSAEK with a short triplanar corneal tunnel and overlap of the inner lip of the wound with the DSAEK graft.

cell count and increasing graft thickness confirmed that graft failure was imminent. A DMEK graft was successfully placed. While the graft did have good central adhesion there was a small, persistent inferior-temporal graft detachment within the borders of the original PK graft (▶ Fig. 19.7). Since this detachment had shown some enlargement in the first 2 weeks after surgery an additional air injection was placed, and the patient resumed supine positioning for 3 days. A surgeon should decide if a DMEK detachment requires additional air or gas injection within the first month after surgery because the detached portion of the graft can become fibrotic and inflexible beyond this time. Additional considerations include the area of intended host Descemet membrane (DM) stripping since retained DM is a risk factor for DMEK graft nonadhesion. DM should not be stripped across an old PK wound because this is one of the strongest points of adhesion between the graft and the host in a healed PK. Also, this can lead to additional posterior stromal irregularities for a DMEK graft to negotiate.

19.5.9 Case 8

In this second example of DMEK under PK a man had a history of DSAEK placed under a failed PK. Several months after surgery the DSAEK graft suffered an immune-related graft failure. The failed DSAEK extended beyond the margin of the old PK. While DSAEK does not require full stripping of the DM, removal of a DSAEK often results in concurrent removal of all DM under the graft and in a margin beyond the original EK. Furthermore, retained DM is a risk factor for DMEK detachment in our experience. To further complicate this case the patient had a previous pars plans vitrectomy and a very well functioning trabeculectomy with an average intraocular pressure of 5 to 8 mm Hg. In eyes with an absent vitreous body the anterior chamber is difficult to shallow during surgery, increasing the intraoperative difficulty of DMEK. Eyes with very low intraocular pressure (IOP) present a challenge in postoperative adhesion of EK grafts. Additionally, in eyes with a well-functioning

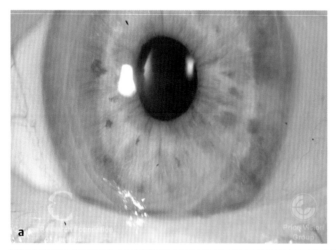

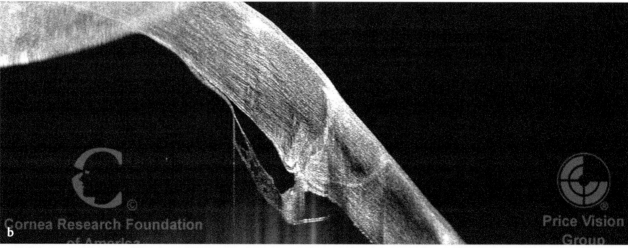

Fig. 19.7 (a) In this postoperative photograph the central cornea is clear, and the Descemet membrane endothelial keratoplasty graft is functioning well. A small inferior-temporal area of haze in the old penetrating keratoplasty represents a stable chronic graft detachment that stabilized after the second air injection. (b) The Optovue Fourier-domain optical coherence tomography (OCT) clearly demonstrates a small piece of tissue at the graft–host interface that is causing the detachment. The OCT also demonstrates the chronic nature of the detachment as Descemet membrane and endothelium have separated and become fibrotic. This stable detachment is unlikely to cause future problems and can simply be observed. Further air injection is unlikely to result in resolution of this detachment.

trabeculectomy the intraoperative air bubble can quickly dissipate via the sclerostomy into the bleb (▶ Fig. 19.8). The choice of air or inert, nonexpansile gas in this setting can be a dilemma. Inert gas may last more than twice as long as air in the normal eye, promoting graft adhesion, but it may occlude the sclerostomy of the trabeculectomy, causing a dangerous elevation in IOP.

19.5.10 Case 9: DMEK: Complete DMEK Detachment

A 38-year-old man with a history of PK presented with endothelial graft failure and cataract. Combined phacoemulsification, IOL placement, and DMEK were performed. On postoperative day 1, the cornea was diffusely edematous, and IOP was 4 mm Hg. At the slit lamp, it was impossible to determine whether or not the DMEK graft was attached. AS-OCT allowed for rapid localization of the fully detached DMEK graft resting against the iris in the anterior chamber (▶ Fig. 19.9a). It was clear from the AS-OCT that an additional air injection was not going to help with graft attachment.

The following day the patient returned to the operating room for repeat DMEK. An attempt could have been made to reposition the existing graft, but out of concern for a decreased cell count after manipulation trauma, the previous graft was removed and a new DMEK graft was placed. On postoperative day 1 after repeat DMEK, the graft showed scattered small areas of detachment and significant nasal detachment. This did not clear on day 2 despite continued supine positioning. The AS-OCT shows a mismatch between the host cornea and the existing PK graft, which interferes with DMEK adherence, resulting in a small temporal and larger nasal DMEK detachment (▶ Fig. 19.9b). Based on the degree of detachment, a repeat air fill to 80% air was performed in the minor procedure room. Three days after the air reinjection, having spent the first 2 days in a supine position with slight left face turn for at least 10 hours per day, AS-OCT demonstrates excellent graft adherence to the PK (▶ Fig. 19.9c). The posterior curvature mismatch continued to discourage complete adherence outside of the graft. Once this degree of attachment is obtained, observation alone is typically sufficient.

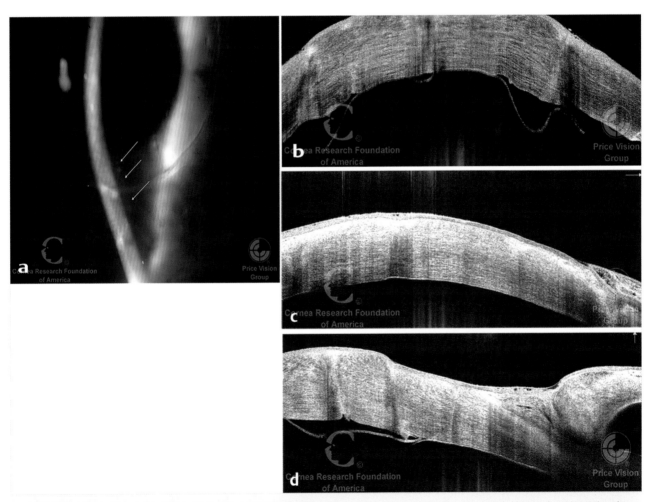

Fig. 19.8 (a) Slit lamp photo of an inferior graft detachment in an early postoperative Descemet membrane endothelial keratoplasty (DMEK) under a penetrating keratoplasty (PK). The air rapidly dissipated due to a well-functioning trabeculectomy. (b) Optovue Fourier-domain optical coherence tomography (FD-OCT) demonstrating a transverse plane view of a superior graft detachment in the early postoperative period due to rapid dissipation of the air bubble. (c,d) Optovue FD-OCT after injection of SF6. This figure demonstrates (b) transverse and (d) vertical planes of the superior cornea. The glaucoma bleb filled with gas can be seen in the vertical plane. (continued)

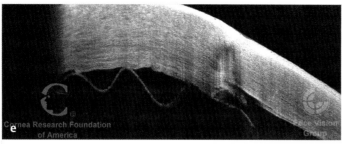

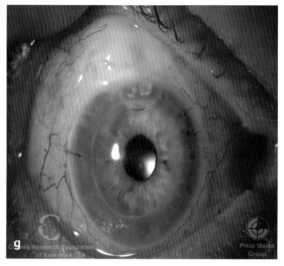

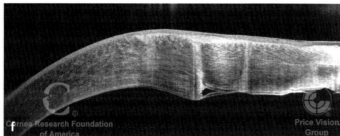

Fig. 19.8 *(continued)* **(e,f)** An undulating temporal graft detachment before SF6 injection **(e)**, and supported by SF6 injection **(f)**. **(g)** The failed PK is now clear with a well attached DMEK graft. The healing time was 2 weeks, and the risk of graft rejection is now < 1%. A small bubble of SF6 is still present in the anterior chamber in this photo.

19.5.11 Case 10: Inverted DMEK Graft

A patient with a history of Fuchs endothelial dystrophy underwent DMEK. On postoperative day 1 he was found to have a posteriorly curling inferior graft detachment. A DMEK graft always scrolls with the endothelium to the outside. A graft curling away from the host cornea indicates that the graft is inverted (▶ Fig. 19.10). This problem is handled in the operating room by re-positioning or replacing the graft.

19.5.12 Case 11: DSAEK Graft Detachment under Prior Corneoscleral Graft

This patient initially presented with a bacterial keratitis involving the cornea, limbus, and limbal sclera that did not respond to aggressive antibacterial therapy. A 15 mm corneoscleral anterior lamellar graft was performed. To decrease the risk of intraocular spread of the infection, the patient's own DM and endothelium were not violated during this procedure. Postoperatively, the infection cleared, and the patient was found to have a dense cataract and retrocorneal membrane. Phacoemulsification, IOL placement, and removal of the membrane—which corresponded to fibrosis surrounding the host DM—was performed without complication. Subsequently, however, the host endothelium failed. The patient underwent DSAEK under the corneoscleral graft.

On postoperative day 2 there was slit lamp evidence of a large supranasal graft detachment of unclear etiology. Conventional management would suggest repeat air injection to float the graft back into position. However, AS-OCT revealed that the graft margin was actually stuck on an iris root remnant from the corneoscleral graft (▶ Fig. 19.11a). Further air injections would not be likely to resolve the detachment. The following day, the patient returned to the operating room where the graft was repositioned. At postoperative week 1, the repositioned

DSAEK graft was well positioned and fully attached (▶ Fig. 19.11b). The corneoscleral graft stroma remained edematous. At 1 year postoperative the graft stroma was clear and of normal thickness (▶ Fig. 19.11c).

19.5.13 Case 12: DSAEK Graft Detachment with Posterior Corneal Fibrosis

A 58-year-old woman had a history of delivery forceps trauma causing chronic childhood corneal clouding. She was wearing bandage contact lenses for painful bullous keratopathy and band keratopathy, which had developed 3 years prior. She underwent combined DSAEK and sodium-EDTA chelation. Descemet stripping was not attempted due to the poor view. After extensive manipulation the graft was unfolded and positioned. A complete air fill for 8 minutes was followed by a reduction to a 50% bubble. On postoperative day 1 the cornea was significantly clearer than preoperatively, but a large inferior and nasal detachment of the graft was visible at the slit lamp. An oblique opacity could also be appreciated, but due to the remaining corneal haze it was unclear if this was a result of host pathology or of a fold in the graft (▶ Fig. 19.12a).

AS-OCT demonstrated a relatively thick, opaque outcropping of tissue consistent with fibrosis of the patient's DM at the site of initial injury (▶ Fig. 19.12b). A laser inferior peripheral iridectomy was made, and the anterior chamber was filled 95% with air. Under air, closer apposition of the graft was achieved, as seen at the slit lamp and on AS-OCT (▶ Fig. 19.12c, d).

19.5.14 Case 13: Intraoperative OCT with the Haag-Streit IOCT

Intraoperative OCT is a promising new technology that has now been integrated into the surgical microscope. In this example a

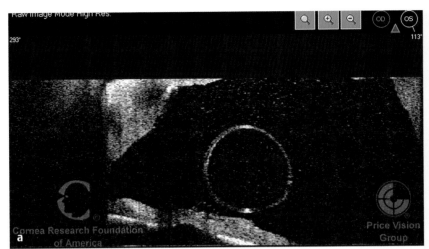

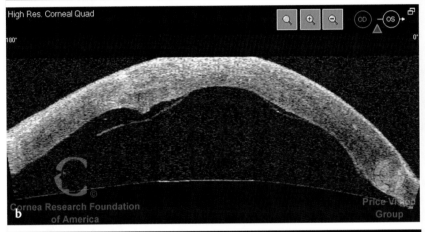

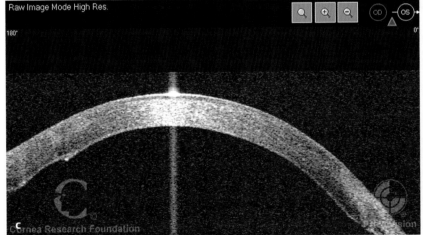

Fig. 19.9 (a) The graft was imaged with time-domain optical coherence tomography in its natural, endothelium-out, scrolled configuration against the iris, en face, with the peripheral cornea visible on the top-left side of the image. (b) The repeat Descemet membrane endothelial keratoplasty (DMEK) graft with a detachment over the graft–host junction of the previous penetrating keratoplasty (PK), a graft detachment requiring repeat air injection is noted. (c) Complete attachment of the DMEK under the PK after air reinjection.

DMEK graft orientation is quickly and positively determined by OCT that is aimed through the main lens of the microscope. This results in real-time information (▸ Fig. 19.13) available to the surgeon without interrupting the surgical process.

19.6 Conclusion

AS-OCT has radically changed the approach to evaluation and management of patients undergoing endothelial keratoplasty. Although preoperative evaluation can help guide surgical planning in difficult cases, postoperative availability of an AS-OCT is critical in managing the inevitable graft detachments that occur in the typical postsurgical course of some patients. Intraoperative OCT is now becoming available, which will further facilitate the surgical process, especially for DMEK. An understanding of the basic concepts, applications, and limitations of different OCT modalities is now a required skill for corneal surgeons. As this technology rapidly advances we should expect further increases in scan width, depth, and resolution. Applying the information gleaned from this amazing technology will help guide corneal surgeons to the correct diagnosis and treatment plan when offering EK to patients.

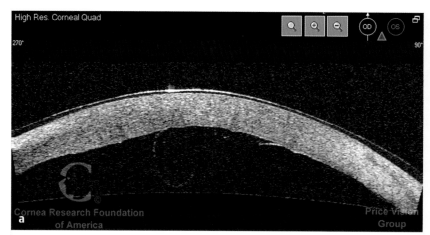

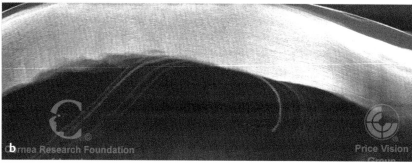

Fig. 19.10 **(a)** Visante time-domain optical coherence tomography (OCT) demonstrated that the graft was curling away from the stroma. **(b)** An Optovue Fourier-domain (OCT) of the inverted graft. The improved resolution but narrower acquisition width of this modality is evident. The ghosting images surrounding the Descemet membrane endothelial keratoplasty graft are the result of movement artifact.

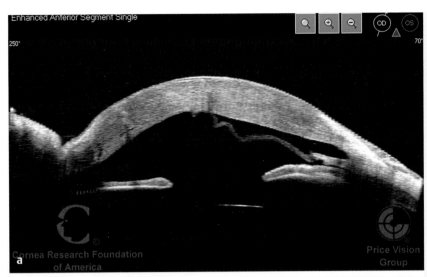

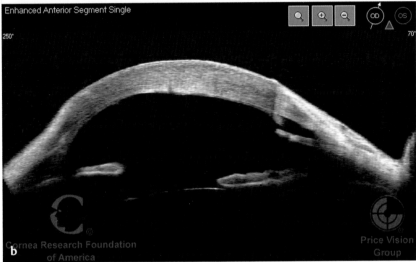

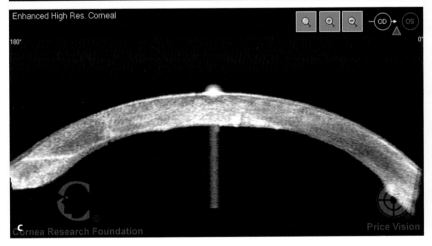

Fig. 19.11 (a) The Descemet stripping automated endothelial keratoplasty (DSAEK) graft edge held out of the proper position by the iris root of the prior corneoscleral graft. (b) Postoperative day 1 from DSAEK reposition. The DSAEK graft is now in good position and fully attached. (c) One year post-DSAEK, the cornea is clear and the graft well attached.

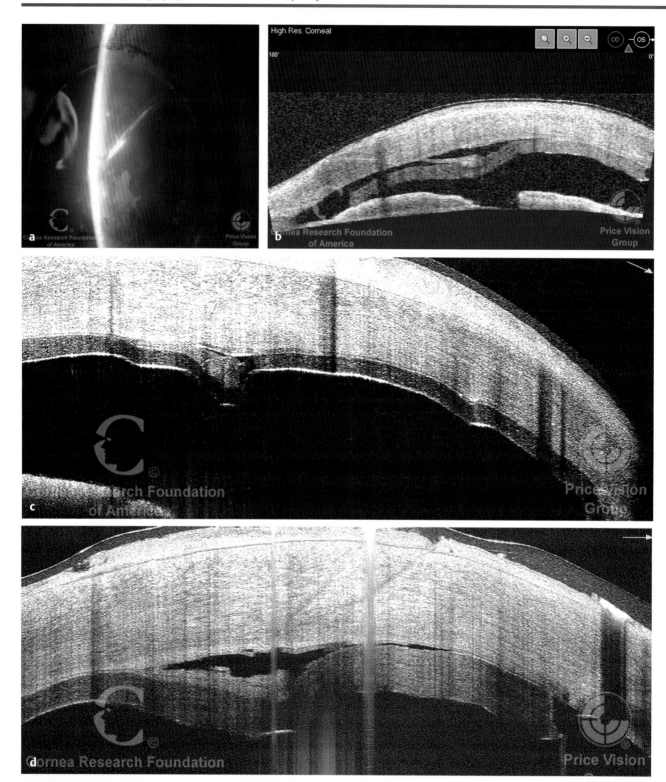

Fig. 19.12 **(a)** Slit beam photo of Descemet stripping automated endothelial keratoplasty (DSAEK) under old forceps delivery injury. **(b)** On postoperative day 1 the graft showed poor apposition to the host cornea, especially in the area of posterior corneal fibrosis. **(c)** Under a 95% air fill the DSAEK graft conformed well to the host corneal deformity. **(d)** One week later, after air was no longer pressing the graft into place, the graft could be seen conforming to the fibrotic Descemet membrane remnant of the host.

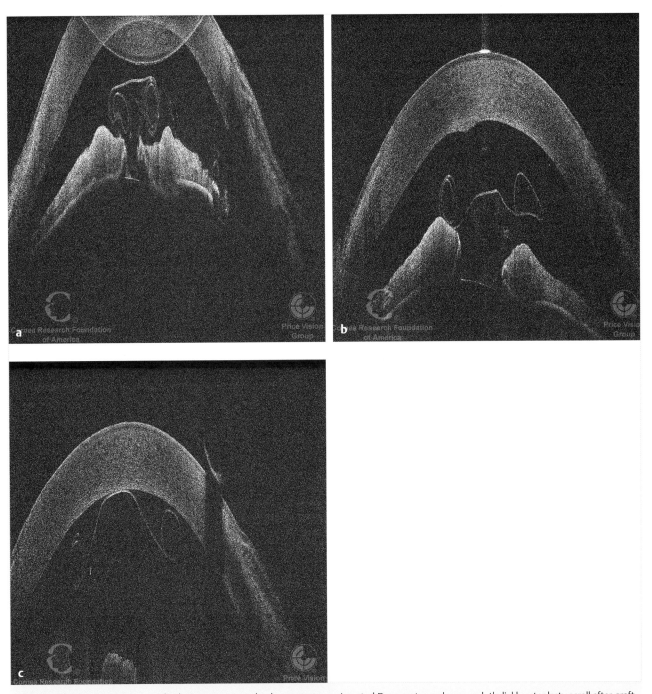

Fig. 19.13 **(a)** Intraoperative optical coherence tomography demonstrates an inverted Descemet membrane endothelial keratoplasty scroll after graft insertion. **(b)** The graft is flipped with a gentle burst of fluid and is now in the proper orientation. **(c)** The graft is suspended against the host stroma by an air bubble, preventing accidental graft inversion and promoting graft opening.

References

[1] Huang D, Swanson EA, Lin CP, et al. Optical coherence tomography. Science. 1991; 254(5035):1178–1181

[2] Melles GR, Eggink FA, Lander F, et al. A surgical technique for posterior lamellar keratoplasty. Cornea. 1998; 17(6):618–626

[3] Anshu A, Price MO, Price FW, Jr. Risk of corneal transplant rejection significantly reduced with Descemet's membrane endothelial keratoplasty. Ophthalmology. 2012; 119(3):536–540

[4] Straiko MD, Terry MA, Shamie N. Descemet stripping automated endothelial keratoplasty under failed penetrating keratoplasty: a surgical strategy to minimize complications. Am J Ophthalmol. 2011; 151(2):233–7.e2

[5] Knecht PB, Kaufmann C, Menke MN, Watson SL, Bosch MM. Use of intraoperative fourier-domain anterior segment optical coherence tomography during descemet stripping endothelial keratoplasty. Am J Ophthalmol. 2010; 150 (3):360–365.e2

[6] Ide T, Wang J, Tao A, et al. Intraoperative use of three-dimensional spectral-domain optical coherence tomography. Ophthalmic Surg Lasers Imaging. 2010; 41(2):250–254

[7] Geerling G, Müller M, Winter C, et al. Intraoperative 2-dimensional optical coherence tomography as a new tool for anterior segment surgery. Arch Ophthalmol. 2005; 123(2):253–257

[8] Steven P, Le Blanc C, Velten K, et al. Optimizing descemet membrane endothelial keratoplasty using intraoperative optical coherence tomography. JAMA Ophthalmol. 2013; 131(9):1135–1142

[9] Moutsouris K, Dapena I, Ham L, Balachandran C, Oellerich S, Melles GRJ. Optical coherence tomography, Scheimpflug imaging, and slit-lamp biomicroscopy in the early detection of graft detachment after Descemet membrane endothelial keratoplasty. Cornea. 2011; 30(12):1369–1375

[10] Saad A, Sabatier P, Gatinel D. Graft orientation, optical coherence tomography, and endothelial keratoplasty. Ophthalmology. 2013; 120(4):871–871.e3

[11] Di Pascuale MA, Prasher P, Schlecte C, et al. Corneal deturgescence after Descemet stripping automated endothelial keratoplasty evaluated by Visante anterior segment optical coherence tomography. Am J Ophthalmol. 2009; 148(1):32–7.e1

[12] Wong MHY, Chew A, Htoon HM, et al. Reproducibility of Corneal Graft Thickness measurements with COLGATE in patients who have undergone DSAEK (Descemet Stripping Automated Endothelial Keratoplasty). BMC Med Imaging. 2012; 12:25

[13] Suh LH, Shousha MA, Ventura RU, et al. Epithelial ingrowth after Descemet stripping automated endothelial keratoplasty: description of cases and assessment with anterior segment optical coherence tomography. Cornea. 2011; 30(5):528–534

[14] de Sanctis U, Brusasco L, Grignolo F. Wave-like opacities at the interface after descemet stripping automated endothelial keratoplasty. Cornea. 2012; 31(11):1335–1338

[15] Suh LH, Yoo SH, Deobhakta A, et al. Complications of Descemet's stripping with automated endothelial keratoplasty: survey of 118 eyes at One Institute. Ophthalmology. 2008; 115(9):1517–1524

[16] Yeh R-Y, Quilendrino R, Musa FU, Liarakos VS, Dapena I, Melles GRJ. Predictive value of optical coherence tomography in graft attachment after Descemet's membrane endothelial keratoplasty. Ophthalmology. 2013; 120(2):240–245

[17] Feng MT, Price MO, Miller JM, Price FW, Jr. Air reinjection and endothelial cell density in Descemet membrane endothelial keratoplasty: five-year follow-up. J Cataract Refract Surg. 2014; 40(7):1116–1121

20 Spectral Domain Optical Coherence Tomography Evaluation of Pre-Descemet Endothelial Keratoplasty Graft

Dhivya Ashok Kumar and Amar Agarwal

20.1 Introduction

Pre-Descemet endothelial keratoplasty (PDEK), a recent modification of endothelial keratoplasty, involves the transplantation of the pre-Descemet layer (Dua layer) along with the Descemet membrane (DM) with endothelium. In this selective tissue transplantation, the pre-Descemet layer provides additional thickness to the thin DM. Dua et al[1] describe the pre-Descemet layer as a tough, fibrous layer about $10.15 \pm 3.6\,\mu m$. The technique allows easy intraoperative tissue handling and less injury to the donor harvested graft. The initial results showed good postoperative outcomes and fewer surgical complications.[2] The technique inherited the basic advantages of early visual rehabilitation and lowered graft rejection similar to DM endothelial keratoplasty (DMEK).[3,4] The postoperative graft position, seen clinically by slit lamp, but high-resolution spectral domain optical coherence tomography (SD-OCT) provides additional information in the configuration of endothelial grafts. This chapter describes the postoperative graft configuration using SD-OCT.

20.1.1 Pre-Descemet Endothelial Keratoplasty

A corneoscleral disc with an approximately 2 mm scleral rim is dissected from the whole globe or obtained from an eye bank. A 30-gauge needle attached to a syringe is inserted from the limbus into the midperipheral stroma (▶ Fig. 20.1a). Air is slowly injected into the donor stroma until a type 1 big bubble is formed (▶ Fig. 20.1a, b). Trephination is done along the margin of the big bubble. The bubble wall is penetrated at the extreme periphery and trypan blue is injected to stain the graft, which is then cut with a pair of corneoscleral scissors and is covered with the tissue culture medium (▶ Fig. 20.1c).

Under peribulbar anesthesia, a trephine mark is made on the recipient cornea respective to the diameter of the DM to be scored on the endothelial side. A 2.8 mm tunnel incision is made at 10 o'clock near the limbus. The anterior chamber (AC) is formed and maintained with saline injection or infusion. The margin of recipient DM to be removed is scored with a reverse Sinskey hook and then peeled (▶ Fig. 20.1d, e). The donor lenticule (endothelium–DM–pre-Descemet layer) roll is inserted in the custom-made injector (▶ Fig. 20.1e, f) and is injected in a controlled fashion into the AC (▶ Fig. 20.1g). The donor graft is oriented endothelial side down and positioned onto the recipient posterior stroma by careful, indirect manipulation of the tissue with air and fluid (▶ Fig. 20.1h). Once the lenticule is unrolled, an air bubble is injected underneath the lenticule to lift it toward the recipient posterior stroma (▶ Fig. 20.1i). The AC is completely filled with air for the next 30 minutes, followed by an air–liquid exchange to pressurize the eye. The eye speculum is finally removed and the AC is examined for air position. The patient is advised to lie in a strictly supine position for the next 3 hours.

20.1.2 Spectral Domain Optical Coherence Tomography

Postoperative SD-OCT scans were performed by an experienced examiner, and the scans were evaluated by expert ophthalmologists. An anterior segment five-line raster pattern in an axis of 0 to 180 degrees and 90 to 270 degrees was used. The raster scan had five lines (length 3 mm) and 250 μm distance between the lines. The scan was centered at the corneal vertex for a central 3 mm scan. Additional inferior, temporal, nasal, and superior positional scans were also taken. Graft thickness (GT) was measured in micrometers with the tool caliper in the SD-OCT. Graft detachment was graded as group I for completely attached grafts or minimal edge detachment; group II for graft detachments less than one-third of the graft surface area, not affecting the visual axis; group III for graft detachments more than one-third of the graft surface area; and group IV for completely detached grafts. Epithelial thickness and recurrence of bulla were noted. The graft–host junction was visualized for interface opacification. A graft split was defined as the separation of the pre-Descemet layer and the DM. Postoperative central corneal thickness (CCT) was also measured in all follow-ups. Twelve eyes of 12 patients with mean age 65 ± 3.8 years were evaluated. There were nine women and three men. The donor age ranged from 1 to 56 years. The graft size ranged from 7.5 mm to 8 mm. All the eyes had preoperative pseudophakic bullous keratopathy as the indication for endothelial transplantation.

20.1.3 Pre-Descemet Endothelial Keratoplasty Graft in Optical Coherence Tomography

The mean GT in PDEK was $37.3 \pm 3.5\,\mu m$ (range 32–44 μm). The graft undergoes minimal dehydration in the postoperative period. The mean GT on day 7, day 30, and day 90 was $35.5 \pm 3.4\,\mu m$ (32–40 μm), $33 \pm 1.8\,\mu m$ (32–36 μm), and $30.3 \pm 2.6\,\mu m$ (28–36 μm), respectively. There was a significant difference in the GT over the time period (Friedman test, $p = 0.000$) (▶ Fig. 20.2). There was no significant difference ($p = 1.000$) between the central (3 mm) and peripheral (4–6 mm) GT. The graft was well adhered (▶ Fig. 20.3) in 9 of 12 eyes on day 1. Two eyes had group II detachment (▶ Fig. 20.4), and 1 eye had group III graft detachment (▶ Fig. 20.5). One eye with grade III detachment underwent air injection. The graft was well apposed on post–air injection day 1; however, there was redetachment on day 12, and bubbling was redone subsequently. In group I eyes with a well-adhered graft, a small, shallow, peripheral detachment was seen in the inferior (2 eyes) and nasal quadrant (1 eye). The mean detachment depth was $24.6 \pm 8.3\,\mu m$. Descemet folds were noted in 2 eyes on day 1 (▶ Fig. 20.6), which resolved on day 7 with medical management and supine position. A smooth, concave configuration of the posterior cornea was obtained in all eyes by 1 month. None of the eyes had complete graft detachment or lenticular drop.

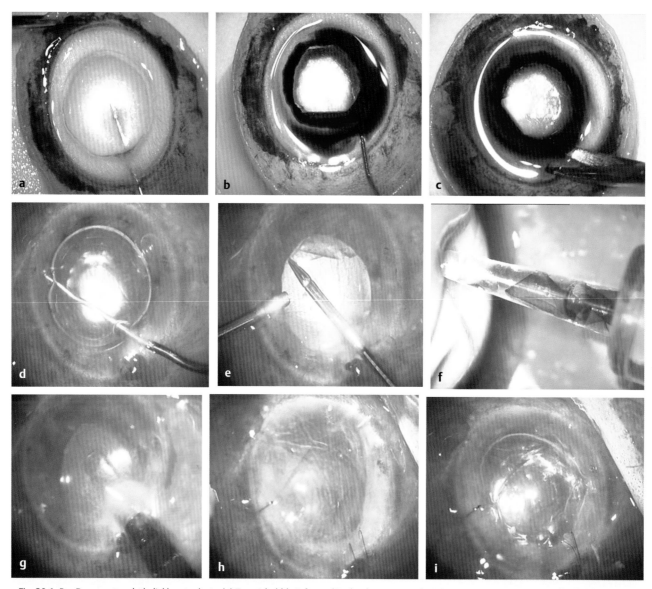

Fig. 20.1 Pre-Descemet endothelial keratoplasty. **(a)** Type 1 bubble is formed in the donor cornea by injecting air via 30-gauge needle. **(b)** Trypan blue is injected into the bubble. **(c)** Trephination is done and the graft is cut with a pair of corneal scissors. **(d,e)** The margin of recipient Descemet membrane to be removed is scored with a reverse Sinskey hook and then peeled. **(f)** Donor lenticule roll is inserted in the custom-made injector and **(g)** is injected in a controlled fashion into the anterior chamber. **(h)** The donor lenticule is positioned onto the recipient posterior stroma and unrolled with air and fluid. **(i)** Finally an air bubble is injected underneath the lenticule to lift it toward the recipient posterior stroma and followed by air–fluid exchange.

Eleven of 12 eyes had a smooth graft–host interface. One eye had minimal interface haze by postoperative 1 month. After a course of intense steroid treatment, the graft–host interface haze decreased in one eye (▶ Fig. 20.7). Separation of the graft into two linear hyperreflective lines was seen with OCT in 2 eyes. The posterior layer was 16 μm and the anterior layer was 12 μm. Both the eyes had mild corneal edema on day 1, which resolved with strict supine position and medical management.

All eyes had central epithelial defect on postoperative day 1. Epithelial healing was complete in all eyes by 48 hours. The mean epithelial thickness was 44.4 ± 9.8 μm in the first week and reduced to 37.5 ± 6.2 μm at the last follow-up. There was significant reduction in the thickness ($p = 0.003$) over the time period. There was no difference in the central and peripheral

epithelium in 11 eyes. The mean day 1 postoperative central corneal thickness was 612 ± 46.4 μm. There was significant resolution of corneal edema by day 7 ($p = 0.001$). A grade 3 cellular reaction was seen in 1 eye, and 1 eye had a grade 4 fibrinous reaction. Shallow detachment was seen in the eye with fibrin (▶ Fig. 20.8). Intense steroid treatment attained good graft adherence by 2 weeks.

20.1.4 Correlations and Associations

There was no significant correlation between the GT and the best corrected vision at day 1 ($p = 0.409$) and day 90 ($p = 0.661$). There was no correlation between the mean central corneal thickness reduction and the GT reduction from day 1 to day 90

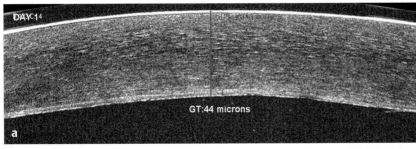

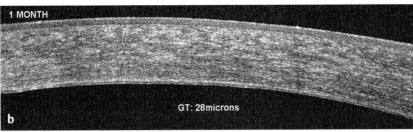

Fig. 20.2 Graft thickness shows significant reduction from the (a) immediate postoperative period to (b) 1 month.

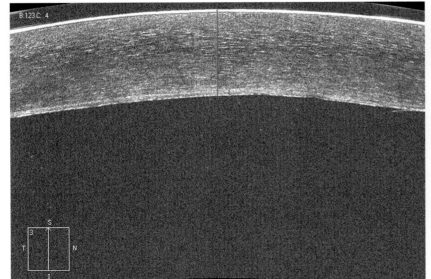

Fig. 20.3 Day 1 postoperative image of a well-adhered graft seen in spectral domain optical coherence tomography.

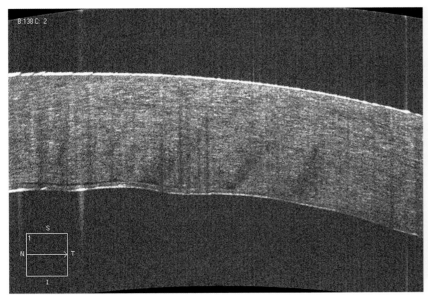

Fig. 20.4 Day 1 postoperative image showing shallow graft detachments in spectral domain optical coherence tomography.

($p = 0.645$, $r = 0.149$). There was no correlation between the corneal edema and GT on day 1 ($p = 0.374$, $r = 0.282$). There was no association between the corneal thickness on day 1 and the graft detachment (Chi square test, p=0.285).There was no association between the GT on day 1 and the graft detachment (Chi square test, $p = 0.167$). There was a strong association with graft adherence and best corrected visual acuity (Chi square, $p = 0.007$) (▶ Fig. 20.9). Eyes with early detachment showed poorer visual outcome.

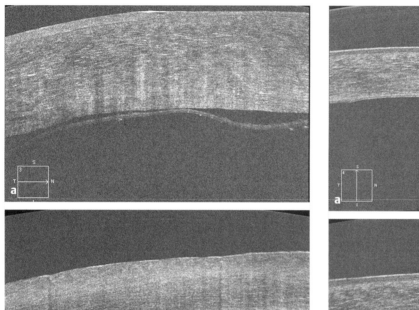

Fig. 20.5 Group III graft detachment after **(a)** Pre-Descemet endothelial keratoplasty and **(b)** reattachment after air injection.

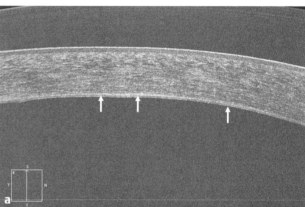

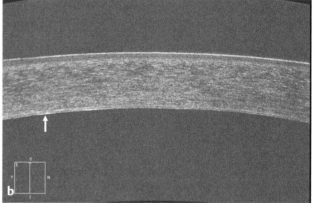

Fig. 20.7 Spectral domain optical coherence tomography showing **(a)** graft interface opacification (arrows) and **(b)** resolution after treatment with intense steroids (arrow).

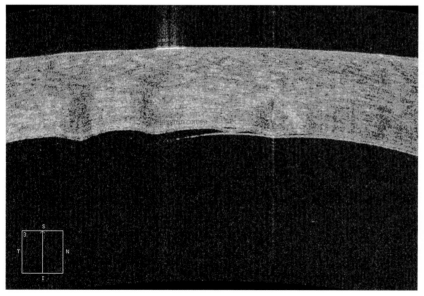

Fig. 20.6 Day 1 postoperative image showing Descemet membrane folds in spectral domain optical coherence tomography.

20.1.5 Optical Coherence Tomography in Endothelial Keratoplasty

Anterior segment OCT has been used in DMEK for predicting the postoperative graft adherence.[5] It has also been used for intraoperative graft positioning.[6] In our study we have shown the behavior of a PDEK graft in vivo in the postoperative follow-up. Yeh et al studied the predictability of an OCT scan for graft attachment in DMEK.[5] They noticed that the initial 1 hour showed the best predictive value in DMEK graft adherence. Because of graft edema and stromal edema in the immediate postoperative period, it might be difficult to localize detachments clinically in slit lamp examinations. Therefore the anterior segment OCT has been used to visualize those endothelial grafts (Descemet stripping automated endothelial keratoplasty [DSAEK] or DMEK) under such situations. Though time domain anterior segment OCT[6,7,8] has been used for evaluating graft status after endothelial keratoplasties such as DSAEK and DMEK, there are no studies on the evaluation of grafts by spectral domain OCT. Clinically undetectable detachments can also be localized by spectral domain OCT because of the higher resolution (5 μm).

20.1.6 Pre-Descemet Endothelial Keratoplasty Graft versus Other Endothelial Grafts

The mean central GT in the Ultrathin Busin DSAEK graft was 78.28 ± 28.89 μm at 3 months postoperative period.[9] Shousha et al reported the thickness of normal DM in elderly patients to be about 16 ± 2 μm (range 13–20 μm) in ultra–high resolution OCT.[10] The mean GT in our study was 37.3 ± 3.5 μm, and it was stabilized by 3 months. From our study we noticed that PDEK grafts are thicker than DMEK grafts and thinner than ultrathin DSAEK grafts. The PDEK grafts were uniform with no difference in the thickness from center to periphery as seen in OCT. Graft adherence has been a single important factor for better functional outcome after successful endothelial keratoplasty.[11,12] Graft detachment has been described as the common complication after endothelial keratoplasty techniques such as DMEK

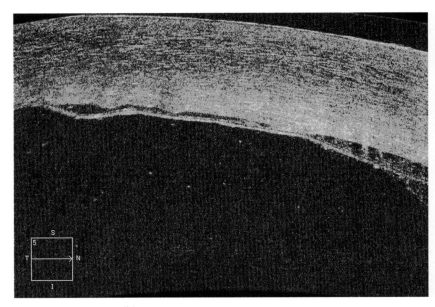

Fig. 20.8 Anterior segment optical coherence tomography showing fibrin reaction with shallow detachment of pre-Descemet endothelial keratoplasty graft.

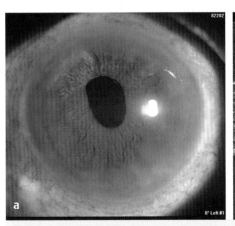
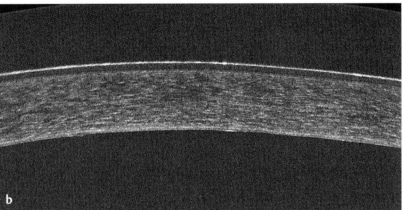

Fig. 20.9 **(a)** Clinical photograph and **(b)** spectral domain optical coherence tomography 6 months after pre-Descemet endothelial keratoplasty with no interface haze.

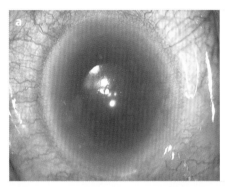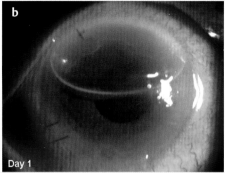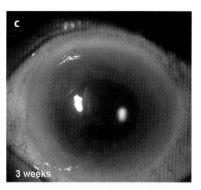

Fig. 20.10 Good postoperative corneal clarity was seen after pre-Descemet endothelial keratoplasty. **(a)** Preoperative image. **(b)** Immediate postoperative image. **(c)** At 3-week postoperative follow-up.

and DSAEK.[11,12,13,14] Though thinner grafts are more susceptible for incomplete graft adhesion after primary positioning, early visual recovery may be possible only with a thin graft.[15] PDEK grafts have the advantage of being thinner, similar to DMEK grafts, which can aid in easy intraoperative manipulation and provide better postoperative adherence.

The two main factors that interfere with graft attachments are the intracorneal pressure and the interposition,[9] and these factors are necessary for the PDEK grafts as well. Precut donor tissue overhydration, stromal edema (both donor or recipient), and an irregular interface prevent graft adherence. In our study, the graft was well adhered in 75% of the eyes. There was no eye with total graft detachment or lenticular drop in the AC.

The possibility of separation of corneal layers by pneumatic dissection has been proven, and it has been technically easier.[16, 17] Hence the preparation of the PDEK lenticule is not difficult in the present clinical setup. The biggest challenge faced in DMEK is the tissue loss in preparation and postoperative attachment. Price and Price reported that the recent advances in instrumentation and technique have reduced the learning curve of DMEK.[18] However, it has been known that DMEK provides faster visual recovery without interface opacification.[19] The absence of interface reaction is one of the advantages with DMEK grafts as compared to DSAEK grafts. Similarly, OCT analysis of PDEK grafts found less or no interface opacification in the postoperative period (► Fig. 20.10). Dua et al reported the absence of keratocytes in the central region of the pre-Descemet layer, and this layer may be the factor that can potentially contribute to reduced haze because air cleavage creates a smooth plane and lessened keratocyte activity.[1] The split in the graft that was seen in two eyes resolved spontaneously with strict supine position. However, those two eyes with graft split did not have graft detachment or corneal edema in the postoperative period. Nevertheless, the additional pre-Descemet layer attached to the DM is expected to provide a splinting effect to the DM in the graft and at the same time preserve the early visual rehabilitation nature of DMEK.

References

[1] Dua HS, Faraj LA, Said DG, Gray T, Lowe J. Human corneal anatomy redefined: a novel pre-Descemet's layer (Dua's layer). Ophthalmology. 2013; 120 (9):1778–1785

[2] Agarwal A, Dua HS, Narang P, et al. Pre-Descemet's endothelial keratoplasty (PDEK). Br J Ophthalmol. 2014; 98(9):1181–1185

[3] Melles GR, Ong TS, Ververs B, van der Wees J. Descemet membrane endothelial keratoplasty (DMEK). Cornea. 2006; 25(8):987–990

[4] Tourtas T, Laaser K, Bachmann BO, Cursiefen C, Kruse FE. Descemet membrane endothelial keratoplasty versus descemet stripping automated endothelial keratoplasty. Am J Ophthalmol. 2012; 153(6):1082–90.e2

[5] Yeh RY, Quilendrino R, Musa FU, Liarakos VS, Dapena I, Melles GR. Predictive value of optical coherence tomography in graft attachment after Descemet's membrane endothelial keratoplasty. Ophthalmology. 2013; 120(2):240–245

[6] Steven P, Le Blanc C, Velten K, et al. Optimizing descemet membrane endothelial keratoplasty using intraoperative optical coherence tomography. JAMA Ophthalmol. 2013; 131(9):1135–1142

[7] Tan GS, He M, Tan DT, Mehta JS. Correlation of anterior segment optical coherence tomography measurements with graft trephine diameter following descemet stripping automated endothelial keratoplasty. BMC Med Imaging. 2012; 12:19

[8] Moutsouris K, Dapena I, Ham L, Balachandran C, Oellerich S, Melles GR. Optical coherence tomography, Scheimpflug imaging, and slit-lamp biomicroscopy in the early detection of graft detachment after Descemet membrane endothelial keratoplasty. Cornea. 2011; 30(12):1369–1375

[9] Busin M, Madi S, Santorum P, Scorcia V, Beltz J. Ultrathin descemet's stripping automated endothelial keratoplasty with the microkeratome double-pass technique: two-year outcomes. Ophthalmology. 2013; 120(6):1186–1194

[10] Shousha MA, Perez VL, Wang J, et al. Use of ultra-high resolution optical coherence tomography to detect in vivo characteristics of Descemet's membrane in Fuchs' dystrophy. Ophthalmology. 2010; 117(6):1220–1227

[11] Dirisamer M, van Dijk K, Dapena I, et al. Prevention and management of graft detachment in descemet membrane endothelial keratoplasty. Arch Ophthalmol. 2012; 130(3):280–291

[12] Guerra FP, Anshu A, Price MO, Giebel AW, Price FW. Descemet's membrane endothelial keratoplasty: prospective study of 1-year visual outcomes, graft survival, and endothelial cell loss. Ophthalmology. 2011; 118(12):2368–2373

[13] Shih CY, Ritterband DC, Rubino S, et al. Visually significant and nonsignificant complications arising from Descemet stripping automated endothelial keratoplasty. Am J Ophthalmol. 2009; 148(6):837–843

[14] Suh LH, Yoo SH, Deobhakta A, et al. Complications of Descemet's stripping with automated endothelial keratoplasty: survey of 118 eyes at One Institute. Ophthalmology. 2008; 115(9):1517–1524

[15] Dapena I, Ham L, Melles GR. Endothelial keratoplasty: DSEK/DSAEK or DMEK—the thinner the better? Curr Opin Ophthalmol. 2009; 20(4):299–307

[16] Anwar M, Teichmann KD. Big-bubble technique to bare Descemet's membrane in anterior lamellar keratoplasty. J Cataract Refract Surg. 2002; 28 (3):398–403

[17] Busin M, Scorcia V, Patel AK, Salvalaio G, Ponzin D. Pneumatic dissection and storage of donor endothelial tissue for Descemet's membrane endothelialkeratoplasty: a novel technique. Ophthalmology. 2010; 117(8):1517–1520

[18] Price MO, Price FW, Jr. Descemet's membrane endothelial keratoplasty surgery: update on the evidence and hurdles to acceptance. Curr Opin Ophthalmol. 2013; 24(4):329–335

[19] Ham L, Balachandran C, Verschoor CA, van der Wees J, Melles GR. Visual rehabilitation rate after isolated descemet membrane transplantation: descemet membrane endothelial keratoplasty. Arch Ophthalmol. 2009; 127(3):252–255

21 Complications of Descemet Stripping Automated Endothelial Keratoplasty

Matthew Shulman, W. Barry Lee, and Bennie H. Jeng

21.1 Introduction

Over the past decade, Descemet stripping automated endothelial keratoplasty (DSAEK) has emerged as the most popular surgical alternative to full-thickness penetrating keratoplasty (PK) in the treatment of corneal endothelial dysfunction, including Fuchs endothelial dystrophy and pseudophakic bullous keratopathy.[1] Because only diseased corneal tissue is targeted with the removal of host endothelium and Descemet membrane (DM) and is replaced with donor endothelium, DM, and a thin posterior stromal layer, all through a small incision, DSAEK offers patients outcomes with faster visual recovery, reduced astigmatism, and decreased risk of wound rupture.[2,3] However, as with any surgical procedure, a number of intra- and postoperative complications can occur. The types of complications that can be encountered with DSAEK are oftentimes distinctly different from any complications seen after PK, and these complications can have significant visual morbidity. Careful attention to potential risk factors identified preoperatively, and understanding of methods and techniques to avoid, manage, and treat the major complications of DSAEK, will be presented herein.

21.2 Donor Dislocation

Despite significant variability in rates reported in the literature, donor graft detachment or dislocation into the anterior chamber is the most commonly encountered postoperative complication of DSAEK.[4] Lenticles may be noted to be free floating within the anterior chamber (▶ Fig. 21.1), centrally detached with some residual peripheral attachment to host tissue or detachment to various degrees in the periphery. Though likely multifactorial, this phenomenon may be attributed to the presence of interface fluid that prevents the development of biochemical adhesions between donor and host stroma.[4] Others

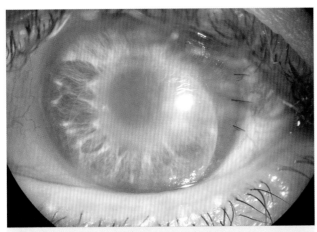

Fig. 21.1 Detached Descemet stripping automated endothelial keratoplasty disc free-floating in the anterior chamber and settled in the inferior angle.

have proposed that incomplete DM stripping with retained DM, intraoperative mechanical trauma to donor tissue (especially damage to donor endothelium and its pump mechanism during graft insertion or iris–cornea touch during removal of the air bubble),[5] retention of viscoelastic within the interface, and even postoperative eye rubbing, may play a role. Though less well understood, postoperative intraocular pressure (IOP) variability, and particularly hypotony, have been cited as contributing to graft dehiscence.[4]

A number of methods and intraoperative techniques have been developed to decrease the risk of graft dislocation and to promote adhesion between donor and host tissue. Recipient peripheral stromal bed scraping (often referred to as stromal roughening) has been used successfully to create more stable and secure points of connection that not only help to prevent detachment but may even facilitate spontaneous reattachment in certain instances of dislocation.[4] Corneal surface massage using a cannula tip or other instrument allows milking of residual graft interface fluid into the anterior chamber. Though not universally practiced, placement of venting incisions in the midperipheral paracentral cornea via beveled stab incisions down to the interface followed by aspiration of residual air or fluid using a 30-gauge cannula can also increase graft stability. A combination of corneal stab incisions with surface sweeping has been demonstrated by Price and Price to significantly reduce dislocation rates,[6] and even further reductions may be seen using the stromal roughening technique.[7,8] Although an uncommon outcome relative to the number of graft detachments, spontaneous reattachments have been documented to occur at higher rates than was previously thought, and this appears to be promoted by positioning following surgery as well as stromal scraping as already described.[4]

If not readily identified postoperatively on slit lamp examination, graft dislocation may be better visualized using anterior-segment optical coherence tomography (OCT)[9] (▶ Fig. 21.2). Graft repositioning and rebubbling can be performed either at the slit lamp or under the operating microscope. It is important to attempt removal of any residual interface fluid during rebubbling, which can be performed either through corneal sweeping or aspiration of fluid via paracentral vents if present.[10] Preoperative and intraoperative recognition of eyes at high risk for graft detachment (as in eyes with glaucoma filters or shunts) may prompt the surgeon to place a retention suture during surgery to facilitate rebubbling should the need arise.

21.2.1 Posterior Segment Dislocation of the Donor Disc

Whereas graft dislocation into the anterior segment remains the most common postoperative complication of DSAEK surgery, dislocation into the posterior segment is comparatively rare. In a retrospective multicenter case series, Afshari and colleagues discuss eight cases of posterior segment dislocation out

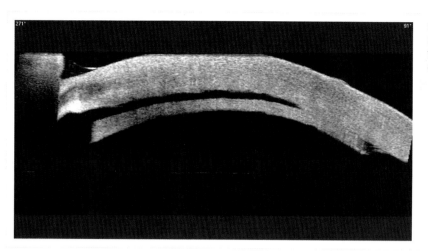

Fig. 21.2 Optical coherence tomography of Descemet stripping automated endothelial keratoplasty disc demonstrating central detachment and peripheral adhesion only.

of 1300 cases reviewed, of which a majority (6 of 8), occurred intraoperatively.[11] They note potential risk factors as prior vitrectomy as well as aphakia or pseudophakia with a sulcus intraocular lens and open communication between the anterior and posterior segments via an open posterior capsule. As with graft dislocation to the anterior chamber, endothelial damage in cases of posterior segment dislocation is likely to occur.[5,11] In fact, in the case series from Afshari and colleagues, all eyes with posteriorly dislocated lenticles required graft replacement following retrieval and removal of the damaged grafts.

Aside from graft failure, other complications of posterior segment dislocation of a donor graft include cystoid macular edema, rhegmatogenous retinal detachment, and epiretinal membrane formation, which may be attributed to the modest inflammatory reaction that can develop, similar to that seen in cases of dropped nuclear fragments during cataract surgery. Given reports of tractional retinal detachment and proliferative vitreoretinopathy in cases of posteriorly dislocated grafts adherent to retinal tissue, it is advisable to attempt graft removal via pars plana vitrectomy by an experienced vitreoretinal surgeon as soon as possible.[12] In cases at high risk for this complication, insertion of the donor graft via a suture pull-through method and immediate placement of a retention suture is advised.

21.2.2 Pupillary Block

Because of the essential role played by the anterior chamber air bubble in tamponading donor graft to host stroma, the surgeon must pay close attention to its size and location at the conclusion of surgery because a large bubble in the anterior chamber or one that has drifted posterior to the iris can cause pupillary block[13] (▶ Fig. 21.3), in turn causing closure of the iridocorneal angle in the immediate term, as well as the later development of peripheral anterior synechiae (PAS), both of which may also injure the graft endothelium and predispose to graft failure.[9,10] The elevated IOP itself can also damage the endothelium.

Once identified by the presence of significant postoperative pain, elevated IOP, and shallow/flat anterior chamber, pupillary block is treated by immediate partial evacuation of the air bubble using needle aspiration and replacement of the lost volume with fluid. This is often only able to be achieved by going through the iris to aspirate the air.

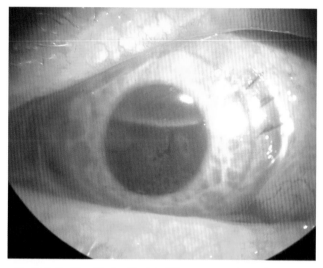

Fig. 21.3 Pupillary block with air bubble seen posterior to the iris.

This complication, however, can be avoided through a number of methods. For example, in a prospective case series of 200 patients in which none developed pupillary block, Terry and colleagues describe a technique in which an initial air bubble is placed comprising ≤ 50% of the anterior chamber after which nearly all is removed. Following this, just enough air is reinjected to cover the graft edges and, to ensure adequate mobility of the bubble, the patient's head is moved from side to side.[13] Pupillary dilation is then achieved with the placement of cyclogyl 1% and phenylephrine 2.5%. This technique did not require the use of prophylactic laser peripheral iridotomy (PI) or intraoperative iridotomy. Alternatively, a surgical PI can be placed at the conclusion of surgery. Some surgeons advocate checking patients 1 hour postoperatively to ensure that pupillary block has not occurred prior to discharge.

21.2.3 Primary Graft Failure

Primary graft failure (PGF) is noted by the presence of persistent corneal edema within the first few weeks following DSAEK and is attributed to graft endothelial dysfunction (▶ Fig. 21.4), which may be iatrogenic or a function of the intrinsic health of the graft tissue.[9,14] Endothelial trauma during graft preparation can occur, but because fewer occurrences of PGF appear to correlate with increasing surgeon experience, it is more likely that endothelial damage incurred during surgery, such as with graft insertion, manipulation, and centration, represents the primary determinant of PGF.[10,13]

Techniques aimed at limiting such endothelial trauma during the preparation phase include preventing artificial anterior chamber collapse during dismounting after cutting the tissue with a microkeratome[9] and storing the graft with the anterior lamellar cap.[15] During insertion, proper care to protect the endothelium and minimizing instrumentation contact with the graft may also decrease the rates of PGF.[13] Removal of the failed graft and replacement with new tissue is the treatment when PGF occurs.

21.2.4 Epithelial Ingrowth

Interface opacification caused by epithelial ingrowth is an uncommon complication after DSAEK surgery. It may be initially detected on slit lamp examination as a hazy lamellar surface with sharply demarcated borders in the early stage or as a homogeneous white mass at the interface in the late stage, and it can even manifest as extension to the iris surface resulting in ectropion uveae and glaucoma.[16,17] The etiology of epithelial ingrowth may be due to dragging of loose host epithelial cells into the interface between the donor and host stroma during graft insertion, or migration of residual donor epithelial cells from eccentrically trephined grafts.[16,18] In addition, epithelial ingrowth can also occur through venting incisions.

Postoperative graft dislocation and subsequent reattachment appear to increase the risk of epithelial ingrowth.[16] Moreover, host conjunctival epithelial ingrowth, in cases of retained vitreous within the surgical wound that can serve as a scaffold for migrating epithelial cells, has also been documented.[16] If not in the visual axis and if not progressing, epithelial ingrowth may not always require surgical intervention. However, in cases of visual compromise from ingrowth in the visual axis, graft removal and repeat DSAEK may be necessary. Some case reports describe using intracameral 5-fluorouracil to inhibit epithelial proliferation, and, in rare instances, PK may be

necessary if the epithelial ingrowth compromises not only the graft interface but the host stroma as well.[16,19]

21.2.5 Graft Rejection

Immunologic graft rejection of the endothelium is characterized by the presence of keratic precipitates on donor endothelium or an endothelial rejection line.[20] Beyond the cornea, other findings of graft rejection include any evidence of anterior chamber cell or flare, conjunctival injection and photophobia, and corneal edema[1] (▶ Fig. 21.5). Though rejection rates appear to vary widely in the literature, the range has been reported as 0.8 to 18%,[21,22,23,24,25] with one study by Anshu and colleagues demonstrating a lower rate of graft rejection for DSAEK compared to PK.[25] Rates of graft failure following episodes of rejection remain relatively low at 6%.[26]

Specific risk factors that increase rejection probabilities include preexisting glaucoma and steroid-responsive ocular hypertension, both of which nearly double the relative risk of initial rejection, and may be related to the need for lower corticosteroid dosing in the postoperative period to improve IOP control.[23] While Ezon and colleagues did not find statistically significant increased rates of rejection in DSAEK eyes with and without glaucoma, they did note higher rates of rejection in eyes with prior incisional glaucoma surgery and in phakic eyes.[20] Whereas age and sex do not appear to influence rejection rates, African American race of the recipient represents a fourfold increase in risk of initial rejection compared with Caucasians, which may necessitate closer follow-up with shorter intervals between visits, as well as higher-dose steroid treatment for longer time periods in this patient cohort.[23]

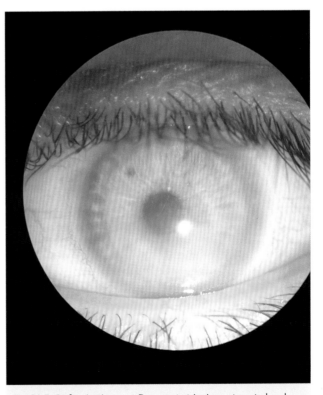

Fig. 21.5 Graft rejection post-Descemet stripping automated endothelial keratoplasty. Note corneal edema inferiorly.

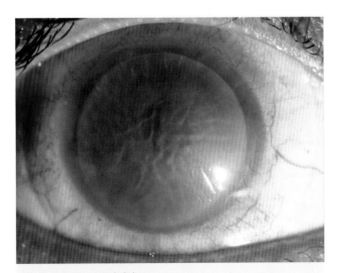

Fig. 21.4 Primary graft failure.

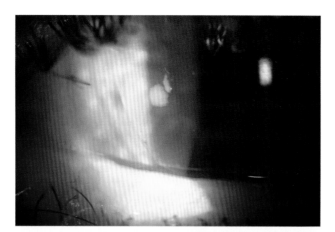

Fig. 21.6 Infiltrate in the interface post-Descemet stripping automated endothelial keratoplasty, which was later found to be *Candida* species.

Posttransplant immunosuppressive dosing regimens are similar among DSAEK and PK patients and typically involve a combination antibiotic–steroid drop four times daily for a week, and then transition to prednisolone acetate 1% four times daily for 1 to 4 months, at which time the dose may be tapered to daily prednisolone acetate 1% indefinitely.[9,23] In instances of graft rejection, it is recommended to increase the topical steroid dosage to hourly, which can then be tapered to the pre-rejection drop regimen over 6 to 12 months if the rejection appears to be improving after a week.[20] The use of systemic steroids or sub-Tenon's capsule triamcinolone is not universally practiced.

21.2.6 Interface Infiltrates and Deposits

The development of infiltrates at the donor–host interface or in the donor lenticle itself is a poor prognostic indicator suggestive of infectious keratitis, which in cases of DSAEK has been shown to be most commonly fungal in origin, with *Candida albicans* as the most common causative organism[27] (▶ Fig. 21.6). Initial development of the infection may occur within the deep stroma, which, in the setting of an already thin cornea with weakly adherent graft in the early postoperative period, may predispose to perforation.[27,28] Donor-to-host transmission has been documented as a potential source of infection; thus it is important to consider culture of the donor corneal rim as well as confocal microscopy in cases of suspected postoperative fungal keratitis.[28] Of note, donor cornea storage solutions in the United States do not routinely include antifungal agents. If there is minimal to no improvement despite aggressive antimycotic therapy with topical, intracameral, and/or oral antifungal agents, removal of the graft is indicated, with possible repeat endothelial keratoplasty or even PK in the more severe cases.[29]

Deposition of blood or retained viscoelastic within the donor–host interface, which may manifest as an interface haze (▶ Fig. 21.7) or subjective visual complaints by the patient, can result in decreased vision. There have also been case reports describing retained metallic particles in the interface, presumably from the metallic microkeratome used for dissection,[30] as well as calcareous degeneration.[31] Repeat grafting may be

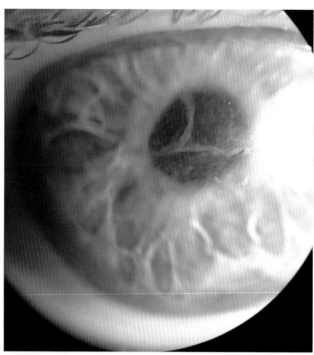

Fig. 21.7 Reticular interface haze presumably from retained viscoelastic in the interface during Descemet stripping automated endothelial keratoplasty.

necessary in cases in which interface deposition does not self-resolve over time.

21.3 Conclusion

With the widespread adoption of posterior lamellar transplantation, including DSAEK, anterior segment surgeons have a robust and highly efficacious method to address endothelial dysfunction with faster rates of visual rehabilitation and fewer refractive complications than experienced with PK. Its ostensible simplicity belies an underlying complexity, as such a highly selective and delicate procedure carries with it attendant challenges and hazards. Some complications have been previously encountered with traditional PK, including PGF, graft rejection, and epithelial ingrowth, whereas others appear to be secondary to the unique and specific graft–host interface found in selective endothelial keratoplasty surgery. Nevertheless, a review of the literature presented in this chapter provides us with a foundation to better recognize complications, both intra- and postoperatively, as well as tools to stratify risk and plan for, prevent, and anticipate surgical challenges, and techniques to correct and manage them as they arise.

References

[1] Jordan CS, Price MO, Trespalacios R, Price FW, Jr. Graft rejection episodes after Descemet stripping with endothelial keratoplasty: part one: clinical signs and symptoms. Br J Ophthalmol. 2009; 93(3):387–390

[2] Price FW, Jr, Price MO. Descemet's stripping with endothelial keratoplasty in 50 eyes: a refractive neutral corneal transplant. J Refract Surg. 2005; 21 (4):339–345

[3] Koenig SB, Covert DJ. Early results of small-incision Descemet's stripping and automated endothelial keratoplasty. Ophthalmology. 2007; 114(2):221–226

[4] Hayes DD, Shih CY, Shamie N, et al. Spontaneous reattachment of Descemet stripping automated endothelial keratoplasty lenticles: a case series of 12 patients. Am J Ophthalmol. 2010; 150(6):790–797

[5] Shulman J, Kropinak M, Ritterband DC, et al. Failed descemet-stripping automated endothelial keratoplasty grafts: a clinicopathologic analysis. Am J Ophthalmol. 2009; 148(5):752–759.e2

[6] Price FW, Jr, Price MO. Descemet's stripping with endothelial keratoplasty in 200 eyes: Early challenges and techniques to enhance donor adherence. J Cataract Refract Surg. 2006; 32(3):411–418

[7] Terry MA, Hoar KL, Wall J, Ousley P. Histology of dislocations in endothelial keratoplasty (DSEK and DLEK): a laboratory-based, surgical solution to dislocation in 100 consecutive DSEK cases. Cornea. 2006; 25(8):926–932

[8] Terry MA, Shamie N, Chen ES, et al. Endothelial keratoplasty for Fuchs' dystrophy with cataract: complications and clinical results with the new triple procedure. Ophthalmology. 2009; 116(4):631–639

[9] Kymionis GD, Ide T, Donaldson K, Yoo SH. Diagnosis of donor graft partial dislocation behind the iris after DSAEK with anterior segment OCT. Ophthalmic Surg Lasers Imaging. 2010;9:1-2.

[10] Suh LH, Yoo SH, Deobhakta A, et al. Complications of Descemet's stripping with automated endothelial keratoplasty: survey of 118 eyes at One Institute. Ophthalmology. 2008; 115(9):1517–1524

[11] Afshari NA, Gorovoy MS, Yoo SH, et al. Dislocation of the donor graft to the posterior segment in descemet stripping automated endothelial keratoplasty. Am J Ophthalmol. 2012; 153(4):638–642, 642.e1–642.e2

[12] Singh A, Gupta A, Stewart JM. Posterior dislocation of descemet stripping automated endothelial keratoplasty graft can lead to retinal detachment. Cornea. 2010; 29(11):1284–1286

[13] Terry MA, Shamie N, Chen ES, Hoar KL, Friend DJ. Endothelial keratoplasty a simplified technique to minimize graft dislocation, iatrogenic graft failure, and pupillary block. Ophthalmology. 2008; 115(7):1179–1186

[14] Wilhelmus KR, Stulting RD, Sugar J, Khan MM, Medical Advisory Board of the Eye Bank Association of America. Primary corneal graft failure. A national reporting system. Arch Ophthalmol. 1995; 113(12):1497–1502

[15] Ide T, Yoo SH, Kymionis GD, Goldman JM, Perez VL, O'Brien TP. Descemet-stripping automated endothelial keratoplasty: effect of anterior lamellar corneal tissue-on/-off storage condition on Descemet-stripping automated endothelial keratoplasty donor tissue. Cornea. 2008; 27(7):754–757

[16] Semeraro F, Di Salvatore A, Bova A, Forbice E. Etiopathogenesis and therapy of epithelial ingrowth after Descemet's stripping automated endothelial keratoplasty. Biomed Res Int. 2014; 2014::906087

[17] Suh LH, Dawson DG, Mutapcic L, et al. Histopathologic examination of failed grafts in descemet's stripping with automated endothelial keratoplasty. Ophthalmology. 2009; 116(4):603–608

[18] Koenig SB, Covert DJ. Epithelial ingrowth after Descemet-stripping automated endothelial keratoplasty. Cornea. 2008; 27(6):727–729

[19] Lai MM, Haller JA. Resolution of epithelial ingrowth in a patient treated with 5-fluorouracil. Am J Ophthalmol. 2002; 133(4):562–564

[20] Ezon I, Shih CY, Rosen LM, Suthar T, Udell IJ. Immunologic graft rejection in descemet's stripping endothelial keratoplasty and penetrating keratoplasty for endothelial disease. Ophthalmology. 2013; 120(7):1360–1365

[21] Shih CY, Ritterband DC, Rubino S, et al. Visually significant and nonsignificant complications arising from Descemet stripping automated endothelial keratoplasty. Am J Ophthalmol. 2009; 148(6):837–843

[22] Lee WB, Jacobs DS, Musch DC, Kaufman SC, Reinhart WJ, Shtein RM. Descemet's stripping endothelial keratoplasty: safety and outcomes: a report by the American Academy of Ophthalmology. Ophthalmology. 2009; 116(9):1818–1830

[23] Price MO, Jordan CS, Moore G, Price FW, Jr. Graft rejection episodes after Descemet stripping with endothelial keratoplasty: part two: the statistical analysis of probability and risk factors. Br J Ophthalmol. 2009; 93(3):391–395

[24] Li JY, Terry MA, Goshe J, Shamie N, Davis-Boozer D. Graft rejection after Descemet's stripping automated endothelial keratoplasty: graft survival and endothelial cell loss. Ophthalmology. 2012; 119(1):90–94

[25] Anshu A, Price MO, Price FW, Jr. Risk of corneal transplant rejection significantly reduced with Descemet's membrane endothelial keratoplasty. Ophthalmology. 2012; 119(3):536–540

[26] Allan BD, Terry MA, Price FW, Jr, Price MO, Griffin NB, Claesson M. Corneal transplant rejection rate and severity after endothelial keratoplasty. Cornea. 2007; 26(9):1039–1042

[27] Araki-Sasaki K, Fukumoto A, Osakabe Y, Kimura H, Kuroda S. The clinical characteristics of fungal keratitis in eyes after Descemet's stripping and automated endothelial keratoplasty. Clin Ophthalmol. 2014; 8:1757–1760

[28] Lee WB, Foster JB, Kozarsky AM, Zhang Q, Grossniklaus HE. Interface fungal keratitis after endothelial keratoplasty: a clinicopathological report. Ophthalmic Surg Lasers Imaging. 2011; 42 Online:e44–e48

[29] Tanaka TS, Mian S. Fungal keratitis after endothelial keratoplasty. Invest Ophthalmol Vis Sci. 1546; 2015(June):56

[30] Kymionis GD, Kankariya VP, Kontadakis GA. Long-term presence of metallic particles in the DSAEK interface. Eye (Lond). 2011; 25(10):1382–1383

[31] Ebrahimi KB, Oster SF, Green WR, Grebe R, Schein OD, Jun AS. Calcareous degeneration of host-donor interface after descemet membrane stripping with automated endothelial keratoplasty. Cornea. 2009; 28(3):342–344

22 Complications of Pre-Descemet Endothelial Keratoplasty

Dhivya Ashok Kumar and Amar Agarwal

22.1 Introduction

The cornea, an exquisite example of physiological engineering, has unique structural characteristics for its very nature. Its normal endothelial cell function is imperative for maintaining transparency. Numerous techniques developed over the last 2 decades have been used to provide vision by endothelial transplantation.[1,2,3,4] Though major complications of penetrating keratoplasties, such as suture inflammation, irregular astigmatism, and keratitis, are prevented after endothelial keratoplasty (EK), they are still not free of complications.[5] Pre-Descemet endothelial keratoplasty (PDEK), a recent modification of EK, involves the transplantation of the pre-Descemet layer (PDL, or Dua layer) along with the Descemet membrane (DM) with endothelium.[6,7] PDEK has many potential advantages over other EKs, such as Descemet membrane endothelial keratoplasty (DMEK) or Descemet stripping endothelial keratoplasty (DSEK); however, learning curve complications are inevitable. These complications are generally manageable, and the risk tends to decline as a surgeon gains experience in the new surgical technique. This chapter discusses the few complications that can arise during the learning curve associated with PDEK and their methods of management.

22.2 Intraoperative Complications

22.2.1 Failure to Form Type 1 Bubble

Type 1 bubble formation is the preliminary step in PDEK surgery for obtaining the donor graft. Failure to form a type 1 bubble can happen intraoperatively, when the correct plane of dissection is not reached. In that case, a small peripheral type 2 bubble or small type 1 bubble is formed (▶ Fig. 22.1). When the small type 1 bubble is formed, it is enhanced by air or viscoelastic injection in a controlled fashion (▶ Fig. 22.2). However, when

a type 2 bubble is formed, DMEK surgery is performed (▶ Fig. 22.3). Double bubble formation is also sometimes noted. Very rarely a bubble may not form on repeated attempts with air, in which case a preservation medium—either McCarey–Kaufman (MK) medium (▶ Fig. 22.4) or Optisol (Chiron Ophthalmics)—can be used for bubble formation. To prevent type 2 bubble formation, one can place multiple peripheral micropunctures on the Descemet membrane before air injection.

22.2.2 Bubble Burst during Pneumatic Dissection

When the bubble bursts early during pneumatic dissection, the size can be enhanced by slow viscoelastic injection via the ostium. Bubble burst usually happens when the surgeon pushes too much air into a small space and the intrabubble pressure raises exponentially faster (▶ Fig. 22.5). Once the bubble bursts after reaching its maximum size, Vannas scissors can be used to excise the graft uniformly along its margin. If the bubble bursts in an early stage (i.e., size < 6 mm), the results are not predictable in smaller grafts; hence rebubbling in another corneal button is preferred.

22.2.3 Small Graft

Similar to any EK, the graft size is vital in PDEK. A small graft is obtained due to the formation of a small type 1 bubble. Whenever a bubble < 4 mm is seen after pneumatic dissection, viscoelastic can be injected into the bubble to enhance the size. However, too much intrabubble pressure should be avoided, which again can lead to bubble burst. The preferred graft size in PDEK is 7.5 to 8 mm. Grafts smaller than 6.5 mm have the risk of late failure. However, a small graft of 6 mm with good endothelial count and morphology can provide good results (▶ Fig. 22.6).

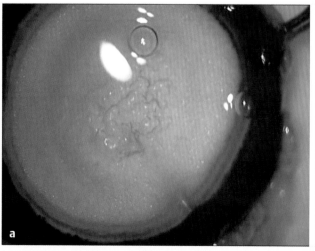 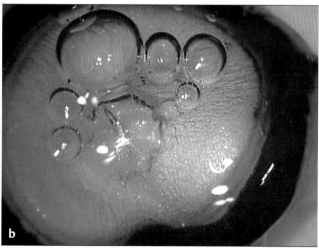

Fig. 22.1 Donor graft preparation. **(a)** Small type 1 bubble formed. **(b)** Type 1 bubble enhanced with air.

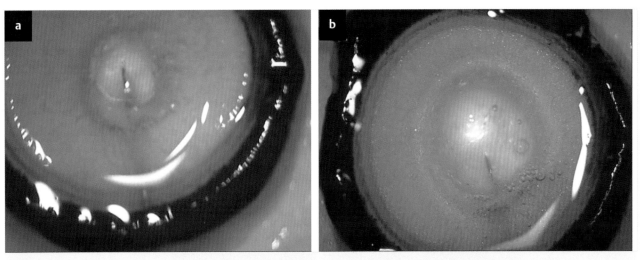

Fig. 22.2 Donor graft preparation. (a) Small type 1 bubble formed. (b) Type 1 big bubble enhanced with viscoelastic substance.

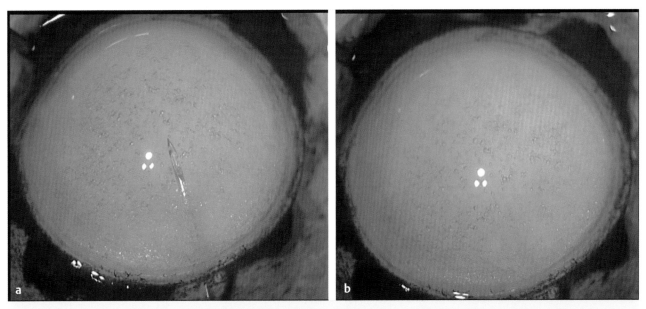

Fig. 22.3 Donor graft preparation. Type 2 bubble formed. (a) During pneumatic dissection. (b) After big bubble formation.

22.2.4 Reverse Graft Unfolding

An endothelial graft always scrolls with the endothelium to the outside. A PDEK graft curling away from the host cornea indicates that the graft is inverted (▶ Fig. 22.7). This is managed by reinversion by saline in the anterior chamber. Intraoperative optical coherence tomography (OCT) can also guide in visualizing the orientation of the graft (▶ Fig. 22.8). Care should be taken to prevent too much manipulation on the endothelium while reinverting.

22.2.5 Chamber Collapse

Loss of anterior chamber pressure can result from a wide incision causing excess fluid outflow. A trocar anterior chamber maintainer (▶ Fig. 22.9) or an air pump–assisted anterior chamber maintainer can help with chamber pressure control. Avoiding too large incisions and proper closure of the main wound immediately after graft injection can prevent intraoperative hypotony.

22.2.6 Poor Graft Visualization

Intraoperative loss of visualization can happen in eyes with chronic corneal decompensation and scarring. Superficial keratectomy or epithelial debridement can be performed in many cases. In eyes with persistent corneal edema visualization can be enhanced by endoilluminator-assisted PDEK (▶ Fig. 22.10).[8]

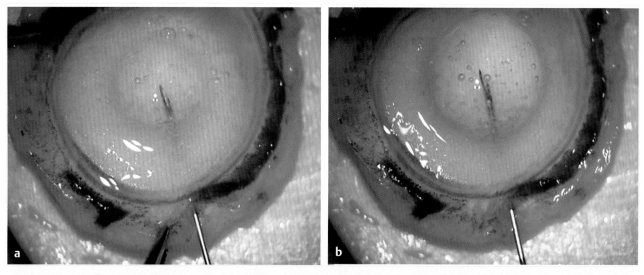

Fig. 22.4 Donor graft preparation by McCarey-Kaufman (MK) medium. **(a)** Small type 1 bubble formed. **(b)** Enhanced with continuous injection of MK medium.

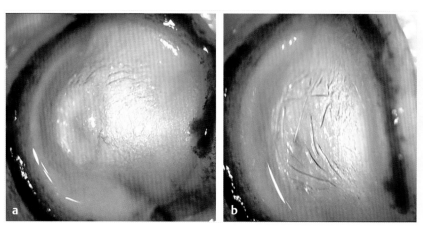

Fig. 22.5 (a) Small type 1 bubble formed. **(b)** Bubble bursts when the surgeon pushes too much air into a small space.

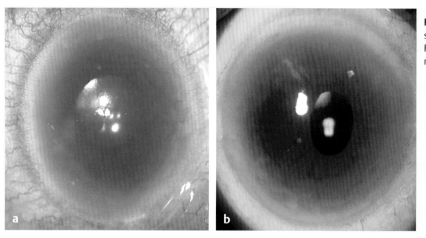

Fig. 22.6 Small donor graft about 6.5 mm showed good corneal clearance. **(a)** Preoperative Fuch's dystrophy. **(b)** Postoperative PDEK at 12 months.

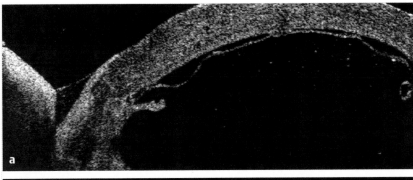

Fig. 22.7 An inverted pre-Descemet endothelial keratoplasty graft in optical coherence tomography. Note the graft curling away from the (a) host cornea and (b) reattached graft.

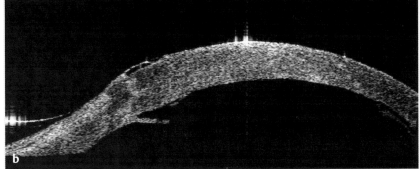

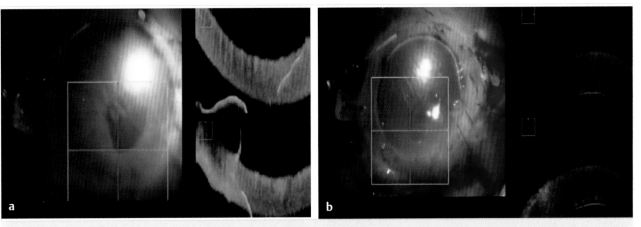

Fig. 22.8 Intraoperative optical coherence tomography–assisted pre-Descemet endothelial keratoplasty. (a) Before air injection. (b) After air injection.

22.3 Immediate Postoperative Complications

22.3.1 Graft Detachment

Due to improper air injection or a leaking wound, the pressure inside the chamber may not be sufficient for graft adhesion. Prolonged graft hydration, which induces change in intracorneal pressure, is known to affect the immediate graft attachment. The initial 30 minutes after air injection is crucial in maintaining the graft attachment. In a short series of PDEKs (n = 12), we noted graft detachment in four eyes.[9] Graft detachment was classified similar to that for DMEK grafts,[10] as grade I when there was a minimal peripheral edge detachment with the remainder of the graft being well attached; grade II when graft detachments were less than one-third of the graft surface area, not affecting the visual axis; grade III when graft

detachment affected more than one-third of the graft surface area; and grade IV when the graft was completely detached. Of four eyes with graft detachment, there were grade I (n = 2), grade II (n = 1), and grade III (n = 1) detachments. In grade I detached grafts, shallow peripheral detachment inferiorly (n = 1) and nasally (n = 1) was observed. Both the grade I and II detachments did not require any further intervention. One eye with grade III detachment underwent air injection on postoperative day 1 (▶ Fig. 22.11). The graft was noted to be apposed after air injection in the one eye with grade III detachment. However, there was redetachment on day 12 in the same eye and rebubbling was done subsequently, with success on day 12.

22.3.2 Lenticule Drop

When there is hindrance for graft attachment or when the chamber pressure is not sufficient to maintain the graft in apposition,

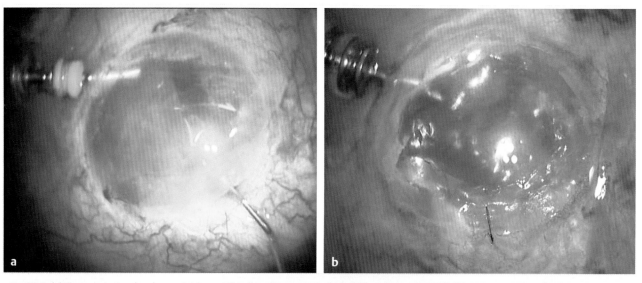

Fig. 22.9 **(a)** Trocar anterior chamber maintainer–assisted pre-Descemet endothelial keratoplasty (PDEK). **(b)** Air pump–assisted PDEK.

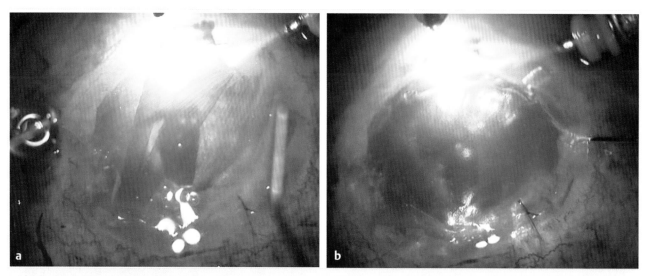

Fig. 22.10 Endoilluminator-assisted pre-Descemet endothelial keratoplasty. **(a)** Before air injection. **(b)** After air injection. Note the illuminator from external source providing good graft visualization.

lenticule drop can result. Especially in eyes with complicated surgery that had posterior capsular rupture or deficient capsule, there is always difficulty in maintaining the air in the anterior chamber. In such eyes one can implant a transscleral fixated intraocular lens (IOL) or a glued IOL and do a pupilloplasty if the pupil was large. Giving strict supine position and following the preceding surgical steps can prevent lenticule drop. By combining a glued IOL procedure with PDEK in eyes with deficient capsules (▶ Fig. 22.12), the posterior capsule IOL aids in maintaining the air in place as compared to an aphakic eye.

22.3.3 Descemet Folds

Smooth concave configuration of the posterior cornea should be obtained in all the eyes with good graft adherence. Descemet folds can occur when there was excess tissue manipulation intraoperatively (▶ Fig. 22.13) or poor intraoperative chamber

pressure for adhesion. Avoiding too much endothelial handling and following the "no touch" technique would definitely reduce the chances for this complication in the immediate postoperative period. This usually resolves with medical management, and no additional treatment is required except for the maintenance of the supine position for the next 24 hours. Air pump–assisted surgery helps in maintaining intraoperative chamber pressure and aids adhesion.

22.3.4 Folded Graft

Improper intraoperative sweeping of the graft can present as postoperative graft fold. Clinically it is seen as marks or striated endothelial lines, and on OCT it can be clearly delineated as folded layers. If it is in the periphery (▶ Fig. 22.14) and there is air filling 80% of the chamber, there is no intervention required. Only supine position maintenance and withholding any

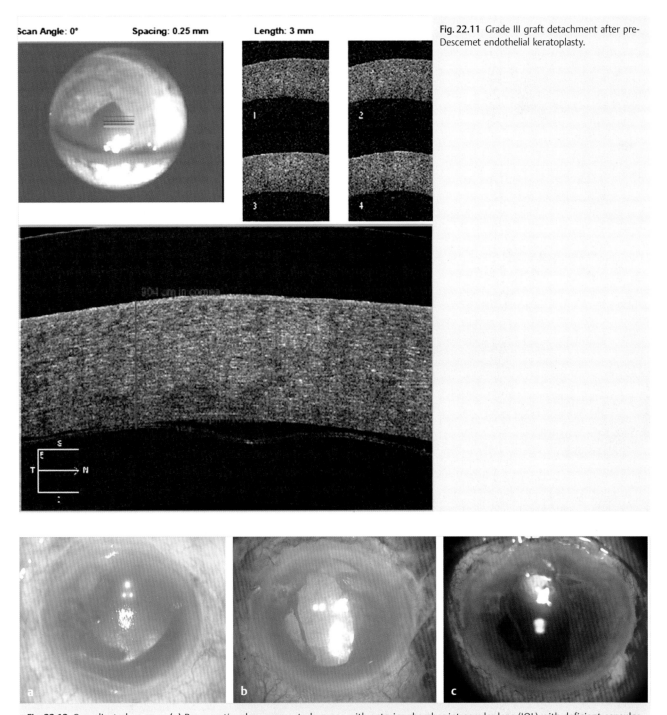

Scan Angle: 0°   Spacing: 0.25 mm   Length: 3 mm

Fig. 22.11 Grade III graft detachment after pre-Descemet endothelial keratoplasty.

Fig. 22.12 Complicated surgery. (a) Preoperative decompensated cornea with anterior chamber intraocular lens (IOL) with deficient capsules. (b) Postoperative image after glued IOL implantation, (c) followed by pre-Descemet endothelial keratoplasty surgery as second sitting.

hypotensive medications can help. When the folded region is larger and there is minimal air fill, surgical repositioning is recommended.

22.3.5 Loss of Air Bubble

We expect 80% of the anterior chamber to be filled with air bubble in the immediate postoperative period. When the surgeon has injected enough air at the end of the procedure and noticed less air on day 1, there could be two reasons. The air has the tendency to move or shift depending on the pressure gradient (either the ocular or the atmosphere). In ocular causes (large pupil, posterior capsular rupture, scleral fixated IOL, or previous iridectomy) the air enters the posterior chamber or the vitreous. In leaky wound or loose sutures, the air escapes into the atmosphere (▶ Fig. 22.15). In both the cases, there is less air in the anterior chamber to aid graft adherence. This can lead to spontaneous graft detachment; hence it is recommended to inject air in cases when there is no air on postoperative day 1 and there is associated detachment.

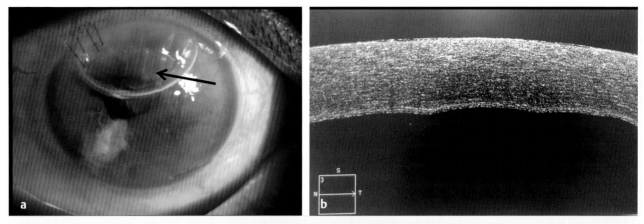

Fig. 22.13 (a) Day 1 postoperative image showing clear cornea and Descemet folds after pre-Descemet endothelial keratoplasty. (b) Spectral domain optical coherence tomography shows folds on the endothelial side.

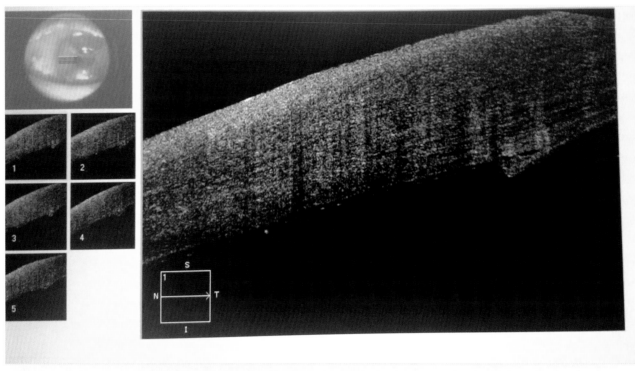

Fig. 22.14 Anterior segment optical coherence tomography showing peripheral graft fold after pre-Descemet endothelial keratoplasty surgery.

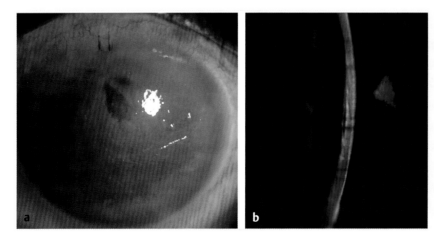

Fig. 22.15 (a) Patient after pre-Descemet endothelial keratoplasty with loss of air due to wound leak on day one and (b) shallow detachment.

22.3.6 Ocular Hypertension

Raised intraocular pressure (IOP) recorded for the first time after PDEK on postoperative day 1 in an eye without any clinical signs of glaucoma is referred to as ocular hypertension due to surgery. The common cause is the high bubble pressure due to 100% air bubble filling the anterior chamber. In that case, anti-osmotic medications (both topical and systemic) should be given. If the IOP is not controlled by these medications the anterior chamber can be decompressed surgically by reducing the air bubble size.

22.3.7 Hyphema

Postoperative hyphema is seen in eyes with intraoperative iris tissue manipulation and combined surgeries. Usually it is mild and resolves spontaneously. Very rarely it can affect graft attachment.

22.3.8 Sterile Hypopyon or Fibrin

This is seen in eyes with prolonged surgeries, especially in eyes with combined procedures (e.g., pupilloplasty) or in eyes with a predisposition to uveitis. It is always sterile and resolves with intense topical steroids and rarely oral steroids. Nonresolving fibrin in the anterior chamber can induce traction and can affect graft adherence. Hence it is essential to treat these eyes emergently. Subconjunctival steroids along with hyalase can help in some cases; topical cycloplegic is required in all these eyes.

22.4 Late Postoperative Complications

22.4.1 Graft Rejection

Graft rejection is identified by the formation of acute-onset endothelial keratic precipitates (Khodadoust line) and sudden anterior chamber reaction with corneal edema. The incidence of rejection in PDEK is expected to be similar to that for DMEK because there is no stroma seen in both the grafts.[11] However, this needs further study. When the endothelial rejection is diagnosed, immediate, intense, topical (1% prednisolone acetate hourly) and systemic steroids (oral prednisolone 1 mg/kg for

first week followed by tapering dose) are recommended. Regular follow-up with good medication compliance is required to prevent rejection in some cases.

22.4.2 Graft Failure

This is a rare complication after EK and is seen in eyes in which donor endothelium was < 2500 cells/mm² or elderly (> 60 years). Because PDEK is performed in both young and adult donor corneas, the risk of primary graft failure due to donor age will be lessened. Nonresolving corneal edema after EK with recurrence of bullous keratopathy is a sign of graft failure (▶ Fig. 22.16). Incidence of graft failure and the factors determining it will be similar to other endothelial keratoplasty.

22.4.3 Graft–Host Interface

Graft–host interface is examined for the presence of haze or opacification. It can be seen clinically in slit lamp and confirmed by OCT (▶ Fig. 22.17) as a hyperreflective region. Eleven out of 12 eyes had a smooth graft–host interface in our series.[9] One

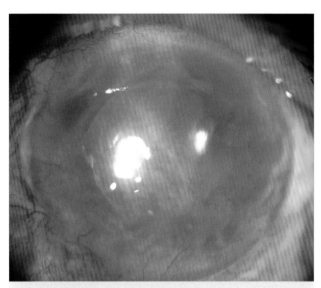

Fig. 22.16 Post–primary graft failure after pre-Descemet endothelial keratoplasty surgery with elderly donor (55 years).

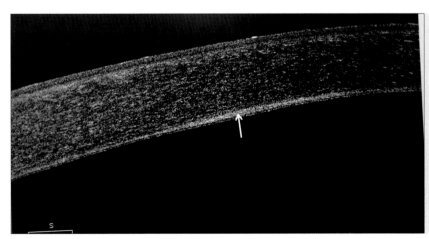

Fig. 22.17 Spectral domain optical coherence tomography showing graft interface opacification (arrow).

eye had minimal interface haze by postoperative 1 month. After a course of intense steroid treatment, the graft–host interface haze decreased in the final follow-up.

22.4.4 Epithelial Change

Central corneal epithelial defect on postoperative day 1 is often seen due to the intraoperative removal of epithelium. Epithelial healing completes in all eyes by 48 hours. In our short series, the mean epithelial thickness of 44.4 ± 9.8 µm on day 7, reduced to 37.5 ± 6.2 µm by day 90. There was no significant change in the thickness ($p = 0.060$) over the time period.[8] There was no difference in the central and peripheral epithelium. Chronic epithelial haze can happen in eyes with too many topical medications with preservatives. In such situations reduce the frequency of medications or change to alternative medications without preservatives. Copious ocular lubricants in the form of drops and gel are recommended for further prevention of symptoms. In some cases autologous serum may be required for a short period.

22.4.5 Intraocular Lens Opacification

IOL opacification after EK has been reported. Intracameral iso expansible gases (e.g., C_3F_8 or SF_6) have been noted to be the etiology in some cases. Though this is a very rare complication (▶ Fig. 22.18), it can happen even after PDEK in those eyes that required repeat gas injection.

22.4.6 Infection

Infections are very rare after EK because there are no sutures or open-sky manipulation as in conventional keratoplasty. However, these patients are on prolonged steroid therapy, and the risk of keratitis cannot be excluded. Hence regular follow-up

and monitoring of symptoms in patients on steroids with or without antibiotics is necessary.

22.5 Conclusion

Graft adherence has been a single important factor for better functional outcome after successful EK. Graft detachment has been described as the common complication after EK techniques such as DMEK and DSAEK. Though thinner grafts are more susceptible to incomplete graft adhesion after primary positioning, early and possibly better visual recovery may be possible only with a thin graft. PDEK has the advantage of thinner grafts similar to DMEK, which can aid in easy intraoperative manipulation and improve postoperative adherence and with fewer complications.

References

[1] Dirisamer M, van Dijk K, Dapena I, et al. Prevention and management of graft detachment in descemet membrane endothelial keratoplasty. Arch Ophthalmol. 2012; 130(3):280–291

[2] Guerra FP, Anshu A, Price MO, Giebel AW, Price FW. Descemet's membrane endothelial keratoplasty: prospective study of 1-year visual outcomes, graft survival, and endothelial cell loss. Ophthalmology. 2011; 118(12):2368–2373

[3] Shih CY, Ritterband DC, Rubino S, et al. Visually significant and nonsignificant complications arising from Descemet stripping automated endothelial keratoplasty. Am J Ophthalmol. 2009; 148(6):837–843

[4] Suh LH, Yoo SH, Deobhakta A, et al. Complications of Descemet's stripping with automated endothelial keratoplasty: survey of 118 eyes at One Institute. Ophthalmology. 2008; 115(9):1517–1524

[5] Nanavaty MA, Wang X, Shortt AJ. Endothelial keratoplasty versus penetrating keratoplasty for Fuchs endothelial dystrophy. Cochrane Database Syst Rev. 2014; 2:CD008420

[6] Agarwal A, Dua HS, Narang P, et al. Pre-Descemet's endothelial keratoplasty (PDEK). Br J Ophthalmol. 2014; 98(9):1181–1185

[7] Dua HS, Faraj LA, Said DG, Gray T, Lowe J. Human corneal anatomy redefined: a novel pre-Descemet's layer (Dua's layer). Ophthalmology. 2013; 120 (9):1778–1785

[8] Jacob S, Agarwal A, Kumar DA. Endoilluminator-assisted Descemet membrane endothelial keratoplasty and endoilluminator-assisted pre-Descemet endothelial keratoplasty. Clin Ophthalmol. 2015; 9:2123–2125

[9] Kumar DA, Dua HS, Agarwal A, Jacob S. Postoperative spectral-domain optical coherence tomography evaluation of pre-Descemet endothelial keratoplasty grafts. J Cataract Refract Surg. 2015; 41(7):1535–1536

[10] Yeh RY, Quilendrino R, Musa FU, Liarakos VS, Dapena I, Melles GR. Predictive value of optical coherence tomography in graft attachment after Descemet's membrane endothelial keratoplasty. Ophthalmology. 2013; 120(2):240–245

[11] Anshu A, Price MO, Price FW, Jr. Risk of corneal transplant rejection significantly reduced with Descemet's membrane endothelial keratoplasty. Ophthalmology. 2012; 119(3):536–540

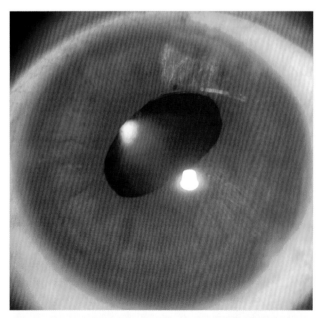

Fig. 22.18 Clinical photograph showing intraocular lens opacification after pre-Descemet endothelial keratoplasty (PDEK). Note the clear cornea after PDEK, vision 20/30.

23 Eye Bank Preparation of Endothelial Keratoplasty Grafts

Michelle J. Kim and Ashiyana Nariani

23.1 Background

23.1.1 Evolution of Eye Banking

The current era of corneal transplantation is marked by tremendous surgical innovation, technological advancement, and expansion in the role of eye banks.[1] The 20th century witnessed the inception of full-thickness penetrating keratoplasty (PK) by Dr. Edward Zirm in 1905[2] and the establishment of the first eye bank by Dr. R. Townley Paton in 1944.[3] Arguably, the greatest step forward in eye banking was the demonstration by Filatov that corneal tissue can be collected and used postmortem in 1937.[4] The Eye Bank Association of America (EBAA) was then established in 1961 to promote medical standards.[5] McCarey–Kaufman (MK) medium was used for corneal tissue storage in the 1970s and was later transitioned to Optisol-GS medium (Bausch & Lomb) in the 1980s, after demonstration of its superiority in maintaining corneal deturgescence, the appearance of the endothelial cells, and overall tissue preservation.[6]

The 21st century then witnessed the subsequent transition to partial-thickness endothelial keratoplasty (EK) with Gerrit Melles, who laid the foundation of modern EK in 1998 with posterior lamellar keratoplasty (PLK),[7] followed by Mark Terry in 2003 with deep lamellar endothelial keratoplasty (DLEK),[8] and Francis Price Jr. in 2005 with Descemet stripping endothelial keratoplasty (DSEK).[9] Mark Gorovoy thereafter, in 2006, introduced the technique known as Descemet stripping automated endothelial keratoplasty (DSAEK), with the use of an artificial anterior chamber and blade microkeratome for cutting donor grafts.[10,11]

Eye banks swiftly excelled in the midst of the multitude of surgical advancements. Though faced with initial surgeon hesitation to allow nonsurgeons to prepare their donor corneal grafts, in 2006, eye banks began supplying precut tissue for DSEK. Early studies further substantiated eye bank efforts with the demonstration of minimal difference in tissue quality and postoperative outcomes with the use eye bank–prepared precut tissue as compared with surgeon-prepared grafts.[12,13,14,15,16]

This shift in paradigm led to the rapid adoption of DSEK. From 2005 to 2014, the EBAA reported an increase in the number of endothelial transplants in the United States from 1429 to 28,961, with a simultaneous decrease in the number of full-thickness PK transplants from 45,821 to 38,919.[17,18] The reduction in surgical time and the increase in graft preparation precision yielded faster visual recovery and lower complication rates than ever before.[16,19]

Today, eye banks are taking their repertoire to the next level with the preparation of Descemet membrane endothelial keratoplasty (DMEK) grafts,[20,21,22] and more recently, in pioneering graft preparation for Amar Agarwal's pre-Descemet endothelial keratoplasty (PDEK) technique.[23,24,25] Thanks to the collaborative efforts of expert eye surgeons and eye banks globally, the world of EK is in the midst of history in the making, with the unified goal to achieve safe and effective tissue for sight restoration and lessen the global burden of corneal blindness.[1,26]

23.1.2 Advantages of Eye Bank–Prepared Grafts

With the concurrent evolutionary advancements in eye banking and in corneal transplantation surgery tissue recovery, corneal quality evaluation, precutting, and, at times, even preloading into a delivery system are seamlessly being taken care of for the surgeon. The advantages are numerous. Eye banks can perform postdissection assessments and use specular microscopy and slit-lamp biomicroscopy to evaluate endothelial health, which cannot be readily performed when a surgeon dissects donor tissue in the operating room.[14]

Additionally, in electing to have the eye bank prepare the EK graft, the surgeon transfers the risk of tissue perforation during preparation to the eye bank, thus minimizing the inherent risks of tissue wastage and potentially needing to cancel surgery. The resulting improvement in operating room efficiency has demonstrated improved postoperative outcomes and has shown financial benefit, eliminating the need for expensive equipment.[27] Notably, the use of eye bank–prepared EK tissue decreases the number of new skills a surgeon needs to learn when adopting the procedure. The experience some eye bank technicians have with EK graft preparation today far surpasses that of many ophthalmic surgeons.[16]

23.1.3 Donor Graft Recovery

In an effort to optimize graft quality, many eye banks aim to remove corneoscleral tissue from the donor and place it into a storage medium within 18 to 24 hours from the time of death. Indeed, a longer death-to-preservation (DTP) time, time from corneal preservation to subsequent transplantation, as well as the donor's cause of death have all been shown to affect graft quality.[28] Thus eye banks quickly need to obtain tissue recovery authorization, conduct a detailed medical and social interview with the surviving family, review the donor's medical record, perform a thorough physical assessment of the body, obtain a qualified blood sample, and recover the donated ocular tissue.[13,18,29] Recovery of the tissue can be performed via whole eye enucleation or, more commonly, via an in situ excision of the corneoscleral rim, and is generally done in the morgue, at the bedside, in the funeral home, or in an operating room. The diameter of the donated corneoscleral button should be > 16 mm, with the scleral rim being 2 to 4 mm wide and uniform. During graft preparation, these margins help to minimize the risk of the tissue being cut too small or asymmetrically with the microkeratome.[13] Gentle manipulation of the tissue is critical, as excessive mechanical trauma of the tissue during recovery and preparation may decrease the viability of the grafts.[30]

23.1.4 Corneal Storage Media

The history of eye banking includes the development of preservation techniques. Once eye banks were established in 1944, the original method used for preservation was the moist chamber for storing entire globes or excised corneas for up to 1 to 2 days. The later development of MK medium in 1974, consisting of a standard culture medium tissue culture (TC) 199, antibiotics, and dextran as an antiswelling agent, provided viable cold corneal storage at 4°C for 3 to 4 days and was the preferred choice[31] for a number of years, until it was taken over by the organ culture method, which not only allowed for long-term preservation (~ 48 days), but also simulated physiological conditions, at storage temperatures of 31 to 37°C.[32]

At the same time, short-term storage media alternatives, such as K-Sol, CSM, and Dexsol were being formulated, which allowed for 7 to 10 days of storage, adding chondroitin sulfate to the MK medium to help minimize donor swelling during storage.[33,34] Optisol (Bausch & Lomb, Irvine, CA), a hybrid of K-Sol and Dexsol,[6] was later introduced in the 1980s to further prolong endothelial survival during storage at 4°C for up to 2 weeks.[34] Optisol GS (Bausch & Lomb, Irvine, CA),[35,36,37] with the addition of antibiotics gentamicin and streptomycin to Optisol, is currently the most widely used cold storage medium (▶ Fig. 23.1) in the United States,[34] though newer products, such as Eusol-C (Al.Chi.mia., Padova, Italy),[38] LIFE4°C (Numendis, Istanti, MN), and Chen Medium (Chen Laboratories, Baltimore, MD)[39,40,41] are proving to be effective alternatives.[13,34]

Researchers have evaluated the impact of culture conditions on visual outcomes in EK. Laaser et al demonstrated that tissue storage in Optisol-GS short-term culture at 4°C and organ culture at 34°C for DMEK tissue storage demonstrated comparable best-corrected visual acuity (BCVA), postoperative endothelial

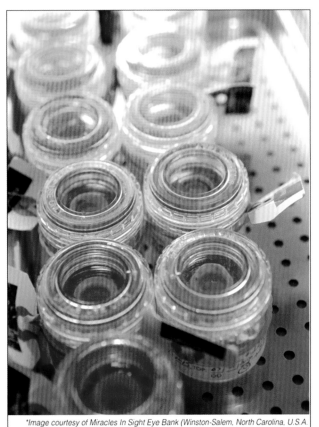

Image courtesy of Miracles In Sight Eye Bank (Winston-Salem, North Carolina, U.S.A.)

Fig. 23.1 Optisol-GS (Optisol with the addition of antibiotics gentamicin and streptomycin) is currently the most widely used cold storage medium in the United States.

cell density (ECD), and central corneal thickness.[42,43] Further evidence suggests that longer storage times may allow better outcomes in high-risk grafts because of the depletion of donor T cells from the donor cornea into the storage media. Thus storage media will need to be optimized for preserving the endothelium for longer periods of time.[34] The addition of fibroblast growth factor-2 and nitric oxide synthase inhibitors is being investigated to further enhance the viability.[34,44,45,46]

Areas of ongoing research include epithelial and limbal stem cell preservation, endothelial preservation, and antimicrobial prophylaxis.[47,48,49]

23.1.5 Graft Eligibility

EBAA has laid out extensive criteria that each donor and associated tissue must meet in order to allow safe and effective transplantation. Endothelial grafts should meet the same criteria as those for PK, except that tissue with noninfectious pathology limited to the anterior stroma is also eligible for use in EK with notification of the surgeon. Although these criteria are in place to prevent potential harm to the recipient, the ultimate responsibility and decision to transplant a particular tissue lie with the surgeon. The lower limit of endothelial cell count for PK is 2000 cells/mm^2 and surgeons often request a density of at least 2500 cells/mm^2, but the optimal density for EK has not been well established.

However, preoperative endothelial cell count does not appear to be correlated with graft dislocation rates or cell counts at 1 year postoperatively.[50] Storage time also does not seem to affect the average percentage of cell loss at time points of up to 2 years postoperatively, and tissue stored for even 14 days appears to be sufficient. Together, these studies may allow for less stringent donor graft selection practices on the surgeon's part, increasing the availability of viable grafts. This can have significant ramifications for the international shipment of donor grafts to areas of shortages; precutting and long-distance overseas transportation of DSAEK have been demonstrated to provide an effective source of tissue with preservation of cell counts at an adequate level.[51]

23.2 Endothelial Keratoplasty Graft Preparation Technique

23.2.1 Descemet Stripping Automated Endothelial Keratoplasty

DSAEK is the most commonly performed type of EK. The DSAEK procedure offers corneal donor graft predictability in the anterior chamber. The transition from manually dissected DSEK grafts to automated dissection with the microkeratome represented a significant advancement for both the surgeon and the eye bank. Today, however, despite the vast improvement in postoperative visual recovery with DSAEK as compared to earlier methods of corneal transplantation, the ophthalmology community continues to look for ways of overcoming what are believed to be the major disadvantages limiting postoperative visual acuity with DSAEK, namely optical degradation associated with the interface between posterior stromal graft tissue and recipient stromal tissue and interface irregularity.[51,52,53]

Microkeratome-Assisted DSAEK

A microkeratome system consists of a blade and an artificial anterior chamber (AAC). Commonly used microkeratome systems include those produced by Moria, Horizon, and Amadeus. In the microkeratome-assisted DSAEK technique (▶ Fig. 23.2), the donor corneoscleral rim is pressurized with balanced salt solution (BSS), Optisol-GS storage medium, or viscoelastic followed by dissection using the appropriately sized microkeratome head, with the goal of leaving approximately 100 to 200 μm of posterior stroma with Descemet membrane and endothelium.[9,10,11,54,55,56,57]

In compliance with EBAA Medical Standards (▶ Fig. 23.3), central endothelial density, graft thickness measurements, and specular microscopy are evaluated before and after the corneal graft is cut.[58] The corneal stroma may be marked peripherally to outline the area of the trephine cut as well as centrally, to allow proper centration of the tissue. Some surgeons also request that an "S stamp" be placed on the anterior aspect of the graft to assist them intraoperatively with graft orientation in the eye (▶ Fig. 23.4). These markings can be done with the ink pen or gentian violet.[13,14,15,55]

The microkeratome blade/head complex is then released and the graft is realigned back with its anterior cap. The proper alignment of the anterior cap with the graft will eliminate gaps in the interface, preventing fluid from leaking in during transit

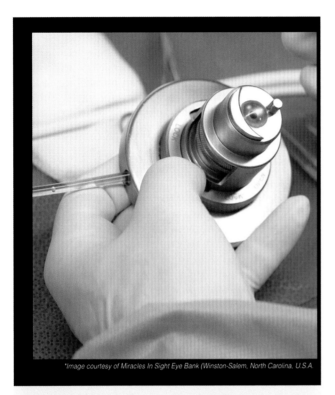

Image courtesy of Miracles In Sight Eye Bank (Winston-Salem, North Carolina, U.S.A.

Fig. 23.2 Reusable artificial anterior chamber (ALTK System, Moria). In 2006, Mark Gorovoy introduced the technique variant known as Descemet stripping automated endothelial keratoplasty (DSAEK), with the use of an artificial anterior chamber and blade microkeratome for cutting donor grafts, a significant advancement for both the surgeon and the eye bank.

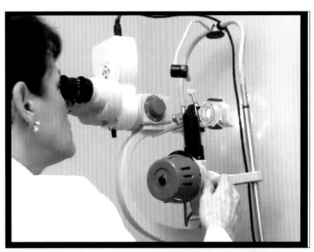

Fig. 23.3 In compliance with the Eye Bank Association of America (EBAA) Medical Standards, DSAEK tissue is evaluated pre– and post–graft preparation with slit lamp microscopy.

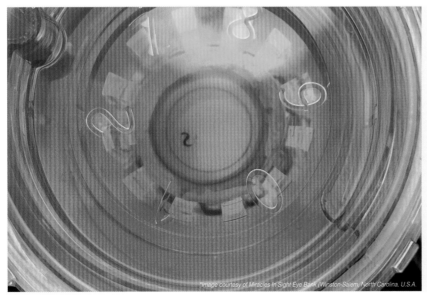

Image courtesy of Miracles In Sight Eye Bank (Winston-Salem, North Carolina, U.S.A.

Fig. 23.4 "S" stamp on an endothelial keratoplasty graft.

to the surgeon. The anterior cap/graft complex can then be safely transferred to its container with fresh cornea storage media.[15,55,59]

Femtosecond Laser-Assisted DSAEK

The efforts to further minimize any interface irregularity in DSAEK brought forward the utility of femtosecond laser innovation for DSAEK graft preparation.[15,60] Compared to microkeratome-prepared tissues, femto-prepared tissues have greater irregularity of the posterior corneal surface, rougher stromal beds, and increased thickness irregularity.[61,62]

No difference was noted in endothelial cell density and viability between the two techniques. The theory behind the irregular stromal dissections is the morph in donor cornea contour upon application by the femtosecond laser applanation cone.[61,62]

Some advocate for use of both the microkeratome and the femtosecond laser together in sequential cuts to yield ultrathin DSAEK grafts. Results have shown promise, with no irregular cuts or perforations during tissue preparation and a reduction in stromal roughness and thickness, with improved contour and symmetry, without endothelial cell damage after excimer laser smoothing passes. However, the clinical significance of these findings has not yet been established.[59,63,64]

23.2.2 Ultrathin Descemet Stripping Automated Endothelial Keratoplasty

Double-Pass Microkeratome Technique

Ultrathin DSAEK (UT-DSAEK) corneal donor graft tissue thickness is generally considered to be < 100 μm. Thinner grafts may improve visual outcomes[65] and possibly reduce the observed postoperative hyperopic shift.[66,67,68,69,70] The rationale behind the double-pass microkeratome technique is that it produces more planar and thinner graft lenticules, though some studies report high perforation rates and increased endothelial cell damage in using this method.[71,72,73]

In an effort to decrease corneal perforation risk, Busin et al hydrated grafts after the initial microkeratome cut by using intrastromal injections of BSS and immersing tissue in hypoosmotic tissue culture medium for 24 hours.[72] Both strategies thickened the residual tissue bed and prevented perforations during the second microkeratome pass. However, the hydration technique in particular was found not to be as clinically useful because there were multiple areas of Descemet detachment.[13,14,15]

Femtosecond Laser-Assisted UT-DSAEK

Ultrathin tissue can also be prepared using a low-pulse energy, high-frequency femtosecond laser, with no increased endothelial cell damage. The current challenge with this technique is the resulting irregular stromal surface, due to the photodisruptive effects of the femtosecond laser, which is thought to be potentially improved with modified laser settings or an inverse cutting approach.[59,74,75]

23.2.3 Descemet Membrane Endothelial Keratoplasty

With DMEK, the transplanted lenticule includes only Descemet membrane (DM) and corneal endothelium with no stromal interface, which may explain the potential improvements in visual acuity reported with this technique. Thinner, well-centered, planar tissue may be associated with less induction of higher-order optical aberrations, although this remains an unproven hypothesis.[21,76]

The challenges associated with DMEK have included both preparing the delicate graft tissue as well as intraoperative handling of the tissue without causing tears or excessive endothelial cell damage. Thus, in current practice, many surgeons delving into DMEK will often have a DSEK corneal graft made available, should the need for conversion to DSEK arise.[76,77,78,79]

Manual Peel

Melles et al described a manual peeling method where a donor corneoscleral rim is initially mounted endothelial side up on a custommade holder with a suction cup. After trephination, a DM was stripped from the posterior stroma with one-point, fine, nontoothed forceps to obtain a 9 mm diameter flap of posterior DM with its endothelial monolayer. Based on the properties of DM, the graft tends to scroll spontaneously with the endothelium on the outer side.[20,56,60,77,78]

Submerged Corneas Using Backgrounds Away Technique

The technique of submerged corneas using backgrounds away (SCUBA) (► Fig. 23.5) was then subsequently described, where a cornea is submerged in corneal storage media or BSS to minimize surface tension and allow for the DM to settle back onto the stroma.[20,77,79] Various other important technique modifications have been trialed since, including the use of a second pair of forceps during peel,[80,81] use of a curvilinear forceps with a half-moon-shaped, nontoothed anterior segment to equally distribute the force needed for DM separation,[82] as well as the use of a microkeratome in combination with a Barraquer sweep to dissect the residual stroma from the DM.[83]

DMEK-S

In DMEK-S, the central graft consists of only DM and endothelium, while an additional layer of posterior stroma is maintained in the periphery.[84] The tissue loss rate was noted to be less with this additional rim of tissue in some studies, whereas others demonstrated an even higher rate secondary to bubble rupture and failure of bubble formation.[85]

DMAEK

The transitions to the DMEK-S and Descemet membrane automated endothelial keratoplasty (DMAEK) techniques parallel the difference between DSEK and DSAEK. With DMAEK, a posterior lamellar dissection is done with a microkeratome[84] or

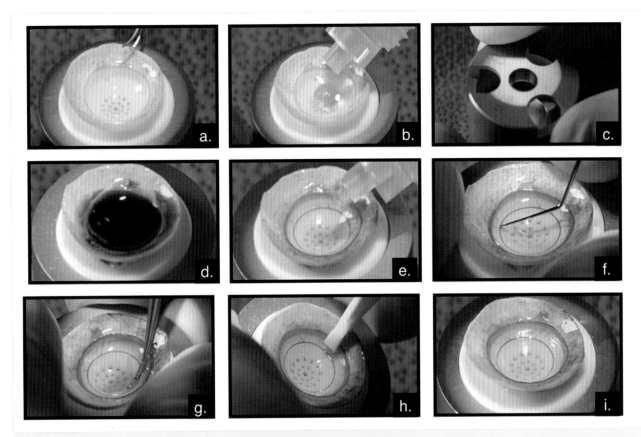

Fig. 23.5 Descemet membrane endothelial keratoplasty (DMEK) prepared using the submerged corneas using backgrounds away (SCUBA) technique. **(a)**The donor corneal tissue is mounted on an artificial chamber, **(b)** irrigated with balanced salt solution (BSS), **(c)** trephined, **(d)** stained with trypan blue, and **(e)** reirrigated with BSS. **(f)** The Descemet membrane is then scored 360 degrees along the trephination line, **(g)** stripped from the posterior stroma, **(h)** laid back down, and **(i)** interface dried with a Weck-cel (Beaver-Visitec) to minimize fluid in the interface.

femtosecond laser.[22] An AAC is used, and mechanical separation of the DM is conducted. This can be done with a 330Æ superficial trephination followed by cannula insertion with BSS injected to detach the DM[86] or with the use of an epi-keratome (Senturium; Norwood Abbey EyeCare).[87,88]

Pneumatic Dissection

Initially used for anterior lamellar keratoplasty, pneumatic dissection is now being used for the preparation of DMEK and PDEK grafts, wherein air is injected into the cornea to create a dissection plane between the donor stroma and the DM.[89] The use of an AAC as well as trypan blue staining of the endothelium to visualize needle positioning have also been described.[90] Notably, less endothelial cell damage was being observed when the bubble was immediately deflated after DM separation. Further modifications being used include the reverse big-bubble technique,[91] and the addition of a superficial keratectomy prior to air injection.[59,92]

23.2.4 Pre-Descemet Endothelial Keratoplasty

PDEK is gaining momentum as an effective alternative to current EK techniques, which combines the advantages of DSEK, allowing use of younger donors and reportedly easier unfolding

of the tissue, with the advantage of having thinner grafts as with DMEK.[24,93,94]

Proficient, well-established eye banks are currently under way in trialing out various methods to adapting PDEK graft preparation into the eye bank setting, using reproducible modalities, as well as alternatives to specular microscopy, for evaluating grafts postpreparation.[23]

With PDEK graft preparation, an innovative method for detaching the DM with air detaches the pre-Descemet layer (PDL), DM, and endothelium from the posterior stroma (▶ Fig. 23.6). Deep stromal air injection with a 30-gauge needle can be used to achieve a type 1 bubble, that is, the separation of the stroma from the PDL, also known as the Dua layer. If a type 1 bubble is created, then BSS can be injected into the bubble to provide additional expansion, and the graft is then cut out (▶ Fig. 23.7).[24,95]

Storage medium or viscoelastic agent can be used for donor graft preparation in specific cases. To measure PDEK graft thickness and endothelial cell loss (ECL), optical coherence tomography (OCT) imaging and Fiji imaging software, respectively, have been trialed pre- and postgraft preparation.[23]

Techniques are being investigated to overcome the current challenges of DM perforations, bubble bursts during BSS expansion, and excess ECL with tissue manipulation. With central endothelial perforation, a more viscous material can be used to prevent leakage from the perforation. Older donors are more

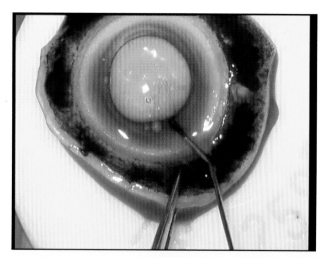

Fig. 23.6 Pneumatic dissection and staining with trypan blue dye for pre-Descemet endothelial keratoplasty graft.

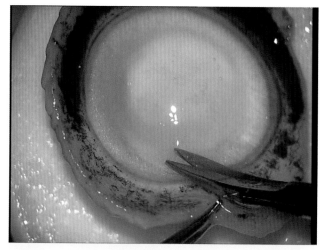

Fig. 23.7 Pre-Descemet layer along with Descemet membrane is dissected for pre-Descemet endothelial keratoplasty procedure using the McCarey–Kaufman (MK) storage medium.

likely to form a type 2 bubble, with the separation lying between the PDL and the DM. If a type 2 bubble forms instead of type 1, it can be prevented from expanding further by puncturing it and allowing air to escape. A small type 2 bubble at the periphery can be sequestered from an expanding central type 1 bubble by applying pressure between the two with a thin blunt instrument and not allowing the type 1 to meet the type 2 bubble.[95,96]

A controversial aspect, thought to be a drawback in PDEK, is the limitation in donor graft diameter to about 7 to 7.5 mm due to the physiological diameter of the PDL. However, given the ability to use young donor tissue in PDEK, which is not possible with DMEK, this potential obstacle has not been problematic in the face of the promising postoperative outcomes that have been noted with regard to corneal clarity and visual acuity. Taking a glimpse into the future, surgeons and eye banks will next need to strategize the transition from PDEK grafts prepared solely by surgeons, to the preparation done in the hands of skilled eye bank technicians (▶ Fig. 23.8).[95,96]

23.2.5 International Eye Banking and Endothelial Keratoplasty Grafts

Corneal disease represents the fourth leading cause of blindness in the majority of developing countries, particularly high in the geographic regions of Africa, Asia, South America, and the Middle East. Due to shortages of corneal tissue, optimally functioning eye bank establishments, funds, corneal storage media, adequate infrastructure, coupled with the lack of public awareness, religious superstition, and governmental negligence, more than 50% of tissues collected by eye banks in some of these regions are either graded as unsuitable for transplant or discarded due to exceeding preservation time.[26,97,98]

Surgeons and eye banks can use EK to introduce unique solutions for sight restoration in developing countries. The widespread adaptation of EK techniques holds promise to improve corneal transplant success rates, providing faster visual recovery while minimizing the risk of infection, than traditional full-thickness PKs. Additionally, in the setting of corneal donor tissue shortages, maximizing efficiency in EK graft preparation

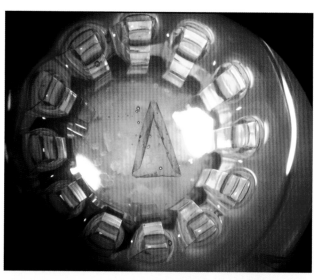

Fig. 23.8 Pre-Descemet endothelial keratoplasty graft prepared in eye bank by pneumatic dissection and stored in medium.

will be critical, wherein one corneal donor tissue can be used, for example, for EK, anterior lamellar keratoplasty, and cadaveric limbal stem cell transplantation.[99] In the pipeline with PDEK, infant corneal grafts, thought to be suboptimal for PK given the rejection risk, are increasingly showing promise, thus potentially expanding the corneal donor pool.[94] However, rapid technological modernization of the eye bank infrastructure and exponential growth in the number of well-run eye banks will be necessary in order to perfect graft preparation to this level of technique. The ascendancy of cataract surgical rates and more robust eye care infrastructure of several Asian and African countries have now provided a base upon which to dramatically expand corneal transplantation rates. Two key factors are the development of professional eye bank managers and the establishment of hospital cornea recovery programs. Adaptation of these modern eye banking models in India has led to corresponding high growth rates in the procurement of transplantable tissues, improved utilization rates, improved operating efficiency, and increased financial sustainability.

Although the challenges are ongoing, the experience and accomplishments of established eye banks suggest that collaborative efforts worldwide, with appropriate adaptations of current methodology and technology, can scale up widespread access to corneal transplantation to meet the needs of the millions who are currently blind.[98,100]

23.3 Conclusion

Since the birth of EK, there have been more advances in corneal transplantation and sight restoration over the past 2 decades than ever before. Microkeratomes are being replaced by femtosecond lasers to prepare corneal donor tissue. DSEK graft preparation is now becoming commonplace in the face of DMEK and PDEK graft preparation by eye banks on the horizon. As new techniques are being developed, requiring transplantation of thinner and thinner layers of the cornea, eye banks continue to perfect their techniques and delve into more complex innovation. The strong, unified collaboration between surgeons and eye banks have allowed for even faster resolutions to new challenges that arise and the zeal to move forward into unknown territory, in order to further optimize the humanitarian efforts for providing sight restoration.[1,26]

References

[1] Macsai MS, Nariani A, Reed C. Eye banking: What the eye bank can do for you. In: Jeng BH, ed. Advances in Medical and Surgical Cornea: From Diagnosis to Procedure. Berlin, Germany: Springer; 2015:133–143

[2] Bock J. The jubilee of the first successful optic keratoplasty by Eduard Zim [in German]. Wien Klin Wochenschr. 1958; 70(21):381–383

[3] Paton RT. History of corneal transplantation. Int Ophthalmol Clin. 1970; 10 (2):181–186

[4] Lee WB, Meinecke E, Varnum B. The evolution of eye banking and corneal transplantation: a symbiotic relationship. Int Ophthalmol Clin. 2013; 53 (2):115–129

[5] Franko-Gazzarari MD. Eye banking in America. J Ophthalmic Nurs Technol. 1991; 10(2):63–65

[6] Lindstrom RL, Kaufman HE, Skelnik DL, et al. Optisol corneal storage medium. Am J Ophthalmol. 1992; 114(3):345–356

[7] Melles GR, Eggink FA, Lander F, et al. A surgical technique for posterior lamellar keratoplasty. Cornea. 1998; 17(6):618–626

[8] Terry MA, Ousley PJ. Replacing the endothelium without corneal surface incisions or sutures: the first United States clinical series using the deep lamellar endothelial keratoplasty procedure. Ophthalmology. 2003; 110 (4):755–764, discussion 764

[9] Price FW, Jr, Price MO. Descemet's stripping with endothelial keratoplasty in 50 eyes: a refractive neutral corneal transplant. J Refract Surg. 2005; 21 (4):339–345

[10] Gorovoy MS. Descemet-stripping automated endothelial keratoplasty. Cornea. 2006; 25(8):886–889

[11] Price MO, Price FW, Jr. Descemet's stripping with endothelial keratoplasty: comparative outcomes with microkeratome-dissected and manually dissected donor tissue. Ophthalmology. 2006; 113(11):1936–1942

[12] Rose L, Briceño CA, Stark WJ, Gloria DG, Jun AS. Assessment of eye bank-prepared posterior lamellar corneal tissue for endothelial keratoplasty. Ophthalmology. 2008; 115(2):279–286

[13] Chen ES, Terry MA, Shamie N, Hoar KL, Friend DJ. Precut tissue in Descemet's stripping automated endothelial keratoplasty donor characteristics and early postoperative complications. Ophthalmology. 2008; 115(3):497–502

[14] Price MO, Baig KM, Brubaker JW, Price FW, Jr. Randomized, prospective comparison of precut vs surgeon-dissected grafts for descemet stripping automated endothelial keratoplasty. Am J Ophthalmol. 2008; 146(1):36–41

[15] Boynton GE, Woodward MA. Eye-bank preparation of endothelial tissue. Curr Opin Ophthalmol. 2014; 25(4):319–324

[16] Kitzmann AS, Goins KM, Reed C, Padnick-Silver L, Macsai MS, Sutphin JE. Eye bank survey of surgeons using precut donor tissue for descemet stripping automated endothelial keratoplasty. Cornea. 2008; 27(6):634–639

[17] 2009 Eye Banking Statistical Report. Eye Bank Association of America. www. restoresight.org

[18] 2014 Eye Banking Statistical Report. Eye Bank Association of America. www. restoresight.org

[19] Price MO, Gorovoy M, Price FW, Jr, Benetz BA, Menegay HJ, Lass JH. Descemet's stripping automated endothelial keratoplasty: three-year graft and endothelial cell survival compared with penetrating keratoplasty. Ophthalmology. 2013; 120(2):246–251

[20] Melles GR, Ong TS, Ververs B, van der Wees J. Descemet membrane endothelial keratoplasty (DMEK). Cornea. 2006; 25(8):987–990

[21] Tausif HN, Johnson L, Titus M, et al. Corneal donor tissue preparation for Descemet's membrane endothelial keratoplasty. J Vis Exp. 2014(91):51919

[22] Jardine GJ, Holiman JD, Galloway JD, Stoeger CG, Chamberlain WD. Eye Bank-Prepared Femtosecond Laser-Assisted Automated Descemet Membrane Endothelial Grafts. Cornea. 2015; 34(7):838–843

[23] Nariani A, Kumar D, Agarwal A, et al. Eye bank graft preparation for pre-Descemet's endothelial keratoplasty. Abstract in 2016 ARVO Annual Meeting. 2016 May 1–5; Seattle, Washington

[24] Agarwal A, Dua HS, Narang P, et al. Pre-Descemet's endothelial keratoplasty (PDEK). Br J Ophthalmol. 2014; 98(9):1181–1185

[25] Altaan SL, Gupta A, Sidney LE, Elalfy MS, Agarwal A, Dua HS. Endothelial cell loss following tissue harvesting by pneumodissection for endothelial keratoplasty: an ex vivo study. Br J Ophthalmol. 2015; 99(5):710–713

[26] Pineda R. Corneal Transplantation in the Developing World: Lessons Learned and Meeting the Challenge. Cornea. 2015; 34 Suppl 10:S35–S40

[27] Silvera D, Goins K, Sutphin JE, Goins ST. Comparison of visual outcomes, O.R. efficiency, and complication rates of eye bank pre-cut tissue versus intraoperatively cut tissue for DSEK. Federated Societies Scientific Session; 2006 December 12; Las Vegas, Nevada

[28] Grabska-Liberek I, Szaflik J, Brix-Warzecha M. The importance of various factors relating to the morphological quality of corneas used for PKP by the Warsaw Eye Bank from 1996 to 2002. Ann Transplant. 2003; 8(2):26–31

[29] Evaluation of Human Corneas for the North Carolina Eye Bank DSAEK Procedures. Cornea Numbers: 1123–05–01 and 1123–05–02. Protocol number 05PHCE-NCEB101. Report number 105. SOP Number 05SHCE-NCEB101. Winston-Salem, NC: North Carolina Eye Bank (Miracles In Sight Eye Bank); 2005

[30] Chang MA, Chuck RS. Total anterior corneal surface and epithelial stem cell harvesting: current microkeratomes and beyond. Expert Rev Med Devices. 2004; 1(2):251–258

[31] McCarey BE, Kaufman HE. Improved corneal storage. Invest Ophthalmol. 1974; 13(3):165–173

[32] Ehlers N, Hjortdal J, Nielsen K. Corneal grafting and banking. Dev Ophthalmol. 2009; 43:1–14

[33] Wilson SE, Bourne WM. Corneal preservation. Surv Ophthalmol. 1989; 33 (4):237–259

[34] Jeng BH. Preserving the cornea: corneal storage media. Curr Opin Ophthalmol. 2006; 17(4):332–337

[35] Lass JH, Gordon JF, Sugar A, et al. Optisol containing streptomycin. Am J Ophthalmol. 1993; 116(4):503–504

[36] Smith TM, Popplewell J, Nakamura T, Trousdale MD. Efficacy and safety of gentamicin and streptomycin in Optisol-GS, a preservation medium for donor corneas. Cornea. 1995; 14(1):49–55

[37] Hwang DG, Nakamura T, Trousdale MD, Smith TM. Combination antibiotic supplementation of corneal storage medium. Am J Ophthalmol. 1993; 115 (3):299–308

[38] Bryan GS, Abdullayev E, Wellemeyer M, et al. Eusol-C effectiveness as a corneal storage media. Abstract in 2005 Federated Societies Scientific Session. Eye Bank Association of America and the Cornea Society. 2005 October 15; Chicago, Illinois

[39] Nelson LR, Hodge DO, Bourne WM. In vitro comparison of Chen medium and Optisol-GS medium for human corneal storage. Cornea. 2000; 19 (6):782–787

[40] Naor J, Slomovic AR, Chipman M, Rootman DS. A randomized, double-masked clinical trial of Optisol-GS vs Chen Medium for human corneal storage. Arch Ophthalmol. 2002; 120(10):1280–1285

[41] Bourne WM, Nelson LR, Maguire LJ, Baratz KH, Hodge DO. Comparison of Chen Medium and Optisol-GS for human corneal preservation at 4 degrees C: results of transplantation. Cornea. 2001; 20(7):683–686

[42] Laaser K, Bachmann BO, Horn FK, Schlötzer-Schrehardt U, Cursiefen C, Kruse FE. Donor tissue culture conditions and outcome after descemet membrane endothelial keratoplasty. Am J Ophthalmol. 2011; 151(6):1007–1018.e2

[43] Woodward MA, Ross KW, Requard JJ, Sugar A, Shtein RM. Impact of surgeon acceptance parameters on cost and availability of corneal donor tissue for transplantation. Cornea. 2013; 32(6):737–740

[44] Rieck PW, von Stockhausen RM, Metzner S, Hartmann C, Courtois Y. Fibroblast growth factor-2 protects endothelial cells from damage after corneal storage at 4 degrees C. Graefes Arch Clin Exp Ophthalmol. 2003; 241 (9):757–764

[45] Jeng BH, Shadrach KG, Meisler DM, et al. Immunohistochemical detection and Western blot analysis of nitrated protein in stored human corneal epithelium. Exp Eye Res. 2005; 80(4):509–514

[46] Meisler DM, Koeck T, Connor JT, et al. Inhibition of nitric oxide synthesis in corneas in storage media. Exp Eye Res. 2004; 78(4):891–894

[47] Kim T, Palay DA, Lynn M. Donor factors associated with epithelial defects after penetrating keratoplasty. Cornea. 1996; 15(5):451–456

[48] Means TL, Geroski DH, L'Hernault N, Grossniklaus HE, Kim T, Edelhauser HF. The corneal epithelium after optisol-GS storage. Cornea. 1996; 15(6):599–605

[49] Spelsberg H, Reinhard T, Sundmacher R. Epithelial damage of corneal grafts after prolonged storage in dextran-containing organ culture medium—a prospective study [in German]. Klin Monatsbl Augenheilkd. 2002; 219 (6):417–421

[50] Terry MA, Shamie N, Straiko MD, Friend DJ, Davis-Boozer D. Endothelial keratoplasty: the relationship between donor tissue storage time and donor endothelial survival. Ophthalmology. 2011; 118(1):36–40

[51] Ruzza A, Salvalaio G, Bruni A, Frigo AC, Busin M, Ponzin D. Banking of donor tissues for descemet stripping automated endothelial keratoplasty. Cornea. 2013; 32(1):70–75

[52] Wacker K, Bourne WM, Patel SV. Effect of graft thickness on visual acuity after Descemet stripping endothelial keratoplasty: a systematic review and meta-analysis. Am J Ophthalmol. 2016; 163:18–28

[53] Taravella MJ, Shah V, Davidson R. Ultrathin DSAEK. Int Ophthalmol Clin. 2013; 53(2):21–30

[54] Hsu M, Hereth WL, Moshirfar M. Double-pass microkeratome technique for ultra-thin graft preparation in Descemet's stripping automated endothelial keratoplasty. Clin Ophthalmol. 2012; 6:425–432

[55] Perry, Isaac. Miracles In Sight Eye Bank DSAEK Graft Preparation. Winston-Salem, NC: Miracles In Sight Eye Bank; 2015

[56] Bhogal MS, Allan BD. Graft profile and thickness as a function of cut transition speed in Descemet-stripping automated endothelial keratoplasty. J Cataract Refract Surg. 2012; 38(4):690–695

[57] Dapena I, Ham L, Melles GR. Endothelial keratoplasty: DSEK/DSAEK or DMEK—the thinner the better? Curr Opin Ophthalmol. 2009; 20(4):299–307

[58] Eye Bank Association of America (EBAA).

[59] Woodward MA, Titus M, Mavin K, Shtein RM. Corneal donor tissue preparation for endothelial keratoplasty. J Vis Exp. 2012; 64(64):e3847

[60] Moshirfar M, Imbornoni LM, Muthappan V, et al. In vitro pilot analysis of uniformity, circularity, and concentricity of DSAEK donor endothelial grafts prepared by a microkeratome. Cornea. 2014; 33(2):191–196

[61] Vetter JM, Butsch C, Faust M, et al. Irregularity of the posterior corneal surface after curved interface femtosecond laser-assisted versus microkeratome-assisted descemet stripping automated endothelial keratoplasty. Cornea. 2013; 32(2):118–124

[62] Mootha VV, Heck E, Verity SM, et al. Comparative study of descemet stripping automated endothelial keratoplasty donor preparation by Moria CBm microkeratome, horizon microkeratome, and Intralase FS60. Cornea. 2011; 30(3):320–324

[63] Cleary C, Liu Y, Tang M, Li Y, Stoeger C, Huang D. Excimer laser smoothing of endothelial keratoplasty grafts. Cornea. 2012; 31(4):431–436

[64] Rosa AM, Silva MF, Quadrado MJ, Costa E, Marques I, Murta JN. Femtosecond laser and microkeratome-assisted Descemet stripping endothelial keratoplasty: first clinical results. Br J Ophthalmol. 2013; 97(9):1104–1107

[65] Neff KD, Biber JM, Holland EJ. Comparison of central corneal graft thickness to visual acuity outcomes in endothelial keratoplasty. Cornea. 2011; 30 (4):388–391

[66] Holz HA, Meyer JJ, Espandar L, Tabin GC, Mifflin MD, Moshirfar M. Corneal profile analysis after Descemet stripping endothelial keratoplasty and its relationship to postoperative hyperopic shift. J Cataract Refract Surg. 2008; 34(2):211–214

[67] Lee WB, Jacobs DS, Musch DC, Kaufman SC, Reinhart WJ, Shtein RM. Descemet's stripping endothelial keratoplasty: safety and outcomes: a report by the American Academy of Ophthalmology. Ophthalmology. 2009; 116 (9):1818–1830

[68] Scorcia V, Matteoni S, Scorcia GB, Scorcia G, Busin M. Pentacam assessment of posterior lamellar grafts to explain hyperopization after Descemet's stripping automated endothelial keratoplasty. Ophthalmology. 2009; 116 (9):1651–1655

[69] Esquenazi S, Rand W. Effect of the shape of the endothelial graft on the refractive results after Descemet's stripping with automated endothelial keratoplasty. Can J Ophthalmol. 2009; 44(5):557–561

[70] Jun B, Kuo AN, Afshari NA, Carlson AN, Kim T. Refractive change after descemet stripping automated endothelial keratoplasty surgery and its correlation with graft thickness and diameter. Cornea. 2009; 28(1):19–23

[71] Waite A, Davidson R, Taravella MJ. Descemet-stripping automated endothelial keratoplasty donor tissue preparation using the double-pass microkeratome technique. J Cataract Refract Surg. 2013; 39(3):446–450

[72] Busin M, Patel AK, Scorcia V, Ponzin D. Microkeratome-assisted preparation of ultrathin grafts for descemet stripping automated endothelial keratoplasty. Invest Ophthalmol Vis Sci. 2012; 53(1):521–524

[73] Sikder S, Nordgren RN, Neravetla SR, Moshirfar M. Ultra-thin donor tissue preparation for endothelial keratoplasty with a double-pass microkeratome. Am J Ophthalmol. 2011; 152(2):202–208.e2

[74] Phillips PM, Phillips LJ, Saad HA, et al. "Ultrathin" DSAEK tissue prepared with a low-pulse energy, high-frequency femtosecond laser. Cornea. 2013; 32(1):81–86

[75] Liu YC, Teo EP, Adnan KB, et al. Endothelial approach ultrathin corneal grafts prepared by femtosecond laser for descemet stripping endothelial keratoplasty. Invest Ophthalmol Vis Sci. 2014; 55(12):8393–8401

[76] Rudolph M, Laaser K, Bachmann BO, Cursiefen C, Epstein D, Kruse FE. Corneal higher-order aberrations after Descemet's membrane endothelial keratoplasty. Ophthalmology. 2012; 119(3):528–535

[77] Lie JT, Birbal R, Ham L, van der Wees J, Melles GR. Donor tissue preparation for Descemet membrane endothelial keratoplasty. J Cataract Refract Surg. 2008; 34(9):1578–1583

[78] Melles GR, Lander F, Rietveld FJ. Transplantation of Descemet's membrane carrying viable endothelium through a small scleral incision. Cornea. 2002; 21(4):415–418

[79] Price MO, Giebel AW, Fairchild KM, Price FW, Jr. Descemet's membrane endothelial keratoplasty: prospective multicenter study of visual and refractive outcomes and endothelial survival. Ophthalmology. 2009; 116 (12):2361–2368

[80] Kruse FE, Laaser K, Cursiefen C, et al. A stepwise approach to donor preparation and insertion increases safety and outcome of Descemet membrane endothelial keratoplasty. Cornea. 2011; 30(5):580–587

[81] Schlötzer-Schrehardt U, Bachmann BO, Tourtas T, et al. Reproducibility of graft preparations in Descemet's membrane endothelial keratoplasty. Ophthalmology. 2013; 120(9):1769–1777

[82] Yoeruek E, Bartz-Schmidt KU. Novel surgical instruments facilitating Descemet membrane dissection. Cornea. 2013; 32(4):523–526

[83] Sikder S, Ward D, Jun AS. A surgical technique for donor tissue harvesting for descemet membrane endothelial keratoplasty. Cornea. 2011; 30(1):91–94

[84] Studeny P, Farkas A, Vokrojova M, Liskova P, Jirsova K. Descemet membrane endothelial keratoplasty with a stromal rim (DMEK-S). Br J Ophthalmol. 2010; 94(7):909–914

[85] Krabcova I, Studeny P, Jirsova K. Endothelial quality of pre-cut posterior corneal lamellae for Descemet membrane endothelial keratoplasty with a stromal rim (DMEK-S): two-year outcome of manual preparation in an ocular tissue bank. Cell Tissue Bank. 2013; 14(2):325–331

[86] Muraine M, Gueudry J, He Z, Piselli S, Lefevre S, Toubeau D. Novel technique for the preparation of corneal grafts for descemet membrane endothelial keratoplasty. Am J Ophthalmol. 2013; 156(5):851–859

[87] Kymionis GD, Yoo SH, Diakonis VF, Grentzelos MA, Naoumidi I, Pallikaris IG. Automated donor tissue preparation for descemet membrane automated endothelial keratoplasty (DMAEK): an experimental study. Ophthalmic Surg Lasers Imaging. 2011; 42(2):158–161

[88] Pereira CdaR, Guerra FP, Price FW, Jr, Price MO. Descemet's membrane automated endothelial keratoplasty (DMAEK): visual outcomes and visual quality. Br J Ophthalmol. 2011; 95(7):951–954

[89] Anwar M, Teichmann KD. Big-bubble technique to bare Descemet's membrane in anterior lamellar keratoplasty. J Cataract Refract Surg. 2002; 28 (3):398–403

[90] Venzano D, Pagani P, Randazzo N, Cabiddu F, Traverso CE. Descemet membrane air-bubble separation in donor corneas. J Cataract Refract Surg. 2010; 36(12):2022–2027

[91] Zarei-Ghanavati S, Khakshoor H, Zarei-Ghanavati M. Reverse big bubble: a new technique for preparing donor tissue of Descemet membrane endothelial keratoplasty. Br J Ophthalmol. 2010; 94(8):1110–1111

[92] Busin M, Scorcia V, Patel AK, Salvalaio G, Ponzin D. Donor tissue preparation for Descemet membrane endothelial keratoplasty. Br J Ophthalmol. 2011; 95 (8):1172–1173, author reply 1173

[93] Lass JH, Gal RL, Dontchev M, et al. Cornea Donor Study Investigator Group. Donor age and corneal endothelial cell loss 5 years after successful corneal transplantation. Specular microscopy ancillary study results. Ophthalmology. 2008; 115(4):627–632.e8

[94] Agarwal A, Agarwal A, Narang P, Kumar DA, Jacob S. Pre-Descemet Endothelial Keratoplasty With Infant Donor Corneas: A Prospective Analysis. Cornea. 2015; 34(8):859–865

[95] Dua HS, Faraj LA, Said DG, Gray T, Lowe J. Human corneal anatomy redefined: a novel pre-Descemet's layer (Dua's layer). Ophthalmology. 2013; 120 (9):1778–1785

[96] Jacob S. PDEK Bubble Challenges. Eurotimes Stories. 2014. http://www.eurotimes.org/node/1661. Accessed February 2, 2016

[97] Whitcher JP, Srinivasan M, Upadhyay MP. Corneal blindness: a global perspective. Bull World Health Organ. 2001; 79(3):214–221

[98] Oliva MS, Schottman T, Gulati M. Turning the tide of corneal blindness. Indian J Ophthalmol. 2012; 60(5):423–427

[99] Vajpayee RB, Sharma N, Jhanji V, Titiyal JS, Tandon R. One donor cornea for 3 recipients: a new concept for corneal transplantation surgery. Arch Ophthalmol. 2007; 125(4):552–554

[100] Rao GN. Eye banking in developing countries. In: Lass JH, ed. Advances in Corneal Research: Selected Transactions of the World Congress on the Cornea IV. New York: Springer; 1997:580–581

Index